The Well-being of Children
in the UK

EDITED BY JONATHAN BRADSHAW

THE UNIVERSITY *of York*

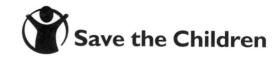 Save the Children

Save the Children is the UK's leading international children's charity. Working in more than 70 countries, Save the Children runs emergency relief alongside long-term development and prevention work to help children, their families and communities to be self-sufficient.

Drawing on this practical experience, Save the Children also seeks to influence policy and practice to achieve lasting benefits for children within their communities. In all its work, Save the Children endeavours to make children's rights a reality.

Published by
Save the Children
17 Grove Lane
London SE5 8RD
First published in 2002
© The Save the Children Fund 2002

Registered charity no. 213890

ISBN 1 84187 060 9

Contents

List of Contributors

Professor Sally Baldwin	Director of the Social Policy Research Unit, University of York
Dr Bryony Beresford	Research Fellow, Social Policy Research Unit, University of York
Professor Jonathan Bradshaw	Professor of Social Policy, University of York
Bob Coles	Senior Lecturer in Social Policy, University of York
Karen Croucher	Research Fellow, Centre for Housing Policy, University of York
Eirean Edwards	Research Student, Department of Social Policy and Social Work, University of York
Naomi Finch	Research Fellow, Social Policy Research Unit, University of York
Dr Ian Gibbs	Senior Research Fellow, Social Work Research and Development Unit, University of York
Dr Michael Hirst	Research Fellow, Social Policy Research Unit, University of York
Dr Carol-Ann Hooper	Lecturer in Social Policy, University of York
Dr Anwen Jones	Research Fellow, Centre for Housing Policy, University of York
Helen Kenwright	Research Student, Department of Social Policy and Social Work, University of York
Suzanne Maile	Research Assistant, Department of Social Policy and Social Work, University of York
Deborah Quilgars	Research Fellow, Centre for Housing Policy, University of York
Gwyther Rees	Research Manager, The Children's Society
Beverly Searle	Research Student, Department of Social Policy and Social Work, University of York
Professor Ian Sinclair	Director of the Social Work Research and

	Development Unit, University of York
Dr Christine Skinner	Lecturer in Social Policy, University of York
Professor Patricia Sloper	Professor of Children's Health Care, Social Policy Research Unit, University of York.
Professor Mike Stein	Professor of Social Work, University of York
Dr Sharon Tabberer	Research Fellow, Department of Sociology, University of York
Alison Wallace	Research Fellow, Social Policy Research Unit, University of York

Abbreviations

ALSPAC	Avon Longitudinal Study of Pregnancy and Childhood
BCS	British Crime Survey
BHPS	British Household Panel Survey
CAPT	Child Accident Prevention Trust
CIPFA	Chartered Institute of Public Finance and Accountancy
CPS	Crown Prosecution Service
CYPU	Children and Young Person's Unit
DETR	Department of the Environment, Transport and the Regions
DfE	Department for Education
DfEE	Department for Education and Employment
DfES	Department for Education and Skills
DHSSPS	Department for Health, Social Services and Public Safety, Northern Ireland
DoH	Department of Health
DSS	Department of Social Security
DTLR	Department for Transport, Local Government and the Regions
DWP	Department for Work and Pensions
ECHP	European Community Household Panel Survey
ELB	Education and Library Board, Northern Ireland
ESRC	Economic and Social Research Council
EU	European Union
FEANTSA	European Federation of National Organisations Working with the Homeless
GCCNI	General Consumer Council Northern Ireland
GLA	Greater London Authority
GMB	Britain's General Union (General and Municipal Boiler-makers)
GMSC	General Medical Services Committee
GNVQ	General National Vocational Qualification

HBAI	Households Below Average Income
HBSC	Health and Behaviour of School Children (WHO survey)
HEA	Health Education Authority
HPA	Health Promotion Agency
HRBQ	Health Related Behaviour Questionnaire
HVA	Health Visitors Association
ICD	International Classification of Disease
ISD	Information and Statistic Division, Scotland
LEA	Local Education Authority
LIS	Luxembourg Income Study
MMR	Measles, Mumps and Rubella (immunisation)
MPO	Managerial and Professional Officers
NACRO	National Association for the Care and Resettlement of Offenders
NEET	Not in Education, Employment or Training
NIHE	Northern Ireland Housing Executive
NISRA	Northern Ireland Statistics and Research Agency
OECD	Organisation for Economic Co-operation and Development
OFSTED	Office for Standards in Education
ONS	Office for National Statistics
OOSC	Out-Of-School Club
OPCS	Office of Population, Censuses and Surveys
OSCE	Organisation for Security and Co-operation in Europe
PHLS	Public Health Laboratory Service
PRILIF	Programme of Research on Low Income Families
RNI	Reference Nutrition Intake
SAT	Standard Assessment Test
SDQ	Strengths and Difficulties Questionnaire
SEU	Social Exclusion Unit
STI	Sexually Transmitted Infection
SoF	Survey of Families with Children
SoLIF	Survey of Low Income Families
TSN	Targeting Social Need
UKCCSG	United Kingdom Children's Cancer Study Group
UNICEF	United Nations Children's Fund
YLS	Youth Lifestyles Survey
YTS	Youth Training Scheme

Social Class Classifications

I	Professional
II	Managerial and technical operations
IIIN	Skilled occupation non-manual
IIIM	Skilled occupation manual
IV	Partly skilled occupation
V	Unskilled occupation

Preface

Jonathan Bradshaw

The United Kingdom does not produce a regular, comprehensive analysis of the well-being of children. Even before the introduction of devolved administrations in Scotland, Wales and Northern Ireland, there was no Ministry for Children (or the Family) in the UK. In the past there has been no body required to publish information on the impact of government policies on children. Of course there are official sources of data on children's well-being and the Office for National Statistics (ONS) published a *Social Focus on Children* in 1994 (Central Statistical Office, 1994) and *Social Focus on Young People* in 2000 (ONS, 2000f). The ONS is currently working on an update of its *Health of Children* (Botting *et al.,* 1996), which is due to be published in 2003.

Now things are changing:

- In England, the Children and Young Person's Unit (CYPU) has been established in the Department for Education and Skills with responsibility for policy co-ordination and for running the Children's Fund. The CYPU has recently begun work to develop a framework for monitoring outcomes for children and young people and in *Building a Strategy for Children and Young People* (CYPU, 2001a) proposes that it will produce a regular State of the Nation's Children and Young Persons' Report.

- The Office of the Children's Rights Commissioner for London has been established and produced an excellent *The State of London's Children Report* (Hood, 2001).

- In Scotland there is a Minister for Education and Young People. The Scottish Parliament is considering a proposal to establish a Children's Commissioner. Social work and education responsibility for children's issues have been brought together within a single Children and Young People's Group within the Scottish Executive Education Department, and every health board in Scotland now has a lead Commissioner for Children's Services.

- The Welsh Assembly has established a Children's Commissioner for Wales and it is envisaged that the annual report that the Commissioner is required to produce will report on children in Wales.

- In Northern Ireland the Office of the First Minister and Deputy First Minister issued a consultation paper in August 2001 on establishing a Commissioner for Children. The plan is to have the Commissioner in post by spring 2002.

There are a variety of sources of data on children's well-being generated by the research community, including the British birth cohort studies of children born in one week in 1949, 1958, and 1970 and with another in progress in 2000/01. There are also the British Household Panel Survey (which includes a young person's questionnaire), PRILIF (Lone Parents Cohort) and SoLIF/SoF (Survey of Low Income Families/Families with Children). Both PRILIF and SoF are being adapted to collect data on children. There is also ALSPAC (a cohort survey of children born in Avon in 1991/92). However, although these sources are useful, none of them are designed to monitor the well-being of children over time.

The Government committed itself to producing an annual report on its progress in reducing child poverty in the Green and White Papers on Welfare Reform (Cm 3805, 1998; Cm 4101, 1998). The New Policy Institute, with the support of the Joseph Rowntree Foundation, has published four model reports, which included children's indicators (Howarth *et al.*, 1999a, 1999b; Rahman *et al.*, 2000; Rahman *et al.*, 2001). The Department of Social Security and the Department for Work and Pensions have also now published three annual reports (DSS, 1999, 2000; DWP, 2001b) which contain data covering a variety of domains of child well-being in England and Wales (and similar reports are being produced in Scotland and Northern Ireland – see web addresses in Chapter 1), which are being used to monitor the success of their anti-poverty strategy.

At the University of York we have been engaged in research on the well-being of children since we were commissioned by UNICEF to write the UK report (Bradshaw, 1990) for its comparative study of the well-being of children in industrialised countries (Cornia and Danziger, 1997). We had originally worked on the UNICEF report as a sub-contractor of the National Children's Bureau (NCB) and the NCB funded an update of that review (Kumar, 1995). Then as part of the ESRC Programme on Children 5–16 we were funded to undertake *Poverty: The outcomes for children* (Bradshaw, 2001a). This project involved:

1   A programme of secondary analysis of large datasets focusing on child poverty. This included British data – the Family Resources Survey, the Breadline Britain Survey and the British Household Panel Survey and

comparative data – the Luxembourg Income Survey and the European Community Household Panel Survey (Whiteford, Kennedy and Bradshaw, 1996; Adelman and Bradshaw, 1998; Bradshaw, 1997b, 1999, 2001b; Clarke *et al.*, 2000).

2   A comparative study to discover how other countries attempt to monitor the well-being of their children.

3   A review of existing evidence on the impact of poverty on the outcomes for children.

The last two elements were published by the Family Policy Studies Centre and the National Children's Bureau (Bradshaw, 2001a).

One of the conclusions of this work is that there is a strong case for a routinely produced and comprehensive national report on the state of children in the UK. We had thought that the Office for National Statistics might undertake this work, or perhaps a coalition of voluntary bodies. But we were delighted to be approached by Save the Children and commissioned to undertake this work.

The agreement with Save the Children is that:

- We produce a report on the state of children in the UK, which focuses on well-being – physical, cognitive, behavioural and emotional.

- It will be based on the most up-to-date data and a thorough review of existing sources. It will not be based on new empirical research, but would include, where it is appropriate, some secondary analysis of national datasets.

- **Age group**: the focus is on children and young people and they, not families or households, are as far as possible the 'unit of analysis'. We focus on children and young people up to age 18 but have to be fairly flexible about the upper age limit where the only data available includes older young people.

- **The UK**: Save the Children is a UK-based agency but organised around the different countries in the UK. Therefore the report seeks to cover the well-being of children in all parts of the UK. Indeed comparisons between children in different countries of the UK are a feature. However, again we have had to be flexible – not all the data is available at UK level, nor is it possible to break down UK data to an England, Wales, Scotland and Northern Ireland basis with any reliability. Indeed, we seek to highlight deficits in sub-national data in order to inform the debate on this issue. As well as the individual chapters making national comparisons within the UK, the concluding chapter summarises and highlights national results within the UK.

- **International perspective:** The main thrust of the work is to explore the well-being of UK children. However, one powerful device for this is to look at British children from a comparative perspective. We have experience of doing this as part of the work we undertook when co-ordinating the European Observatory on National Family Policies (Ditch *et al.*, 1995, 1996, 1998) and have used the Luxembourg Income Survey and the European Community Household Panel Survey with the child as the unit of analysis (Bradshaw, 2001a). We are also associated with two international collaborative studies of child well-being: The COST Action 19 on Child Welfare and the *Multi-National Project: Measuring and Monitoring Children's Well-Being*. This review contains comparative data where it is available and appropriate in order to view UK children in a comparative perspective.

- **Content:** Our previous work has focused on the outcomes for *poor* children. Save the Children wanted us to continue to emphasise their outcomes but also to report on children in the UK from all walks of life as well as the dispersion in well-being – by gender, ethnicity, age, family type and socio-economic group. The report focuses on outcomes – on well-being. From time to time we reflect on inputs – policies. But this report is not designed to report on or to evaluate specific policy initiatives.

The work in this report has been undertaken by a team of researchers, all actively engaged in research on children, at the University of York, mainly drawn from the Department of Social Policy and Social Work and its research units – Social Policy Research Unit, Centre for Housing Policy and the Social Work Research and Development Unit.

This is the first report of its kind, and is therefore somewhat experimental. The content, scope and coverage will be reviewed and possibly changed for any future reports. Comments and suggestions are invited (jrb1@york.ac.uk).

Acknowledgements

This project was steered by a Save the Children Advisory Group. We are grateful for the comments and suggestions that they made on drafts. We also acknowledge Didi Alayli, and then Kath Pinnock, our liaison officers in Save the Children.

At York, Emese Mayhew provided editorial support in the final stages. The final manuscript was prepared by Sally Pulleyn with her usual calm efficiency.

1 Children and Poor Children

Jonathan Bradshaw

Key statistics:
- In 1999 there were just over 12 million children under 16 in the UK, or 20 per cent of the population.
- In 2000/01, 32 per cent of these children were living in relative poverty.

Key trends:
- The number of children in the UK has declined since the mid-1970s and is expected to fall over the next 30 years by over 800,000.
- The child poverty rate increased more than threefold in the last 20 years, but has now begun to decline.

Key sources:
- *Population Trends*
- *Households Below Average Incomes*
- *Opportunity for All*

Introduction

This report is about all children in the UK, not just poor children. However, perhaps the best indicator of the well-being of children generally is the prevalence of poor children, and the best measure of public concern for children is the extent to which children are protected from poverty. Since the Prime Minister's historic commitment in March 1999 to end child poverty in 20 years, the abolition of child poverty has become a key objective of the Government. The fact that it was not an objective of governments before that is an outrage. This chapter will trace how we are doing in pursuit of the objective of abolishing child poverty and Chapter 2 will review some of the comparative evidence. But first we review the demography of UK children.

The child population

The latest population estimates (better estimates will emerge with the results of the 2001 census) give a child (under 16) population for the UK of 12,114,000. That number has declined by over 2 million since 1971, though the number has risen very slightly since 1996. Table 1.1 gives the numbers of children in each constituent country of the UK and as a proportion of their populations. Children under 16 represent just over 20 per cent of the UK population, with a slightly larger proportion in Northern Ireland. Over 80 per cent of UK children live in England.

There are more boys than girls under 16 in the child population – 308,000 more in the UK in 1999.

Chart 1.1 gives trends (actual and projected) in numbers of children under 16 for each constituent country up to 2031. Between 1999 and 2031 the number of children in the UK is expected to fall by over 800,000.

Table 1.1: Numbers and proportion of children under 16 by country, 1999, thousands

	England	Wales	Scotland	Northern Ireland	UK
Children under 16	10,097	597	1,008	411	12,114
% of the total population	20.3	20.3	19.5	24.3	20.4
% of children in the UK	83.3	4.9	8.3	3.4	100

Source: Population Trends

Chart 1.1: Children under 16 (actual and projected)

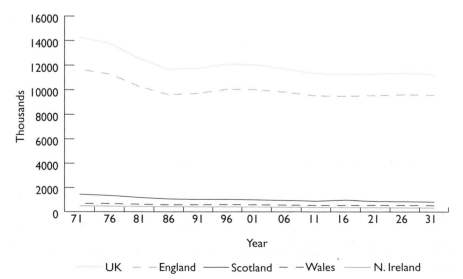

Chart 1.2: Birth rate and fertility rate

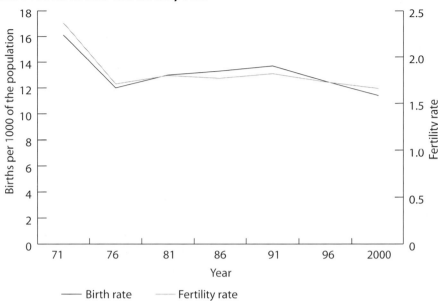

The main factors that determine changes in the child population are the birth rate and the fertility rate. Chart 1.2 shows for the UK that the birth rate (births per 1,000) fell from the early 1970s but began to pick up in the mid-70s as the 60s 'baby boomers' began to have their children. However, the birth rate began to fall again from the early 90s. The fertility rate (the number of children each woman will have) is a better indicator of long-term trends and it has been below replacement level (2.1 children per woman) since the mid-70s, fluctuating around 1.7 (in 2000 it fell to 1.66).

These variations lead to changes in the age composition of children over time. As can be seen in Table 1.2 the number of preschool-age children in the UK has been falling since 1991, but the number of school-age children has been rising since 1986.

Table 1.2: Number of children by age, UK, thousands

	1971	1976	1981	1986	1991	1996	1999
Under 1	899	677	730	749	794	719	708
1–5	3,654	3,043	2,726	2,892	3,094	3,044	2,916
6–14	8,916	9,176	8,147	7,161	7,175	7,596	7,763

Source: Population Trends, various years

Child poverty

It can be seen in Chart 1.3 that during the 1980s Britain experienced a huge surge in child poverty. The proportion of children living in households with incomes less than 50 per cent of the average equivalent (after controlling for the needs of families of different size) income after housing costs increased from 10 per cent in 1979 to 31 per cent in 1990/91. During the 1990s there was a further slight increase and the child poverty rate peaked in 1998/99 at 35 per cent. The latest data available is for 2001/01 and this contains welcome evidence that child poverty has begun to fall.

The latest data only goes up to April 2001 and therefore only covers six months after the big real increases in Child Benefit and Income Support in October 2000. It is to be hoped that the next edition of *Households Below Average Income* (HBAI) will show a more substantial reduction in child poverty. There is certainly evidence from other sources that indicate that the government's efforts to abolish child poverty are beginning to bite. I will briefly rehearse some of these.

As Chart 1.4 shows, the proportion of children in families dependent on Income Support in Britain has been falling from over 25 per cent between 1993

Chart 1.3: Percentage of children in poverty, contemporary terms (after housing costs)

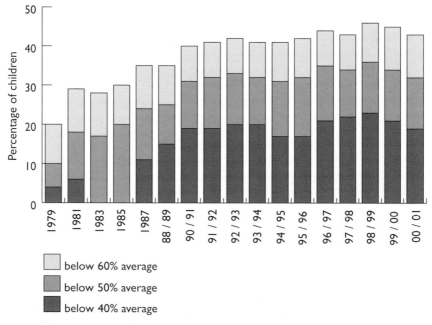

below 60% average
below 50% average
below 40% average

Source: DSS, Households Below Average Income, various years

Chart 1.4: Percentage of all children who are in families receiving Supplementary Benefit/Income Support

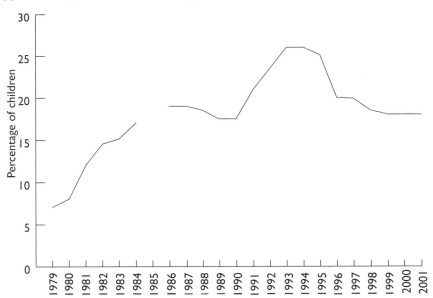

and 1995 to 18.1 per cent in May 2001. As about half of all children in poverty in Britain are in families receiving Income Support, this is a good indication that the numbers are moving in the right direction. One reason for the substantial decline in the numbers of children on Income Support is that the number of lone parent families on Income Support has been falling since 1995, when it reached over a million, to 888,000 in May 2001 (DWP, 2001b). This is despite the fact that the number of lone parents continues to rise.

Another source of evidence on trends in child poverty is the microsimulation analysis undertaken by the Cambridge Microsimulation Unit using POLIMOD. This has the advantage of being up to date and indeed being able to predict the results of policies that have been announced but not yet implemented. The latest analysis, which takes into account the impact of policies announced in the five Labour budgets 1997–2001 (Sutherland, 2001; see also Piachaud, 2001) estimates that 1 million children had been lifted out of 'current' poverty (less than 60 per cent of current median equivalent income before housing costs)[1]. It can be seen in Table 1.3 that if a constant relative poverty line is used (less than

---

[1] This may prove to be too high an estimate. The latest HBAI (DWP 2002) gives a reduction of only 600,000 children in households with equivalent income below 60 per cent of contemporary median before housing costs between 1996/7 and 2000/01. The Institute for Fiscal Studies have sought to explain the discrepancy between the modelled estimates and the survey evidence (Brewer *et al.*, 2002).

Table 1.3: The impact of five Labour budgets on child poverty, POLIMOD analysis

	All persons	All children	Children in lone parent families	Children in two parent families
Poverty rate, April 1997 policy (%)	19.4	25.9	41.9	21.5
'Constant' relative poverty rate in 2001 (%)	14.0	15.8	18.8	15.0
Net reduction (thousands)	3,090	1,330	650	680
'Current' relative poverty rate (%)	15.9	18.3	23.7	16.8
Net reduction (thousands)	2,020	1,000	520	480

Source: Sutherland (2001)

60 per cent of median equivalent income in April 1997 before housing costs), the proportion of children lifted out of poverty is 1.33 million.

These modelled reductions only take account of the impact of policy changes. A further number of children will have been lifted out of poverty as a result of their parent(s) obtaining employment. Between 1997 and 2001 the proportion of children living in workless families fell from 17.9 per cent to 15.3 per cent, and there has been a similar fall in the number of families with dependent children claiming out-of-work benefits.

The government published the third annual report *Opportunity for All* in September 2001 (DWP, 2001b). This latest annual report on progress in its anti-poverty strategy contains (now) 15 indicators relating to children and young people. Table 1.4 summarises the results. On all the indicators the latest results show an improvement on the baseline data.[2] So, for example, the proportion of children living in workless households is falling, as is relative, real terms and persistent poverty. There are small improvements in all the indicators of educational outcomes and a welcome fall in teenage pregnancies.

Of the indicators given here, some are for Great Britain and some are for the UK. Each devolved administration has its own strategies and targets.

- *Social Justice: A Scotland where everyone matters* (November 1999) and the *Social Justice Annual Report 2001* (November 2001) can be found at www.scotland.gov.uk/socialjustice. Scotland has developed its own social justice milestones and targets, which are somewhat different from those below.

---

[2] The proportion of children experiencing persistent poverty (2c) is likely to change very slowly as it is a running total. There is as yet no data for the educational outcomes of children in Sure Start areas (3) and no data, after the base year, on the housing conditions of children (8) because the English House Conditions Survey on which the data is based is only undertaken every six years. There is only a base observation for the educational level of children leaving care (11) and for smoking during pregnancy (15).

Table 1.4: Summary of the *Opportunity for All* indicators for children and young people

---

1. % children living in workless households

17.9	17.8	17.3	15.7	15.3
(1997)	(1998)	(1999)	(2000)	(2001)

2a. % children living in households with income below 60% of the contemporary median before housing costs

26	25	24	23	21
(1996/97)	(1997/98)	(1998/99)	(1999/00)	(2000/01)

2a. % children living in households with income below 60% of the median after housing costs

34	33	33	32	31
(1996/97)	(1997/98)	(1998/99)	(1999/00)	(2000/01)

2b. % children living in households with income below 60% of the 1996/97 median held constant in real terms before housing costs

26	24	22	19	16
(1996/97)	(1997/98)	(1998/99)	(1999/00)	(2000/01)

2b. % children living in households with income below 60% of the 1996/97 median held constant in real terms after housing costs

34	32	31	28	23
(1996/97)	(1997/98)	(1998/99)	(1999/00)	(2000/01)

2c. % of children experiencing persistent low income – below 60% median household income in at least 3 out of 4 years

19	16	17	16
(1991/94)	(1994/97)	(1995/98)	(1996/99)

2c. % children experiencing persistent low income – below 70% median household income – in at least 3 out of 4 years

28	25	26	26
(1991/94)	(1994/97)	(1995/98)	(1996/99)

---

3. % of 7-year-old children in Sure Start areas achieving Key Stage 1 English and maths tests

---

4. % of those aged 11 achieving level 4 or above in Key Stage 2 tests for literacy

57 (1996)	63 (1997)	65 (1998)	71 (1999)	75 (2000)	75 (2001)

---

4. % of those aged 11 achieving level 4 or above in Key Stage 2 tests for numeracy

54 (1996)	62 (1997)	59 (1998)	69 (1999)	72 (2000)	71 (2001)

---

5. % of 16-year-olds with at least one GCSE A*-G

92.2 (1996)	92.3 (1997)	93.4 (1998)	94.0 (1999)	94.4 (2000)

---

6. % of 19-year-olds with at least a level 2 qualification or equivalent

79.7 (1996)	72.3 (1997)	73.9 (1998)	74.9 (1999)	75.3 (2000)

---

7. % truancies and school exclusions

0.17	0.17	0.16	0.14	0.11
(1995/96)	(1996/97)	(1997/98)	(1998/99)	(1999/00)

8. % of children who live in a home which falls below the set standard of decency
    23 (1996)

---

9. Admission rates (per 1,000) to hospital as a result of an unintentional injury resulting in a stay of longer than 3 days for children aged under 16

1.20	1.12	1.02	1.02
(1996/97)	(1997/98)	(1998/99)	(1999/00)

---

10. % of 16–18-year-olds in learning
    76.3 (1996)   74.9 (1997)   74.9 (1998)   75.0 (1999)   75.8 (2000)

---

11. % of young people leaving care with one or more GCSE (grade A*-G) or a vocational qualification
                                31 (1999)

---

12. Under 18 conception rates per 1,000 aged 15–17
    45.9 (1996)   45.5 (1997)   46.5 (1998)   44.7 (1999)

---

12. % of teenage parents who are not in education, employment or training
    83.5 (1996)   82.1 (1997)   72.6 (1998)   72.9 (1999)   68.4 (2000)   71.0 (2001)

---

13. % re-registered on the child protection register
            19 (1997/98)   15 (1998/99)   14 (1999/00)

---

14. The gap in mortality for children under 1 year between manual groups and the population as a whole (difference in infant mortality rates per 1,000)
    0.50 (1996)   0.42 (1997)   0.49 (1998)

---

15. Smoking rates (%)
During pregnancy   18 (2000)

Among children 11–15
    13 (1996)   11 (1998)   9 (1999)   10 (2000)

Source: DWP (2001b) and DWP (2002)

- The National Assembly for Wales draft strategic statement on the preparation of a *Plan for Wales 2001* can be found at www.planforwales.wales.gov.uk
- *New Targeting Social Need* (December 2000) for Northern Ireland can be found at www.newtsnni.gov.uk.

Country and regional variations in child poverty

There are two sources of data on spatial variations in child poverty – survey evidence and evidence derived from administrative statistics. The Family Resources Survey is the only survey at present large enough to provide reasonably reliable comparisons of child poverty rates within Great Britain[3] (Northern

---

[3] The British Household Panel Survey is in the process of enhancing the size of its samples in Wales, Scotland and Northern Ireland and that will, in time, enable country comparisons to be made.

Table 1.5: Child poverty rate, various indicators (excluding the self-employed), 2000/01

Country	Bottom quintile	<40% mean	<50% mean	<60% mean
Before housing costs				
England	25	8	20	35
Wales	31	9	26	41
Scotland	30	10	24	38
Great Britain	25	8	21	35
After housing costs				
England	27	16	30	41
Wales	31	20	33	43
Scotland	26	14	30	41
Great Britain	27	16	30	41

Source: DWP (2002)

Ireland was not included but it will be included from 2002). Table 1.5 provides a comparison of various indicators of child poverty for countries within Great Britain. There is very little variation at the 40 per cent threshold before housing costs. However, after housing costs Scotland has a lower rate than England and Wales. At the other thresholds Wales has the highest child poverty rate both before and after housing costs.

Table 1.6 presents the same data for the English regions. It is important to note the position of London, which before housing costs has a lower child poverty rate than the North East, but after housing costs has by far the highest child poverty rate. The Eastern Region has the lowest child poverty rate both before housing costs and equal lowest with the South East after housing costs.

Table 1.6: Variations in child poverty rates (excluding the self-employed) between the English regions 2000/01

English Region	Below 50% mean equivalent income before housing costs	Below 50% mean equivalent income after housing costs
North East	34	38
North West and Merseyside	21	31
Yorkshire and the Humber	23	29
East Midlands	23	27
West Midlands	24	35
Eastern	10	22
London	25	41
South East	11	22
South West	15	27
England	20	30

Source: DWP (2002)

Table 1.7: Highest and lowest child poverty rates by ward in each country in the UK. Figures in brackets are national rank (out of 11,090 wards in the UK)

England	Wales	Scotland	N. Ireland
(11,083) 88.7 Bidstone, Wirral	(11,048) 81.7 Tredegar Park,	(11,090) 96.1 Whitfield South,	(11,088) 92.4 Shantallow East, Derry
(11,082) 88.7 Princess, Knowsley	(11,045) 81.2 Townhill, Swansea	(11,089) 94.4 Keppochhill, Glasgow City	(11,087) 91.4 Brandywell, Derry
(11,074) 85.5 Smithdown, Liverpool	(11,031) 79.9 Marchog, Gwynedd	(11,086) 90.2 Drumry, Glasgow City	(11,085) 89.4 Creggan South, Derry
(11,073) 85.4 Blackwall, Tower Hamlets	(11,000) 77.4 Penderry, Swansea	(11,084) 89.1 Wellhouse, Glasgow City	(11,081) 88.4 Falls, Belfast
(11,072) 85.2 Beechwood, Middlesborough	(10,996) 77.2 Pembroke: Monkton, Pembrokeshire	(11,080) 87.7 Royston, Glasgow City	(11,064) 83.8 New Lodge, Belfast
(1) 0.5 Gerrads Cross, N. Bucks	(86) 3.3 Killay North, Swansea	(2) 0.7 Kilmardinny, E. Dunbartonshire	(43) 2.4 Cultra, North Down

Source: Social Deprivation Unit, University of Oxford

The other source of data on the spatial variation in child poverty is administrative statistics. Thanks to the work of the Oxford Social Deprivation Unit we now have a fairly up-to-date indicator of the prevalence of child poverty at area level. The index is based on administrative statistics on the number of children in households receiving Income Support, income-based Jobseeker's Allowance, Family Credit or Disabled Working Allowance, as a proportion of the number of children receiving Child Benefit. The addresses of the households are allocated to wards using postcodes.

Table 1.7 lists the five highest child poverty wards and the lowest ward in each country in the UK. There are 11,090 wards in the UK. Whitfield South in Dundee has the highest proportion of poor children, at 96.1 per cent. Then for Scotland come four wards in Glasgow City each with child poverty rates well over 80 per cent. The top three wards in Northern Ireland are all in Derry. The top three wards in England are all in the North West region. Despite Wales having the highest child poverty rate nationally, their highest wards come a little further down the overall distribution, with the highest ward being Tredegar Park in Newport. The ward with the lowest child poverty rate in the UK is Gerrards Cross in North Buckinghamshire, England, with only 0.5 per cent poor children.

Chart 1.5: Distribution of child poverty rates by wards

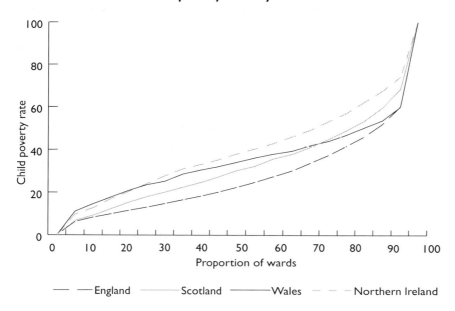

For the UK as a whole the highest 20 per cent of wards have poverty rates of 44 per cent or above while the lowest 20 per cent of wards have child poverty rates of 12.5 per cent or less. Thus child poverty is not evenly distributed between wards in the UK – there are a small proportion of wards with very high rates and a small proportion with very low rates. This variation in the concentration of child poverty in wards is compared for countries within the UK in Chart 1.5. In the chart, this inequality is represented as a curve in which the cumulative percentage of wards is plotted against the rank order of the proportion of children in poverty. It is possible to compare the intensity of poverty between countries using the chart. It shows that there is most inequality in the child poverty rates of wards in England, with a higher proportion of poverty concentrated in fewer wards. In Northern Ireland, by contrast, there are relatively high rates of child poverty in all wards.

A rather different perspective is provided in Table 1.8 where the comparison is made by local authority. By far the highest concentration of child poverty is found in Tower Hamlets in London, and five English local authority areas have higher rates of child poverty even than the highest in Northern Ireland or Scotland and 16 with higher rates than the highest in Wales.

Table 1.8: Child poverty rates by local authority: the top local authority child poverty rates in each country

England	%	Wales	%	Scotland	%	Northern Ireland	%
Tower Hamlets	73.5						
Hackney	61.7						
Newham	58.9						
Liverpool	58.6						
Knowsley	58.6			Glasgow	57.7	Derry	58.0
Manchester	56.8			Dundee Central	47.4	Strabane	54.8
Nottingham	53.5			West Dundee	44.8	Belfast	52.9
Kingston upon Hull, City of	52.7			North Ayr	42.8	Moyle	49.4
Islington	52.7			Inverclyde	41.6	Cookstown	48.1
Middlesborough	51.3			East Ayr	39.9	Newry and Mourne	45.8
Salford	50.3					Dungannon	42.7
Penwith	49.9						
Lincoln	48.9						
Haringey	47.6						
Birmingham	47.5						
Hastings	47.3	Merthyr	47.1				
Southwark	47.0	Blaenau	45.2				
Blackburn with Darwen	47.0	Caerphilly	42.1				
Newcastle upon Tyne	46.9	Rhondda	41.5				
		Newport	41.4				
		Anglesey	39.3				
		Neath Port Talbot	38.2				

Source: Social Deprivation Unit: University of Oxford

The characteristics of children in poverty

Table 1.9 provides a summary of the characteristics of poor children in Britain[4] – both their composition and their rate. So, for example:

- 49 per cent of poor children live in households with no one employed and 80 per cent of children in such households are poor. However, 22 per cent of poor children live in households with someone working full time.
- 44 per cent of poor children live in lone parent households, 55 per cent of children in lone parent households are poor but only 12 per cent of children are poor if the lone parent is employed full time.

---

[4] The sub-samples for Scotland and Wales in the FRS are not large enough to allow for reliable disaggregation at national level.

- 25 per cent of children in couple families are in poverty if there is only one full-time worker.
- The risk of poverty is much higher for younger mothers but mothers under 24 include only 7 per cent of all poor children.
- The risk of child poverty is much higher when there are four or more children in the household. However, 53 per cent of poor children live in one or two child families.
- A child is more likely to be poor if the youngest child in the family is aged under five and 48 per cent of poor children are found in such families.
- The presence of a disabled adult or a disabled child also increases the risk of child poverty.
- Half of all poor children are living in families receiving Income Support or Jobseeker's Allowance and the risk of poverty is highest in such families.
- Over 80 per cent of poor children are white. However, the risk of child poverty is higher in all minority ethnic groups, but especially in households of Pakistani or Bangladeshi ethnic origin.

Table 1.9: Characteristics of children in poverty (<60% median after housing costs)

	Composition (% of children in poverty who live in a household of this type)	Rate (% of children living in a household of this type who are poor)
Economic status of the household		
Households with one or more workers	51	19
Workless households	49	80
Economic status – Lone parent		
Working full-time	2	12
Working part-time	5	32
Not working	36	77
Couples		
Self employed	11	31
Both in full-time work	1	2
One in full-time work, one in part-time work	5	6
One in full-time work, one not working	14	25
One or more in part-time work	8	54
Both not in work	17	96
Family type		
Couples	56	23
Lone parent	44	55

Age of mother in the family

Under 20	1	63
20–24	6	49
25–29	15	41
30–34	27	36
35–39	25	27
40–44	16	25
45–49	7	21
50–-54	2	19
55 and over	1	27

Number of children

One	18	24
Two	35	25
Three	27	36
Four or more	20	56

Age of youngest child in the family

Under 5	48	35
5–10	34	31
11–15	15	25
16–18	3	17

Disability

No disabled adult	74	28
Disabled adult	26	43
No disabled child	86	30
Disabled child	14	36

Benefit/tax credit receipt of family

Disability Living Allowance	5	24
Jobseeker's Allowance	6	85
Incapacity Benefit	6	48
Working Families Tax Credit	17	37
Income Support	44	76
Housing Benefit	50	75
Not in receipt of any benefits/tax credit listed	29	14

Ethnic group

White	81	28
Black Caribbean	2	37
Black other	3	55
Indian	3	37
Pakistani and Bangladeshi	8	73
Other	3	44

All	100	31

Source: DWP (2002)

The dynamics of child poverty

We have seen in Table 1.4 that the proportion of children experiencing persistent poverty (below the poverty threshold in at least 3 of the 4 years) fell from 19 per cent in 1991/94 to 16 per cent in 1996/99. This indicator is derived from longitudinal analysis of the British Household Panel Survey. It can be complemented by more detailed analysis by Hill and Jenkins (2001) from the same source. They traced child poverty experiences of children over six years (1991–1996). They found that 62 per cent of children under 17 had never been poor during that period, 24 per cent had been poor once or twice, 12 per cent three to five times and 1 per cent six times. Children 0–5 had the greatest risk of being poor more than three times. They identified 9 per cent of children under 17 in chronic poverty, where their family income over the six years was below the poverty threshold. Again children 0–5 were most likely to be living in chronic poverty.

Conclusions

This chapter has been concerned with the demography of children and child poverty in the UK. Over the last 20 years the overall size of the child population has been fairly stable with some variations in the age composition. However, after the 1960s baby boomers have completed their families, the impact of sub-replacement fertility will begin to bite and the child population will decline – in number and as a proportion of the overall population.

The relative child poverty rate more than trebled in the 1980s, and in the 1990s there was no reduction. However, welcome evidence of a decline in child poverty in Britain is just beginning to emerge and government indicators of child poverty appear to be moving in the right direction. However, there are huge national, regional and local variations in child poverty and the risks of child poverty are heavily concentrated in certain types of household.

The data sources at UK and country level are adequate for observing trends in the child population. The Family Resources Survey provides an excellent source for monitoring income measures of child poverty in England, Wales and Scotland and the results, although not as up-to-date as one would like, are being published in the *Households Below Average Income* statistics more quickly than in the past. Northern Ireland is not yet covered by this survey and at the moment we have to rely on administrative statistics to compare child poverty in Northern

Ireland with the rest of the UK. The extension of the Family Resources Survey and the British Household Panel Survey to Northern Ireland (and the BHPS enhanced sample in Wales and Scotland) might help this situation. Also, administrative data at local level is extremely valuable in making comparisons between areas and over time. All the countries in the UK have developed their own child poverty indicators and have begun to monitor their own progress in reaching targets to abolish child poverty.

2 Comparisons of Child Poverty and Deprivation Internationally

Jonathan Bradshaw

Key statistics:
- Britain has the third highest child poverty rate out of 25 countries in the Luxembourg Income Study.
- Britain has the highest child poverty rate in the European Union.

Key trends:
- Between the mid-1980s and mid-1990s child poverty in Britain increased more than in any other country.

Key sources:
- Luxembourg Income Study
- European Community Household Panel Survey

Introduction

The preoccupation of the UK government with child poverty has reflected an international concern about the impact of social and economic change for children. Thus, for example, UNICEF, for the first time in its history, launched a study on the impact of social and economic change on children in industrialised countries (Cornia and Danziger, 1997) and more recently followed it up with the report *A League Table of Child Poverty in Rich Nations* (UNICEF, 2000). Following the Lisbon summit, the European Union (EU) has begun to focus on social inclusion. Under the Belgian presidency, Atkinson *et al.* (2001) have produced an authoritative report that sets a standard for the measurement of social inclusion within the EU. At the same time Esping-Anderson *et al.* (2001) have designed *A New Welfare Architecture for Europe* with the battle against child poverty at the heart of it. Meanwhile Eurostat has been publishing reports on social exclusion which focus on children and families with children (European Union, 2001). Even the OECD has been applying its resources to poverty measurement and particularly child poverty in comparisons of child poverty in a selection of member countries (Oxley *et al.*, 2001).

In the last decade our capacity to analyse child poverty comparatively has been greatly enhanced by the availability of new data. Thus the Luxembourg Income Study (LIS) has included more countries and more sweeps, and has become the vehicle for very detailed analysis of child poverty (Bradbury and Jantti, 1999; Bradshaw, 1999). The OECD (Oxley *et al.*, 2001) has obtained data from national sources on child poverty in 16 countries and undertaken a detailed analysis of child poverty rates and trends over time. At last, the results of the European Community Household Panel Survey (ECHP) (European Union, 2001) are emerging more quickly, and the survey is becoming a rich source of comparative analysis within the EU.

But there are limitations. With the exception of the ECHP, poverty and child poverty in these datasets is defined as an arbitrary point on the general distribution of income (albeit equivalised). Thus the LIS analysis generally employs a 50 per cent of median equivalent income threshold, as does the OECD. Eurostat has recently adopted a threshold of 60 per cent of equivalent median income. Most analysis has settled for the modified OECD equivalence scale, despite the fact that research based on budget standards suggests that it (and most other scales) underestimate the real costs of children (Bradshaw, 1993).

These measures of a relative lack of income are not by themselves particularly good indicators of poverty.

- Poverty rates (and the composition of the poor) vary with different definitions of income, especially whether it is before or after housing costs.
- The results are sensitive to the general shape of the income distribution.
- Income tends to misrepresent the real living standards of farmers, the self-employed and students.
- Income 'lumping' at points of the distribution where large numbers of households are receiving the (same) minimum income creates big variations in the poverty rate for small changes in the threshold.
- A household income measure fails to take account of the distribution of in-come within families – especially problematic for those (southern EU) countries with significant minorities of children living in multi-unit households.
- Most analyses report poverty rates, not poverty gaps – ie, how far below the poverty line children are.
- The cross-sectional datasets do not allow an analysis of how often or how long children are in poverty (though see below).

- Finally because they are based on survey data, these estimates take time to emerge – currently researchers are working on the LIS data for circa 1995 (http://lisweb.lu/keyfigures.htm); the OECD data is for 1993–95; and the latest published ECHP analysis of poverty is for the fourth 1998 sweep (1997 income data).

Nevertheless, we know from this work that:

- The UK has a comparatively high child poverty rate. LIS data ranks the UK third from the top (out of 25 countries) – only less than the USA and Russia in the child poverty league table in the mid-1990s (UNICEF, 2000). The most recent data on child poverty is from the 1998 ECHP (income data for 1997) and this finds the UK with the highest child poverty rate in the EU by some margin (Table 2.1 column 1).
- If a less relative threshold is used, such as the proportion of children below the US Poverty Standard, then the UK position improves, with a child poverty rate that is lower than the southern EU countries and Ireland but still considerably higher than all our northern European partners (UNICEF, 2000).

Table 2.1: Relative poverty rates (60% median equivalised income) for children and families with children, 1997

	Children 0–15	Single Parent with at least 1 child	2 adults, 1 child	2 adults, 2 children	2 adults 3+ children
Belgium	15	30	7	12	18
Denmark	3	9	0	3	6
Germany	24	48	8	12	*38
Greece	21	24	13	14	26
Spain	25	30	14	21	33
France	24	*31	7	8	30
Ireland	28	40	14	12	38
Italy	24	25	15	21	34
Luxembourg	*17	*27	*8	*9	*23
Netherlands	13	40	7	6	17
Austria	16	28	11	9	26
Portugal	29	40	12	13	58
Finland	7	9	5	4	9
Sweden	10	16	6	7	12
UK	39	41	12	16	*36

* 1996

Source: European Union (2001)

Table 2.2: Long-term poverty (< 50% median equivalent disposable income) in the first four waves of the ECHP

	All households	Households with children
Austria	2.5	–
Belgium	4.3	6.0
Denmark	0.7	0.1
Finland	1.6	–
France	2.4	1.7
Greece	7.3	5.9
Ireland	3.8	4.3
Italy	4.8	5.3
Netherlands	2.5	2.2
Portugal	8.7	6.4
Spain	3.6	4.6
Sweden	10.5	–
UK	6.5	4.3

Source: Calculations from Koen Vleminckx on the ECHP

- It is very likely to be the case that where child poverty is persistent, it will be worse – a harsher experience and with longer-term consequences. Table 2.2 presents an analysis of the long-term poverty for all households and for households with children based on the ECHP. Long-term poverty is defined here as being in poverty (below 50 per cent of median equivalent disposable income) in each of the first four sweeps (income data 1993–96) of the ECHP. On this definition long-term poverty is very rare in Denmark and rare in France and the Netherlands but it is higher in the UK, Ireland, Belgium and the southern EU countries. Bradbury *et al.* (2001) have compared the dynamics of child poverty in seven countries (the UK, Germany, Hungary, Ireland, Russia, Spain and the USA). The results are summarised in Table 2.3. They found that, among the countries with a consistent income definition, the UK had the highest proportion of children always in poverty in two waves (10 per cent) and five waves (3 per cent) and also the highest proportion ever in poverty in two waves (after Russia) (23 per cent) and in five waves (39 per cent). However, the USA had a larger proportion of children always in poverty than the UK. The UK also had the highest entry rate to poverty and the lowest exit rate from poverty among lone parent families.
- Nine out of the 15 EU countries, including the UK, have a higher child poverty rate than over-65 poverty rate (see Chart 2.1).[1] Britain is special in

---

[1] These results are highly sensitive to the equivalence scale used.

Table 2.3: Persistence of poverty among children

	% children with household income always below half median income				% children with household income ever below half median income			
	In wave 1	2 out of 2 waves	5 out of 5 waves	10 out of 10 waves	In wave 1	In 2 wave	In 5 wave	In 10 wave
Britain	16.8	10.1	3.3	16.8	22.9	39.3		
Germany	7.7	4.1	1.5	7.7	11.9	15.6		
West Germany	6.8	4.3	1.7	2.2	6.8	10.0	14.5	21.3
Hungary	9.7	4.6	2.1	9.7	11.2	19.5		
Russia	24.1	9.6	24.1	33.5				
Spain	11.9	7.6	11.9	18.1				
Ireland*	15.6	8.3	15.6	21.3				
USA**	24.7	19.3	13.0	6.8	24.7	30.4	37.6	44.7

Note: Ireland and USA income definitions not comparable: *annual net income, ** annual gross income
Source: Bradbury et al. (2001)

Chart 2.1: Child and over-65 poverty rates, 1997

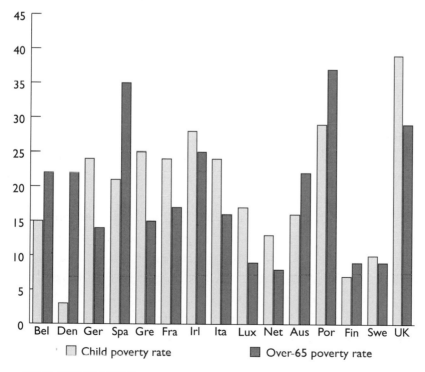

Source: ECHP 1998 (EU 2001)

having comparatively high poverty rates for both children and the over-65s. There need not be a trade-off between child and older people poverty – Luxembourg, the Netherlands, Finland and Sweden achieve low rates of both. However, in some countries there may have been a trade-off – Denmark has a much lower child poverty rate than older poverty rate and Germany and Britain both have a big gap between their over-65 and child poverty rates. The living standards of their pensioners may have been sustained at the expense of children.

- Not all countries experienced an increase in child poverty between the mid-1980s and the mid-1990s; indeed about half have experienced a reduction (Chart 2.2). This demonstrates that it is not the case that changes in family form, particularly the increase in cohabitation and lone parenthood inevitably result in an increase in child poverty. Nor does pressure on the economy from globalisation inevitably result in a deterioration in the living standards of children.

Chart 2.2: Trends in child poverty (% point change)

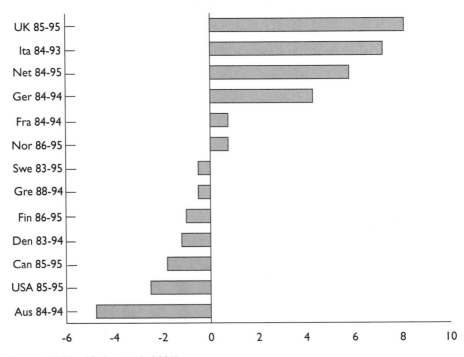

Source: OECD (Oxley et al., 2001)

- Variations in child poverty are to some extent explainable by variations in *demographic patterns*. It is generally the case that children are more likely to be poor if they live in:
    - *A lone parent family*. It can be seen in Table 2.1 column 2 that the poverty rates of lone parent families are higher in all countries than for two-parent families with one or two children. The differential in the poverty rate (between a lone parent and a couple with one child) is largest in Germany, the Netherlands and Britain.
    - If there are *many children in the family*.[2] It can be seen in Table 2.1 that the poverty rates are higher in all countries when there are three or more children in couple families.
- Variations in child poverty are also explainable by variations in the *labour supply of parents*. It is generally the case that children are more likely to be poor if they live in:
    - A *workless family*. Table 2.4 shows that along with Ireland, the UK has the highest rate of worklessness among lone parent families and comes

Table 2.4: Worklessness among families with children, 1998

	Rate of worklessness among lone parent families, %	Rate of worklessness among couple families with children, %
Belgium	51	6
Germany	38	6
Greece	35	3
Spain	39	9
France	34	6
Ireland	61	12
Italy	29	7
Luxembourg	30	2
Netherlands	55	6
Austria	24	3
Portugal	25	3
Finland	42	7
UK	61	11

Source: OECD (1998) Table 1.7 Data for Denmark, Norway and Sweden not available

---

[2] *Age of the youngest child*: In Britain the child poverty rates in couple families are higher if there is a pre-school child in the family. However, in other countries there is little or no difference in the child poverty rate in couple families by the age of the youngest child. However, in lone parent families the child poverty rate in most counties is higher if the youngest child is a pre-school child (Bradshaw, 1999).

Table 2.5: Child poverty rates (%) (children in families with income below 50 per cent of median income), by number of earners, mid-1990s

| | Type of family and number of earners | | | | |
	Couple, no earner	Couple, 1 earner	Couple, 2+ earners	Lone parent, no earner	Lone parent, 1+ earners
Australia	18	9	5	42	9
Belgium	16	3	1	23	11
Canada	74	18	4	73	27
Denmark	6	4	–	34	10
Germany	45	6	1	62	33
Greece	22	15	5	37	16
France	38	7	2	45	13
Finland	4	4	2	10	3
Italy	70	21	6	79	25
Netherlands	51	5	1	41	17
Norway	31	4	–	30	5
Sweden	10	6	1	24	4
UK	50	19	3	69	26
USA	82	31	7	93	39

Source: Oxley et al. (2001)

close to Ireland with the highest rate of worklessness among couple families.

- A *single earner* family. Table 2.5 gives the child poverty rates by the number of earners in the family. In all countries there are very low child poverty rates if there are two earners in a couple family. After Italy, the UK has the highest child poverty rate among couples with only one earner.

However the impact of the demographic patterns and the variations in employment rates on child poverty can be mitigated by social policies, crucially the tax and cash benefit systems. We have seen that the poverty rate for children living in workless families is much lower in some countries than in others. This is because the system of social protection for workless families is so much better in those countries – it protects children more effectively. Similarly we have seen that the poverty rate for children living in families with one or even two earners is much lower in some countries than in others. This is partly a function of variation in the level of earnings. However, it is also the consequence of variations in the level of the tax and benefit package which exists in each country to support the incomes of families raising children. We know from international comparisons that there are major variations in this child tax/benefit package

Chart 2.3: Impact of transfers on child poverty rates, mid-1990s

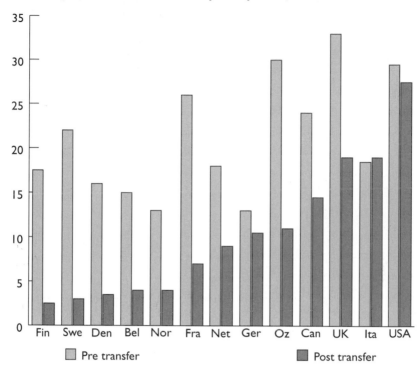

Source: Oxley *et al.* (2001)

(Bradshaw *et al.*, 1993, 1996; Ditch *et al.*, 1998; Kilkey, 2000). One way of illustrating the importance of the transfer mechanisms is to estimate child poverty rates before transfers – that is, the poverty rate that would exist as a result of the market and before any intervention by the state; and after transfers – that is, after the impact of taxes and cash benefits (but not services in this example). The results of such a comparison are presented in Chart 2.3. The UK starts with a pre-transfer poverty rate that is highest of the countries in the comparison. This is a function of our demographic pattern, in particular the large number of children in lone parent and workless households. After the impact of transfers, the child poverty rate in the UK falls by 43 per cent to the third highest of the countries in the chart. The UK's transfer package is more successful at reducing pre-transfer poverty than that in the US and certainly Italy (where the tax system results in an increase in child poverty). However, the UK tax and benefit systems are much less successful in preventing child poverty than, for example, Finland and Sweden, which reduce their pre-transfer child poverty by 88 per cent, or France with a 73 per cent reduction.

Conclusion

It is important to emphasise again that this chapter gives a largely historical picture. Only the ECHP analysis provides any data for after the election of the Labour government in 1997 and none of the data provides evidence of the impact of any of the changes the Labour government began to make after 1999, which might be expected to make a difference to the comparative position of the UK. The next LIS sweep will cover the situation of countries around 2000 but it will probably not be until the 2005 sweep that we see the impact of the government's anti-poverty strategy in a comparative perspective. As part of this project, and the *International Comparative Project on Child Well-being*, we have produced a database, which collects together comparative indicators of the economic well-being of children (http://www-users.york.ac.uk/~jrb1/).

3 Mortality

Patricia Sloper and Deborah Quilgars

Key statistics:

- In 1999, the UK infant mortality rate was 5.7 per 1,000 live births, compared to the EU average of 5.2.
- Mortality rates are highest at and just after birth, falling in the post-neonatal period and during childhood.

Key trends:

- Across the UK, rates of infant and child mortality have decreased substantially over the last 20 years.
- Higher mortality rates are found in social class IV and V; in areas of social deprivation; for children born to lone or teenage mothers; for children whose mothers were born in the New Commonwealth; and in boys compared to girls. Many of these factors are associated with poverty.
- Social deprivation is more strongly linked to mortality rates for deaths at over 28 days after birth. Improved health care around and following birth appears to have reduced social differentials for deaths in the neonatal period.

Key sources:

- Office for National Statistics
- Northern Ireland Statistics and Research Agency
- General Register Office for Scotland

Introduction

In modern UK society, the death of a child is seen as an unnatural event, and 'the loss of a child is every family's worst nightmare' (UNICEF, 2001a, p. 7). A key target in the United Nations Convention on the Rights of the Child is that States Parties should aim to 'diminish infant and child mortality' (Article 24). The second half of the 20th century saw a marked decline in infant and child mortality rates in both advanced economic and developing nations. Although the rate of decline has decelerated in recent years, there is no evidence of any rise (Ahmad *et al.*, 2000). Consistently with international trends, mortality rates in the UK fell substantially during the 20th century. However, comparisons with other European countries indicate considerable room for improvement. In order to understand why this may be the case, it is important to examine the factors associated with higher or lower mortality rates. Concentrating mainly on the UK, this chapter sets out to review evidence on infant and child mortality over time and in relation to age at death, causes of death, gender, social class, family type, age of mother, ethnicity, and area and other deprivation indicators.

Definitions and sources of data

Mortality statistics are produced annually in all countries in the UK, by the Northern Ireland Statistics and Research Agency, General Register Office for Scotland and Office for National Statistics (covering England and Wales). These are based on information recorded on registration of deaths. Official publications categorise five types of infant mortality:

    Early neonatal deaths: deaths at up to 6 completed days of life

    Perinatal: stillbirths plus early neonatal deaths

    Late neonatal: deaths at 7–27 completed days of life

    Post-neonatal: deaths at 28 days and over but under 1 year

    Infant deaths: deaths at ages under 1 year.

Early and late neonatal deaths are usually presented together as *neonatal deaths*, and *stillbirths* are often presented separately. *Child mortality* is commonly presented in three age groups: 1–4, 5–9 and 10–14 years.

Annual mortality statistics are the main data source for examination of infant and child mortality. At the time of writing, the most recent statistics available for all four countries of the UK are for 1999. A number of detailed analyses of factors related to mortality have been carried out, particularly by staff at the Office for National Statistics (ONS). These will be referred to throughout the chapter, but many of these analyses cover figures only for England and Wales or the whole of the UK, without disaggregation by country. One of the reasons for this is the difficulty of carrying out reliable analysis for categories where figures are very small when disaggregated.

Information contained in birth and death records

Information recorded on the death of a child comes from a number of sources: details supplied by the doctor certifying the death, by the informant to the registrar and/or by a coroner. Occupation is recorded for the father and details of whether the mother is in employment are recorded, but a description of mother's occupation is not obligatory. The effect of these differences in recording of mothers' and fathers' occupations means that there are considerable difficulties in using mothers' occupation in analysis of mortality rates (Botting and Cooper, 1993).

In England and Wales, a number of other details are recorded at birth, but not at death. These include birth weight, age of mother, country of birth of mother and marital status. In order to utilise this information in mortality statistics, ONS links the death records of infants (under the age of 1) to birth records using the child's NHS number. Since 1994, ONS has also started linking records for child deaths at ages 1, 2 and 3 years.

When registering a child's birth, there is a legal requirement for the father's current occupation, or last occupation if unemployed, to be recorded when the birth is 'joint' registration (ie, registered by both mother and father). Details of employment status, whether economically active or not, are also collected. Since 1986, registrars have been encouraged to collect details of mother's occupation and employment status, but this is not a legal requirement.

The information collected on occupation is classified according to the Standard Occupational Classification Codes for social class used in the census. However, this classification is approximate, as not all the questions used in the census to inform classification are covered in birth and death records. In addition, although details obtained on parents' occupation are coded for all stillbirths and infant deaths, for live births they are only coded for a 10 per cent sample.

Age and time trends

In all four UK countries, mortality rates are highest at and just after birth. They then fall in the post-neonatal period and during childhood, with the lowest rates between the ages of 5 and 9 years (Table 3.1).

Rates for all types of childhood mortality decreased substantially between 1981 and 1999 in England and Wales. Infant deaths decreased by almost 50 per cent: from 11.1 to 5.8 per 1,000 live births. There has also been a decrease of almost half in child mortality, but the rates for ages 5–9 showed a larger drop during the 1990s than those for 10–14.

Figures for Scotland and Northern Ireland show a similar pattern over time. Infant deaths in Northern Ireland decreased from 10.5 to 6.4 per 1,000 live births between 1984 and 1999, and in Scotland from 10.5 in 1981–85 to 5.0 in 1999. Table 3.2 shows rates for stillbirths, neonatal, post-neonatal, infant and child mortality for the UK as a whole and separately for England, Wales, Scotland and Northern Ireland, for the period 1995–1999. These figures show a general trend of a reduction over this time period in mortality rates for all four countries. Due to the smaller populations of Wales, Scotland and Northern Ireland, mortality rates show greater variation from year to year than for England and the UK as a whole, but no distinct pattern emerges to suggest that rates are consistently different between the countries.

Table 3.1: Stillbirths, infant and child mortality rates, 1981–1999, England and Wales

Year of death	*Still-births	**Neo-natal deaths	**Post-neonatal deaths	**Infant deaths	***Ages 1–4	***Ages 5–9	***Ages 10–14
1981	6.6	6.7	4.4	11.1	50	23	24
1982	6.3	6.3	4.6	10.8	47	21	23
1983	5.7	5.9	4.3	10.1	44	23	22
1984	5.7	5.6	3.9	9.5	42	21	22
1985	5.5	5.4	4.0	9.4	45	20	23
1986	5.3	5.3	4.3	9.6	42	19	19
1987	5.0	5.1	4.1	9.2	42	18	20
1988	4.9	4.9	4.1	9.0	42	19	20
1989	4.7	4.8	3.7	8.4	40	19	19
1990	4.6	4.6	3.3	7.9	38	17	19
1991	4.6	4.4	3.0	7.4	36	18	19
1992	4.3	4.3	2.3	6.6	32	16	17
1993	5.7	4.2	2.2	6.3	32	14	18
1994	5.7	4.1	2.1	6.2	29	14	17
1995	5.5	4.2	2.0	6.1	26	14	17
1996	5.4	4.1	2.0	6.1	28	12	15
1997	5.3	3.9	2.0	5.9	27	13	16
1998	5.3	3.8	1.9	5.7	28	12	14
1999	5.3	3.9	1.9	5.8	27	11	14

* Stillbirth rates per 1,000 total births. Up to 1992 these figures represent foetal deaths at or over 28 weeks gestation, and from 1993 at or over 24 weeks gestation.
** Neonatal, post-neonatal and infant deaths per 1,000 live births
*** Childhood deaths per 100,000 population of the same age
Source: ONS (2001a)

Table 3.2: Stillbirths, infant and child mortality rates 1995–1999: UK, England, Wales, Scotland and Northern Ireland

Year	Stillbirths per 1,000 total births					Neonatal deaths per 1,000 live births				
	95	96	97	98	99	95	96	97	98	99
UK	**5.6**	**5.5**	**5.3**	**5.4**	**5.3**	**4.2**	**4.0**	**3.9**	**3.8**	**3.9**
England*	5.5	5.4	5.3	5.3	5.3	4.2	4.1	3.9	3.8	3.9
Wales*	5.0	4.9	5.1	5.4	4.8	3.9	3.5	3.9	3.6	4.0
Scotland**	6.6	6.4	5.3	6.1	5.2	4.0	3.9	3.2	3.6	3.3
Northern Ireland***	61	6.3	5.4	5.1	5.7	5.5	3.7	4.2	3.9	4.8

Year	Post-neonatal deaths per 1,000 live births					Infant deaths per 1,000 live births				
	95	96	97	98	99	95	96	97	98	99
UK	**2.0**	**2.0**	**2.0**	**1.9**	**1.9**	**6.2**	**6.1**	**5.9**	**5.7**	**5.8**
England*	1.9	2.0	2.0	1.8	1.9	6.1	6.0	5.9	5.6	5.7
Wales*	2.0	1.9	2.0	2.0	2.1	5.9	5.4	5.9	5.6	6.1
Scotland**	2.2	2.2	2.1	2.0	1.7	6.2	6.2	5.3	5.6	5.0
Northern Ireland***	1.6	2.0	1.4	1.7	1.6	7.1	5.8	5.6	5.7	6.4

Year	Ages 1–4 Deaths per 100,000 population of the same age					Ages 5–9					Ages 10–14				
	95	96	97	98	99	95	96	97	98	99	95	96	97	98	99
UK	**26**	**28**	**27**	**27**	**27**	**14**	**12**	**13**	**13**	**12**	**17**	**16**	**16**	**15**	**14**
England*	26	27	26	27	26	13	12	13	12	11	17	15	16	14	14
Wales*	26	35	34	18	33	10	10	10	12	9	13	14	13	14	15
Scotland**	24	25	22	26	24	14	17	15	19	13	17	21	15	18	15
Northern Ireland***	29	18	25	26	33	20	12	16	13	18	24	17	16	15	14

* excluding non-residents of England and Wales
** including non-residents of Scotland
*** including deaths of non-residents of Northern Ireland
Sources: ONS (1997; 1998; 1999; 2000; 2001a)

The average 1998 infant mortality rate for the EU was 5.2 per 1,000 live births. The UK rate for 1998 of 5.7 was above the average, and considerably higher than those for Iceland (2.6), Sweden (3.5), Norway (4.0), Finland (4.2), Switzerland (4.4), Germany (4.7), France (4.8), and Austria (4.9) (Eurostat, 2000).

Causes of death

Causes of death are different at different ages. Conditions related to immaturity were recorded as causes of nearly 50 per cent of neonatal deaths in 1999 (ONS, 2001a). The next most common cause was congenital anomalies. Rosano *et al.* (2000) show a decrease over time in the proportion of infant mortality attributable to congenital anomalies for the UK. In 1980–84, this proportion was 29 per cent, declining to 21 per cent by 1994. Sudden infant deaths (that is, deaths of infants under 1 year old and defined as 'the sudden or unexpected death of any infant or young child which is unexpected by history and in which a thorough post-mortem examination fails to demonstrate an adequate cause of death' (Dattani, 2001)) have also declined during the 1990s. The sudden infant death rate for England and Wales was 0.69 per 1,000 live births in 1993 (Dattani, 2001), decreasing by 42 per cent to 0.40 per 1,000 live births by 2000 (ONS, 2001b). In Northern Ireland, 15 sudden infants deaths were recorded in 1996, reducing to three in 1999 (NISRA, 2000a). This decrease has been observed in many countries and has, at least in part, been attributed to more babies being placed to sleep on their backs (eg, Mehanni *et al.*, 2000).

In all four UK countries, injury and poisoning are the most common cause of death for boys over 1 year and girls over 4 years, with the most common injury deaths being due to motor vehicle traffic accidents (see Chapter 6). This pattern of causes is similar in other European countries (Morrison *et al.*, 1999). There has been a significant fall in the rate of child injury deaths in the UK from 14.3 per 100,000 children aged 1–14 in 1971–75 to 6.1 per 100,000 in 1991–95 (UNICEF, 2001a). Comparable reductions have been observed in most industrialised nations, with the UK now having one of the lowest injury death rates.

Deaths from cancer accounted for 27 per cent of deaths in 1991 for 5–9-year-olds and 19 per cent for 10–14-year-olds (Botting and Crawley, 1995). Although there has been little change in the incidence of childhood cancer over the past 40 years, the mortality rate from cancer has decreased over this time, with improvements in treatment leading to higher survival rates. Ten year survival rates have increased from less than 30 per cent in 1962–66, to almost 60 per cent in 1982–86, and 70 per cent in 1992–96 (UKCCSG, 2000).

In recent years, AIDS and HIV have emerged as causes of concern. By 2001, 1,100 cases of HIV infection in children had been recorded in the UK and 310 of these children had died (see Chapter 4).

Multiple births

The incidence of multiple births has increased dramatically in the UK in recent years. In England and Wales, the proportion of pregnancies resulting in multiple births increased from 9.9 per 1,000 in 1975 to 13.6 per 1,000 in 1994. The rise in the rate of triplet and higher order births was even greater: from 0.13 per 1,000 to 0.41 per 1,000 (Dunn and Macfarlane, 1996). Much of this increase has been linked to methods of infertility treatment. Mortality rates are much higher for multiple births than for singletons: in 1991 neonatal mortality rates were seven times higher for twins and over 20 times higher in triplets and higher order births (Doyle, 1996). This increase in risk is directly related to increases in risk of pre-term delivery and low birth weight for multiple gestation pregnancies (Warner et al., 2000).

Sex differences in mortality rates

Boys show higher mortality rates than girls at all ages, as illustrated in Table 3.3 for the UK as a whole. Figures for the four countries show the same basic pattern. From the age of 1 to 15 years, boys also show a higher proportion of deaths due to injury or poisoning than girls, with the proportion of deaths due to such causes for boys being almost half as much again as that for girls from age 5–9 (ONS, 2001a).

Table 3.3: Stillbirths, infant and child mortality rates for UK, 1999, by sex

Sex	*Still-births	**Neo-natal deaths	**Post neonatal deaths	**Infant deaths	***Ages 1–4	***Ages 5–9	***Ages 1–14
Male	5.4	4.3	2.1	6.4	31	13	16
Female	5.2	3.4	1.6	5.1	24	10	13

* Stillbirth rates per 1,000 total births
** Neonatal, post-neonatal and infant deaths per 1,000 live births
*** Childhood deaths per 100,000 population of the same age
Source: ONS (2001a)

Social class

As noted earlier, data recorded on social class are only approximate and, particularly for mothers, are incomplete. However, a number of analyses of social class trends in infant and child mortality rates have been undertaken, and

Table 3.4: UK infant mortality rates* by father's social class (babies born inside marriage)

Social class	1981	Year of birth 1991	1996	1997
All classes	10.4	6.3	5.4	5.2
Social class I	7.8	5.0	3.6	4.4
Social class II	8.2	5.3	4.4	4.0
Social class IIIN	9.0	6.2	5.4	5.4
Social class IIIM	10.5	6.3	5.8	5.3
Social class IV	12.7	7.2	5.9	6.4
Social class V	15.7	8.4	7.8	6.8
Other	15.6	11.8	8.3	8.8

* Deaths within 1 year of birth per 1,000 live births
Source: ONS (2000a)
I: Professional. *II*: Employers and managers. *IIIN*: Skilled occupation non-manual.
IIIM: Skilled occupation manual. *IV*: Junior non-manual. *V*: Skilled manual & own account non-professional. *VI*: Semi-skilled manual and personal service.
VII: Unskilled manual.
Source: 2000 General Household Survey.

results consistently show a class gradient, with highest mortality rates in social classes IV and V for both infant and child deaths.

The ONS (2000a) recently examined data on father's social class and infant mortality rates in the UK for births inside marriage registered in 1981, 1991, 1996 and 1997. The infant mortality rate for babies born in 1997 was one-and-a-half times higher for those with fathers in unskilled occupations than for those with fathers in professional occupations. Although infant mortality rates decreased for all social classes over the period, there was no decrease in the class differential (Table 3.4).

In the above table, rates for the 'other' category are comparatively high. There is a lack of information for parents classified as 'other', and it is likely that many lone mothers will be included in this category. Mortality rates for children of lone mothers will be discussed later in this chapter.

Whitehead and Drever (1999) analysed perinatal, neonatal and infant mortality rates combining social classes I and II, and IV and V, to increase the numbers in the analysis, and using 3-year moving averages to observe changes over time. Table 3.5 shows that infant mortality declined between 1975 and 1996 for every social class, with a slight decrease in the differential between IV and V compared to I and II from 64 per cent in 1975–7 to 52 per cent in 1994–6. The differentials were greater for post-neonatal mortality rates (78 per cent in 1994–6) than for perinatal mortality rates (41 per cent in 1994–6). Botting (1997) suggests that perinatal deaths are more likely to be linked to factors

Table 3.5: Trends in infant mortality rates for couple registrations by father's social class, England and Wales, 1975–1996

Year and category	Class I–II	Class IV-V	Excess mortality classes IV–V over II–I (%)
Perinatal mortality per 1,000 total births			
1975–7	13.8	20.6	50
1982–4	8.2	12.4	51
1989–91	6.5	9.5	47
1994–6	7.2	10.2	41
Neonatal mortality per 1,000 total births			
1975–7	7.6	11.3	48
1982–4	4.7	7.0	50
1989–91	3.7	5.2	40
1994–6	3.4	4.8	42
Post-neonatal mortality per 1,000 total births			
1975–7	3.0	6.1	105
1982–4	2.9	5.2	78
1989–91	2.0	4.3	118
1994–6	1.3	2.2	78
Overall infant mortality per 1,000 total births			
1975–7	10.6	17.5	64
1982–4	7.6	12.2	61
1989–91	5.7	9.6	67
1994–6	4.6	7.0	52

Source: Whitehead and Drever (1999), Table 4.

related to the birth, whereas later deaths may be more affected by external influences in the infant's home environment.

In general, infant mortality rates show clear class gradients which have persisted over time. The patterns for all four UK countries are similar. For example, for Northern Ireland in 1996–2000, the rate for social class V (7.5 per 1,000 live births) was 1.6 times higher than that for social class I (4.2 per 1,000 live births) (NISRA, 2001a). Figures for deaths in 1999 in England and Wales (ONS, 2001a) show infant mortality rates for registrations inside marriage to be more than double for social class V compared with social class I (8.4 compared with 3.8 per 1,000 live births) and 1.5 times higher for joint registrations outside marriage (8.7 compared with 5.8 per 1,000 live births).

Child mortality rates show a slightly different pattern. Botting (1997) compared child mortality rates for 1979–80 and 1982–3 with those from 1991–3, using population denominators from 1981 and 1991 census data (Table 3.6). In both time periods and in each age group, the mortality rates for children in class V were higher than for children in classes I–IV. For most observations, the

Table 3.6: Childhood mortality rates per 100,000 by age and social class, England and Wales

	1979–80, 82–83	*1991–93*
Age 1–4		
Social class I	34	27
Social class II	34	23
Social class IIIN	41	23
Social class IIIM	47	37
Social class IV	57	30
Social class V	98	71
All classes	*48*	*34*
Age 5–9		
Social class I	21	14
Social class II	19	12
Social class IIIN	22	11
Social class IIIM	23	19
Social class IV	28	14
Social class V	42	30
All classes	*25*	*16*
Age 10–14		
Social class I	19	14
Social class II	19	13
Social class IIIN	18	15
Social class IIIM	23	22
Social class IV	24	20
Social class V	30	29
All classes	*23*	*18*
Age 5–9		
Social class I	24	18
Social class II	22	16
Social class IIIN	25	16
Social class IIIM	28	26
Social class IV	33	22
Social class V	49	42
All classes	30	23

Source: Botting (1997) Table 7.6.
I: Professional. *II*: Employers and managers. *IIIN*: Skilled occupation non-manual. *IIIM*: Skilled occupation manual. *IV*: Junior non-manual. *V*: Skilled manual & own account non-professional. *VI*: Semi-skilled manual and personal service. *VII*: Unskilled manual.
Source: 2000 General Household Survey.

main differences do not show a consistent gradient of increased mortality over the class distribution, as is largely seen for infant mortality, but a marked increase between class IV and V. For instance, the 1991–93 overall child mortality rate is 1.9 times higher for class V compared with class IV. Ages 1–4 show the greatest differentials in both time periods.

Class gradients are seen for most of the causes of infant and child mortality, with the exception of cancer (OPCS, 1988; Fear *et al.*, 1999). Sudden infant death syndrome shows a particularly strong relationship with social class. Figures for England and Wales for 2000 show that the rates in social class V were over four times those in social class I (ONS, 2001b). In childhood, accidental deaths show the strongest class gradients across all ages (OPCS, 1988; see also Chapter 6).

Family type

The traditional method of analysing social trends in infant and child mortality statistics by social class of the father has limited examination of the position for children of lone mothers. However, analysis of linked birth and death records for England and Wales has shown that mortality rates for births outside marriage are relatively high. It is likely that this group will contain a high proportion of lone mothers.

The most recent study of mortality trends for babies registered solely by their mothers is that of Whitehead and Drever (1999), using linked birth and death records from 1975 to 1996 to compare infant mortality for couple registrations with sole registrations. Sole registrations were chosen on the assumption that most will be made by lone mothers. For sole registrations, infant mortality had fallen to less than a third of the 1975 level and the gap between mortality rates for couple and sole registrations had reduced: the excess mortality of 79 per cent in 1975 had reduced to 33 per cent in 1996 (Table 3.7). The reduction was greatest for the neonatal period (improved from 81 per cent to 2 per cent by 1996) and the perinatal period (improved from 100 per cent to 24 per cent). By contrast, excess mortality figures for the post-neonatal period rose from 74 per cent in 1975–77 to 103 per cent in 1994–96. The post-neonatal period is when factors associated with the infant's home environment are likely to be more influential, and the authors suggest that the improvements in the neonatal and perinatal periods may therefore be due to improved health care around and following the birth, rather than socio-economic factors.

An even more pronounced effect is seen for sudden infant deaths: in 2000,

Table 3.7: Trends in infant mortality for sole and couple registrations, England and Wales, 1975–1996

Year and category	Sole registrations	Couple registrations	Excess sole/couple (%)
Perinatal mortality per 1,000 total births			
1975–7	34.2	17.2	100
1982–4	17.8	10.1	77
1989–91	11.5	7.8	47
1994–6	10.6	8.6	24
Neonatal mortality per 1,000 total births			
1975–7	17.1	9.5	81
1982–4	8.2	5.7	43
1989–91	5.3	4.4	19
1994–6	4.2	4.1	2
Post-neonatal mortality per 1,000 total births			
1975–7	7.6	4.4	74
1982–4	7.5	3.9	91
1989–91	6.6	3.0	123
1994–6	3.7	1.8	103
Overall infant mortality per 1,000 total births			
1975–7	24.7	13.9	79
1982–4	15.7	9.6	63
1989–91	11.9	7.4	61
1994–6	7.8	5.9	33

Source: Whitehead and Drever (1999), Table 3.

the rate for babies born outside marriage and registered only by the mother was six times greater than for babies born inside marriage. Again, the difference was greater for post-neonatal than neonatal deaths (ONS, 2001b).

Comparisons between data in Table 3.5 and 3.7 indicate that sole registrations have higher mortality rates than social class IV and V couple registrations. For example, infant mortality in 1994–96 was 7.0 for social class IV and V and 7.8 for all sole registrations. It is possible that poverty is a factor influencing mortality rates in lone parent families: as we have seen in Chapter 1 the child poverty rate in lone parent families is 2.7 times the rate in couple families.

Age of mother

Children born to teenage mothers have higher mortality rates than those of other mothers. Schuman (1998) showed that for the years 1993–95, mothers under 20 at the time of birth had the highest infant mortality rates of all age groups (see Table 3.8), with the next highest rates being for mothers over 40. Mortality at ages 1 and 2 showed similar patterns, although babies dying at age

Table 3.8: Infant and child mortality rates by mother's age, England and Wales, 1993–1995

Mother's age	Year of birth	Infant deaths*	Age 1**	Age 2**
Total	1993	617	45	29
	1994	599	46	–
	1995	609	–	–
Under 20	1993	909	60	65
	1994	1,007	79	–
	1995	947	–	–
20–24	1993	692	64	28
	1994	709	65	–
	1995	730	–	–
25–29	1993	530	37	25
	1994	520	39	–
	1995	544	–	–
30–34	1993	557	35	25
	1994	511	29	–
	1995	502	–	–
35–39	1993	656	39	27
	1994	622	48	–
	1995	627	–	–
40+	1993	874	58	48
	1994	597	47	–
	1995	822	–	–

* Rates for infant deaths are per 100,000 live births
** Rates for ages 1 and 2 are per 100,000 population of the same age
Source: Schuman (1998), Table 4.

1 year whose mothers were in the 20–24 age group had similar rates to those of mothers under 20.

Mortality rates for 1999 (ONS, 2001a) show an overall drop, but a similar pattern in relation to mother's age to the above table. The rate for deaths under 1 year old of babies born to mothers under 20 was 8.7 per 1,000 live births, while that for mothers aged 30–34 was 5.0. The rate for mothers 40 and over was 6.3.

Recent analysis of sudden infant death rates for England and Wales (ONS, 2001b) shows a particularly steep gradient by age of mother: 1.05 per 1,000 live births for mothers under 20 compared with 0.30 for 25–29 and 0.21 for 30–34. The biggest differences are for deaths during the post-neonatal period.

Younger mothers tend to be disproportionately represented in manual social class groups and this may account for some of the findings on infant and child mortality and maternal age. Higher rates for mothers aged 40 or over are likely to be at least partly related to medical factors associated with late births.

Ethnicity

Data on ethnic background, births and childhood deaths are not recorded in a manner that can reliably link child mortality rates with ethnic origin. Although data on mothers' country of birth are collected at the registration of the birth of a child, this is an inadequate indicator of ethnic background, since an increasing proportion of the minority ethnic population of the UK are born in this country (Soni Raleigh and Balarajan, 1995). This should be born in mind when considering figures on mortality rates. Despite these caveats, it is possible to ascertain some patterns in rates by mothers' country of birth. Soni Raleigh and Balarajan (1995) analysed 1989–91 perinatal, neonatal and post-neonatal mortality rates. These were higher for infants of mothers born outside the UK, with the highest rates being for mothers born in Pakistan followed by the Caribbean and 'Rest of Africa' (Table 3.9). For infants of mothers born in India, Bangladesh and East Africa, the higher perinatal rates are followed by lower post-neonatal mortality rates than those for infants of mothers born in the UK. The authors suggest that the differences in mortality rates are partly, but not wholly, explained by social class and biological factors, such as the mother's age. Other contributory factors are nutritional differences, attitudes to antenatal screening, and quality and uptake of health care.

Figures for infant mortality rates for England and Wales in 1999 indicate that these differences have persisted. Mothers born in the New Commonwealth show a higher infant mortality rate (7.9) than mothers born in the UK (5.6), with Pakistan (10.1) and Rest of Africa (10.8) still showing the highest rates (ONS, 2001a).

Table 3.9: Perinatal, neonatal and post-neonatal mortality per 1,000 live births by mother's country of birth, England and Wales, 1989–1991

Mother's country of birth	Perinatal mortality	Neonatal mortality	Post-neonatal mortality
UK	7.9	4.4	3.2
East Africa	10.0	5.1	2.3
Bangladesh	10.9	3.8	2.3
India	9.9	5.9	2.7
Rest of Africa	13.2	7.6	3.5
Caribbean	13.3	6.5	4.3
Pakistan	14.2	7.4	5.5

Source: Soni Raleigh and Balarajan (1995)

Area and other deprivation indicators

The association between social class and mortality rates suggests links between poverty and infant and child deaths. Other indicators of deprivation add to this picture. Mortality rates vary by geographical area (Table 3.10), with higher rates in economically depressed areas (Woodroffe *et al.*, 1993).

A number of studies have examined the relationship between geographical area and mortality rates in more detail, looking at smaller areas and using standard measures of deprivation, such as the Townsend Deprivation Index (Townsend *et al.*, 1988). Bambamg *et al.* (2000) studied perinatal death rates in the West Midlands from 1991–93. Positive linear trends were found with increasing deprivation for perinatal death rates associated with different causes: congenital anomaly, antepartum events, intrapartum events and immaturity. Only deaths classified as 'other causes' failed to show this trend. Calculating relative risks of dying for each cause in relation to deprivation indices, they concluded that 'nearly 30 per cent of perinatal deaths were statistically "attributable" to social inequality' (p. 76).

Guildea *et al.* (2001) investigated the relationship between social deprivation and causes of stillbirths and infant deaths in Wales for the period 1993–98. They found that the relative risk of combined stillbirth and infant death was 1.53 for the most deprived compared with the least deprived districts. This relationship persisted across a number of causes of death and was particularly strong for sudden infant death syndrome, although early neonatal mortality was not significantly associated with deprivation. Within London, Hood (2001) shows that infant mortality rates for 1999–2000 range from 0 in City of London and 2.0 in Richmond to 9.0 and 9.1 in Waltham Forest and Hackney respectively.

Table 3.10: Regional variations in infant mortality rates*

	England 1998	Wales 1997–99	Scotland 1997–99	Northern Ireland 1997–99
Lowest	South East: 4.4	Powys and Merthyr Tydfil: 3.8	East Lothian: 2.6	Eastern Health and Social Services Board: 4.2
Highest	Yorkshire and Humber: 6.9	Blaenau Gwent: 8.4	West Dumbartonshire: 8.1	Western area: 8.1

*Per 1,000 live births
Source: ONS (2000a)

Areas with the highest levels on the deprivation index have some of the highest mortality rates. Earlier studies showed similar findings. For instance, Carstairs and Morris (1991) found associations between area deprivation and deaths in childhood at all ages in Scotland in 1980–82.

Bambamg et al's (2000) findings of a social gradient for different causes of death suggest that factors which operate from conception through to labour exert an effect. They note that the findings are consistent with suggestions that socio-economic effects are mediated through poor nutrition and ill health in the mother's foetal period and early childhood (Baird, 1980; Lumey, 1992) and through poor nutrition, stress and smoking during pregnancy (Brooke et al., 1989; Blair et al., 1996; Sheehan, 1998).

These observations indicate the need for detailed investigation of the more specific factors which underlie associations between mortality rates and broad-based variables such as social class and area deprivation. One such factor which has been investigated in considerable detail is parental smoking. The link between maternal smoking during pregnancy and perinatal mortality is well established (eg, Tuthill et al., 1999), and smoking during pregnancy shows a clear association with deprivation. For example, nearly 40 per cent of women in the most deprived areas of Scotland smoke during pregnancy, compared to only 14 per cent in the least deprived areas (Scottish Executive, 2001e). However, smoking shows effects independent of social deprivation. Blair et al. (1996) showed an increased risk of sudden infant death syndrome associated with maternal smoking during pregnancy, and additive effects of paternal smoking and daily exposure to tobacco smoke postnatally. These effects remained significant after controlling for maternal age, lone parenthood, short gestation, birth weight, sleeping position, and socio-economic status.

Conclusions

Rates of infant and child mortality have shown clear improvements over time in the UK. However, comparisons with other European countries show that there is potential for further improvement. The links between proxy indicators of poverty, such as social class and area deprivation, and higher mortality rates are well established. However, the factors underlying these links are complex. Boys, children of teenage mothers, infants born outside marriage and those from minority ethnic backgrounds are also at higher risk. Many of these additional factors are associated with social deprivation, but as yet there is no analysis which investigates the inter-relationship between different factors in order to inform more targeted interventions to decrease childhood mortality. The strongest associations between social factors and mortality rates are for the post-neonatal period, when factors in the home environment are likely to have more effect. This suggests that improvements in the neonatal and perinatal periods may be due to improved health care around and following the birth, rather than socio-economic factors. Opportunities for more detailed analysis are limited by the lack of reliable and comprehensive data which would enable mortality rates to be linked to variables such as income, minority ethnic background and family lifestyle factors.

The data available suggest that further reductions in childhood mortality rates require policies which address the effects of child poverty and social deprivation. Countries that have the lowest child mortality rates, such as Sweden, have pursued social policies of reducing income inequalities (Wallace *et al.*, 1982). Mitchell *et al.* (2000) estimate that if child poverty was eradicated across Britain, 1,407 child lives per year would be saved. However, Bradshaw (2001d) points out that the slowing down of the UK rate of improvement in infant mortality seen after 1980, and attributed by some commentators to the effects of increasing inequality, has also occurred in more equal countries such as Sweden. He suggests that reducing infant mortality beyond a certain level is not only about reducing poverty.

It is clear from the evidence so far available that a multi-faceted approach is needed to improve the current position. The decrease in mortality rates seen over the last half of the 20th century can be attributed to many different factors. These include: better nutrition contributing to better health of the population in general and so mediating the effects of mothers' health which impinge on conception and the foetus; improved ante- and postnatal care; immunisation programmes resulting in decreases in deaths from infectious diseases such as measles and whooping cough; public education campaigns resulting in a reduction in smoking during pregnancy and the reduction in sudden infant death syndrome following the campaign to educate parents about the risk to babies placed in the prone sleeping position; better forms of treatment resulting in a reduction in deaths from childhood cancer; and accident prevention and child protection policies contributing to a fall in deaths due to injury. In recent years, new challenges and causes of concern are emerging, including the fall in uptake of immunisation, the rise in cases of AIDS and HIV in children, and the increase in multiple births linked to infertility treatment.

In many ways, the fall in infant and child mortality during the 20th century is a success story, and our understanding of the factors associated with death in childhood has increased greatly. Nevertheless, the true effects of childhood mortality are not measured simply in numbers, but in the depth of the distress involved for families on the death of a child. Reduction in mortality rates is still a pressing problem, requiring action in many different arenas and government agencies, and covering policies and practice in public health and clinical care, education, poverty and living standards, social care, environmental issues and accident prevention. In order to inform such action, more detailed investigation is required of how a range of factors interact to produce the current patterns in the deaths of children in the UK.

4 Diet and Nutrition

Beverley Searle

Key statistics:
- The most popular consumed foods reported by children aged 18 months to 18 years are chips and savoury snacks (81 per cent) and drinks and confectionery (62 per cent).
- Less than half of children regularly consume cereals, milk and dairy products, meat, fish, fruit and vegetables.
- On average 58 per cent of males and 61 per cent of females fail to reach Reference Nutrient Intake (RNI) levels for vitamin A.
- On average 64 per cent of males and 83 per cent of females fail to reach RNI levels for minerals.

Key trends:
- The diets and nutrition intake of British school children have failed to improve over the past two decades. Young people still consume too much fat and sugar and not enough fruit and vegetables.
- Children from lower socio-economic households are more likely to experience food poverty, resulting in a less balanced diet which is lacking in energy, vitamins and minerals.
- International analysis shows that among industrialised nations, the poorest diets are among young people in UK nations, especially in Scotland.
- Eating practices in general are increasingly influenced by the 'fast food' culture. Changes in eating habits and less active lifestyles have been associated with the increase in obesity among school-aged children in the UK.

Key sources:
- World Health Organization – Health Behaviour in School-Aged Children

- National Diet and Nutrition Surveys of Young People in Great Britain
- Survey of eating habits among children and young people in Northern Ireland

Introduction

Food is a major contribution to basic survival and long-term health. Growth and development in early years and prevention of chronic disease in later life is dependent upon the intake of adequate nutrients. Eating patterns developed at a young age often remain very influential in adult diets. The adoption of a healthy lifestyle, which includes diet and physical activity (see Chapter 16), is seen as a key aspect of resisting ill-health throughout life (DoH, 1999). This chapter will review the evidence in respect of the difference in diet and nutrient intake of young people in the UK. Differences are examined in respect of age, gender and household circumstances. Evidence will be reviewed in respect of regional and international variations, as well as trends in food intake of young people. The chapter will also discuss the implications of these variations for present and future health risks.

Data sources

The main sources of data for this chapter are the reports of the National Diet and Nutrition Survey programme (Gregory *et al.*, 1995; Gregory and Lowe, 2000). This research is a representative sample of the dietary intake of young people in Great Britain. A survey of 1,859 children aged 1½–4½ years was carried out during 1992/93 (Gregory *et al.*, 1995) and of 2,127 young people aged 4–18 years during 1997 (Gregory and Lowe, 2000). They are the first national representative surveys of children's and young people's diets in Great Britain since 1967/68 for children under 5 years and 1983 for children aged 5–18.[1] The Reference Nutrient Intake (RNI) of food energy and nutrients referred to by the surveys are based on those set in 1991 (DoH, 1991). Information on young people in Northern Ireland is provided from the Health Promotion Agency's (HPA) report on children's eating habits

---

[1] Department of Health and Social Security (1975) 'Report on Health and Social Subjects 10', *A Nutrition Survey of Pre-school Children 1967–68*, London: HMSO; Department of Health (1989) *The Diets of British School Children: 1983*, London: HMSO.

as reported by their parents in 2,050 households in 1999 (HPA, 2001). This survey provides information on the frequency of food consumption of 5–17 year olds.

International comparisons are made using data from the Health Behaviour in School-Aged Children (HBSC) Survey. This is a cross-national survey conducted by the World Health Organization of the health and well-being of young people aged 11, 13, and 15. The survey was established in 1985/86 and has been conducted at 4-yearly intervals (Currie *et al.*, 2000). The data used in this chapter relates to the latest survey conducted in 1997/98, which included 120,000 children in 28 countries.

Food consumption

The National Diet and Nutrition Surveys and the HPA survey showed that children and young people in the UK have excessive fat and sugar intake, while not eating enough fruit, vegetables and high fibre products. As will be shown below, for school-aged children (4–18 years) this is consistent with the diets of British school children in 1983 (Holden and MacDonald, 2000; Gregory and Lowe, 2000). The latest surveys showed that the most popular foods consumed by all children in Great Britain were chips and savoury snacks (81 per cent), and confectionery and soft drinks (62 per cent). Less than half of young people regularly consume cereals, milk and dairy products (with the exception of 1½–3½ year olds), meat, fish, fruit and vegetables. There is a higher consumption of saturated fats (26 per cent of boys and 27 per cent of girls) than polyunsaturated fats (18 per cent of both boys and girls) (Table 4.1).

Food consumption varies with age among young people. Consumption of high fibre or wholegrain cereal is more likely among younger children aged 18 months to 4½ years (61 per cent) than adolescents aged 15–18 years (38 per cent) (Gregory *et al.*, 1995, Table 4.14; Gregory and Lowe, 2000, Table 4.11). In Northern Ireland 86 per cent of children ate breakfast on all five weekdays. However, this dropped to 70 per cent among girls aged 12–17 years (HPA, 2001). The use of whole milk also reduces with age. However, this is in line with nutritional requirements that recommend the use of semi-skimmed milk from the age of 5 years (Local Authority Caterers Association, 2000). While younger children consumed more chips and savoury snacks (90 per cent of 4–6 year olds and 81 per cent of 15–18 year olds), they were also more likely to eat fruit, nuts and seeds than older children (25 per cent of 4–6 year olds and 15 per cent of

15–18 year olds). Sugar product consumption remains fairly constant across both sexes and all age groups, although this is mainly through the consumption of sugar confectionery and preserves in the younger age group (57 per cent) and carbonated soft drinks as children get older (67 per cent) (Gregory *et al.*, 1995, Table 4.14; Gregory and Lowe, 2000, Table 4.11).

Country and regional variations

Regional variations in consumption of food are also evident. The National Diet and Nutrition Surveys divide information into four regions containing government offices as follows:

Scotland

Northern (Yorkshire and Humberside, North East, North West and Merseyside)

London and South East

Central (West Midlands, East Midlands, Eastern), South West and Wales.

Children in the Northern region (28 per cent) and Scotland (27 per cent) were more likely to eat saturated fats, while those in London and the South East (23 per cent) and Scotland (22 per cent) were more likely to consume polyunsaturated fats. Sugary confectionery was more likely to be consumed by children in Scotland and the Central, South West and Wales region (both 67 per cent), than in the Northern region, London and South East (both 64 per cent). Chips and savoury snacks were most popular in Scotland (80 per cent) and the Northern region (79 per cent), with the lowest levels of consumption in London and the South East (74 per cent) (Table 4.1). In Northern Ireland only 10 per cent of children were reported as eating the recommended five portions of fruit and vegetables every day, and 47 per cent were reported as eating confectionery at least once per day (HPA, 2001).

Food consumption and poverty

Variations in average food consumption patterns in differing socio-economic circumstances are also evident. In Great Britain children in couple households are more likely to consume sugary foods (90 per cent) compared to single parent households (67 per cent). Breads, cereals and pasta are more likely to be consumed by children in couple households (59 per cent), households in the top quintile (50 per cent) or not receiving benefits (51 per cent) than in single parent households (49 per cent), households in the bottom quintile (47 per cent) or receiving benefits (49 per cent). Fruit and vegetables are also more likely to be consumed by children in households in the top quintile (43 per cent) or not receiving benefits (40 per cent) than are children in households in the bottom quintile or receiving benefits (both 35 per cent) (Table 4.1). Separate research also shows the quality and variety of foods consumed in poorer households is lower than for the population generally. Although food preferences may not be affected by income levels, there is a tendency for such households to adopt a 'cheaper imitation of conventional eating patterns' (Dobson *et al.*, 1994). Children from lower socio-economic households are less likely to consume a variety of foods, resulting in a less balanced diet which is lacking in energy, vitamins and minerals (as will be shown), and having poorer eating patterns whereby they are more prone to eating sweets and snacking between meals (Acheson, 1998; HPA, 2001).

Poor diet, however, is not necessarily a consequence of lack of knowledge within poorer households. Family budgeting and access to food outlets are also important. Over one-third of children now live in poverty (see Chapter 1) and benefit levels are too low to afford a healthy diet (GCCNI, 2001), meaning 'many people on low incomes simply do not have enough money or other resources to be able to eat a healthy balanced diet' (Lobstein, 1997). For example, the Family Budget Unit have shown that a family of two parents and two children received £121.75 per week in Income Support, but needed £160.82 for a low cost but acceptable standard of living, leaving a weekly shortfall of £40 (Parker, 1998). The gap between the Family Budget Unit low cost but acceptable budget and the Income Support scales has since been reduced as a result of the welcome real increases in the Income Support scales (Bradshaw, 2001a). The food budget is often seen as flexible and is more likely to be squeezed in order to meet fixed costs such as rent or utility bills (Dowler and Leather, 2000). Changes in physical and commercial environments have also made access to food difficult for those on low incomes. A reduction in the number of food outlets – mostly local shops and markets – has been matched by an increase in the number of large out-of-town stores (DoH, 1996). Access to such food outlets is often only possible by car or bus and 'those in the poorest households are less likely to have access to cars, and public transport to better shopping centres is often inadequate' (Dowler and Leather, 2000). The food budget may therefore be under further pressure where additional transport costs need to be met (GCCNI, 2001).

Table 4.1: Percentage of young people consuming food types by sex, age, region and socio-economic circumstances (reported over a 7 day period)

	Milk and dairy (not butter/marg)	Breads cereals and pasta	Saturated fats (butter and marg)	Polyun-saturated fats (marg. and other spreads)	Meat and fish (not meat/fish products)	Meat/fish products (inc. pasties, burgers, coated meat/fish)	Fruit and veg	Chips and savoury snacks	Sugars (confec-tionary and soft drinks)
	%	%	%	%	%	%	%	%	%
Males and females									
1½–3½ years	52	42	22	18	24	32	37	73	60
Males									
Total	47	45	26	18	30	44	35	87	65
3½–4 ½ years	46	42	22	17	23	34	31	78	66
4–6 years	52	47	25	19	28	50	40	91	65
7–10 years	48	48	27	20	32	48	37	91	70
11–14 years	44	44	26	20	34	43	34	89	67
15–18 years	43	43	31	15	35	43	34	84	57
Females									
Total	43	48	27	18	28	39	37	83	62
3½–4 ½ years	47	43	24	17	23	37	33	79	66
4–6 years	42	58	30	21	29	46	42	88	66
7–10 years	46	47	25	18	32	44	39	89	66
11–14 years	41	47	26	17	28	36	35	83	61
15–18 years	41	46	31	18	29	32	37	78	53

Region									
Scotland	47	42	27	22	25	39	34	80	67
Northern	47	45	28	21	28	41	38	79	64
Central, South West + Wales	48	46	25	19	29	37	39	77	67
London + South East	48	45	26	23	28	36	40	74	64
Socio-economic circumstances									
couples*	47	59	28	21	41	47	39	88	90
single parent*	46	49	29	23	26	45	37	87	67
Head of household									
manual	47	46	27	17	27	38	38	83	66
non-manual	40	53	25	19	28	38	38	81	65
Gross weekly household income*									
bottom quintile (<£160)	45	47	26	20	30	45	35	91	68
top quintile (£600+)	49	50	34	18	34	42	43	85	67
receiving benefits*	44	49	28	20	30	45	35	91	69
not receiving benefits*	49	51	29	18	33	44	40	89	69

* 4–18 year olds only

Sources: Gregory et al. (1995) Tables 4.14–4.16, 4.18; Gregory and Lowe (2000), Tables 4.11, 4.14–4.18

In addition to the physiological affects of a poor diet (discussed below) it is argued that there are also psychological consequences of food poverty where people 'cannot afford to eat in ways acceptable to society; for whom shopping is a stressful experience because they have insufficient money or the shops they can reach are inadequately stocked with poor quality goods; whose children cannot have a packed lunch similar to their friends; [and] who cannot invite friends or family to a meal' (Dowler and Leather, 2000). Food poverty can therefore have significant consequences on the physical and mental development of children. It

Table 4.2: International comparison of nutritional intake of young people (11–15 years), 1997/98

	Average % of young people (11–15 years) consuming selected food every day								Nutrition Score (Fruit & milk) – (crisps & sweets)	Rank (inc UK)	Rank (inc UK regions)
	Fruit		Low-fat milk		Crisps & chips		Sweets or chocolate and soft drinks				
	*f	m	f	m	f	m	f	m			
Denmark	65	55	73	75	3	5	22	29	211	1	1
Norway	56	47	67	70	3	7	19	27	183	2	2
Canada	70	65	68	74	10	14	32	40	181	3	3
Sweden	74	65	32	33	3	6	20	27	149	4	4
Czech Republic	85	80	37	36	9	11	43	48	128	5	5
Poland	84	82	44	49	18	24	42	48	127	6	6
France	56	56	57	63	12	17	36	43	124	7	7
Belgium	52	44	41	47	6	9	35	40	93	8	8
Hungary	82	72	36	41	16	18	53	56	88	9	9
Austria	75	62	17	20	7	11	33	38	84	10	10
Germany	69	62	28	34	8	12	43	50	81	11	11
Greece	81	81	21	26	22	30	40	48	70	12	12
USA	62	58	58	62	26	30	58	60	66	13	13
Portugal	94	92	15	18	22	29	50	56	62	14	14
UK	67	59	60	64	45	50	61	67	27	15	
Ireland	78	74	27	27	37	43	65	74	−12	16	18
England	63	58	67	74	40	48	55	63	56		15
Wales	58	48	50	55	30	34	48	54	46		16
N Ireland	77	69	70	73	59	62	76	76	17		17
Scotland	68	61	51	56	50	56	66	75	−10		19

* f = female, m = male

Source: Currie et al. (2000) and author's own calculations

could be argued that this is in contravention to the United Nations Convention on the Rights of the Child.[2]

International comparisons

International comparisons show that among the 28 nations studied in the HBSC, in general girls eat a healthier diet than boys. Girls are more likely to report eating fruit or drinking low-fat milk every day than boys, while boys are more likely to report eating chips, crisps, sweets or chocolate and soft drinks every day (Currie *et al.*, 2000) (Table 4.2). By using a very crude nutrition score, based on the percentage of young people reporting consuming healthy food daily (fruit and low-fat milk), and subtracting the percentage that report consuming unhealthy food every day (chips, crisps, sweets or chocolates and soft drinks), it can be seen that the most healthy diets are consumed in Scandinavian countries and Canada, with the worst diets being among young people in USA, Portugal, UK and Ireland. Including individual UK countries, the poorest diets are among young people in England, Wales and Northern Ireland, with the worst diets of all nations included in this analysis being in Scotland (Table 4.2).

Diet and health

Dietary habits established at a young age provide the basis of eating habits through life. Poor diets in young people can lead to difficulties in resisting infection, increasing the risk of illness. Under-nourishment can also lead to irritability in young people causing problems in concentration which may inhibit educational capacity (Miles and Eid, 1987). An unbalanced diet has implications for physical and mental health, affecting skeletal, muscle and neurological growth and development in adolescence and throughout adult life.

Energy intake

The 1992/93 and 1997 surveys showed that energy intake was below the Estimated Average Requirement (EAR) for both sexes of all ages. The highest intake is by boys aged 7–10 (91 per cent) and girls aged 4–6 (91 per cent).

---

[2] In particular Articles 24 and 27 (http//eurochild.gla.ac.uk/documents/UN/Rights/Unconvention/htm)

Table 4.3: Energy intake by age (in years) and gender

Energy Intake	Mean Energy Intake (Mj)	EAR	Intake as % EAR
Males (average)			
3½–4½	5.36		75
4–6	6.39	7.16	89
7–10	7.47	8.24	91
11–14	8.28	9.27	89
15–18	9.6	11.51	83
Females (average)			
3½–4½	4.98		77
4–6	5.87	6.46	91
7–10	6.72	7.28	92
11–14	7.03	7.92	89
15–18	6.82	8.83	77

Source: Gregory and Lowe (2000), Tables 5.3, 5.15.

Lowest energy intake is for girls aged 3½–4 ½ and 15–18 (both 77 per cent) (Table 4.3). Energy intake also shows regional variations. For females (4–18 years) the lowest energy intake is in Scotland (84 per cent) and the highest in the Northern region (89 per cent), for males (4–18 years) the lowest energy intake is in London and the South East (87 per cent) and the highest is in Central and South West England and Wales (90 per cent) (Chart 4.1).

Chart 4.1: Energy intake by region as percentage of RNI, 4–18 year olds

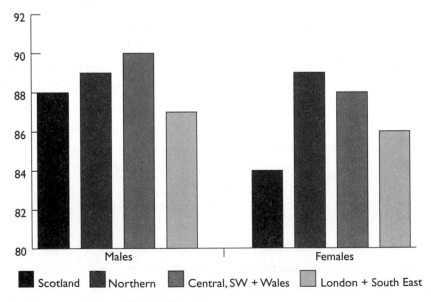

Source: Gregory and Lowe (2000), Table 5.8

Table 4.4: Trends in energy intake during the 1980s and 1990s

Sex and age of young person		Survey year	Average daily energy intake (Mj)	Intake as % EAR*
Males (years)	3½–4½	1992/93	5.36	75
	4–6	1997	6.39	89
	10–11	1983	8.67	105
	10–11	1997	7.98	97
	14–15	1983	10.40	112
	14–15	1997	9.13	98
	16–24	1986/87	10.29	89
	15–18	1997	9.60	83
Females (years)	3½–4½	1992/93	4.98	77
	4–6	1997	5.87	91
	10–11	1983	7.69	106
	10–11	1997	7.04	96
	14–15	1983	7.85	99
	14–15	1997	6.90	87
	16–24	1986/87	7.11	81
	15–18	1997	6.82	77

* Based on Dietary Reference Values for 1991
Sources: Gregory and Lowe (2000), Table 5.15 [1983 – DoH (1989); 1986/87–
Gregory et al. (1990); 1992/93 – Gregory et al. (1995)]

Comparisons with previous research shows that for pre-school children average energy intake was 17 per cent lower in 1992/93 than in 1967/68, with the main source of energy coming from cereal and cereal products and milk food types. However, the proportion of energy derived from biscuits, buns, cakes and pastries, and sugars, preserves and confectionery in 1992/93 was only about half that in the 1996/67 survey (Gregory et al., 1995). For school-aged children, energy intake of boys and girls reduced between the early 1980s and late 1990s (Table 4.4). The main sources of energy in diets in 1997 are broadly similar to those identified in 1983 and include bread, chips and savoury snacks, milk, biscuits/buns and pastries, meat products and sugar preserves and confectionery (Bradshaw, 1997b; Gregory and Lowe, 2000; Holden and MacDonald, 2000).

Energy intake and poverty

School-aged children from families of lower socio-economic status (ie, manual head of household, single parents, households on benefits and households in the bottom quintile of the survey, with less than £160 average income per week) are on average more likely to have lower energy intake (Charts 4.2a and b). The

Chart 4.2a: Energy intake as % of EAR by socio-economic circumstances Males aged 4–18

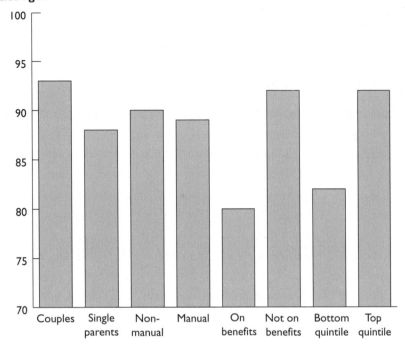

Chart 4.2b: Energy intake as % of EAR by socio-economic circumstances Females aged 4–18

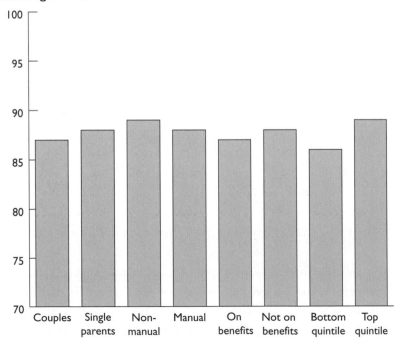

Sources: Gregory and Lowe (2000), Tables 5.10–5.13

variation is most notable among males: for example, boys living in families on benefits achieve 80 per cent of EAR compared to 92 per cent of those in families not on benefits (Chart 4.2a).

Energy intake and health

Energy intake is important for hormonal activity and the growth and development of young people. However, behavioural changes and changes in eating patterns are posing risks for young people. The increase in consumption of energy-dense fast foods (discussed below) is being matched with an increase in sedentary behaviour (eg, watching television, playing computer games, being driven to school) and a reduction in physical activity (eg, playing sports) (National Audit Office, 2001b). There are also problems where children are failing to reach estimated average requirements for energy intake. Low energy levels can limit physical activity, which, together with high fat/high energy food choices and snacking, puts young people at increased risk of obesity, cardiovascular diseases, diabetes, high blood cholesterol and high blood pressure, throughout their adult life (Currie *et al.*, 2000).

Vitamins and minerals

The 1992/93 and 1997 surveys showed that, on average, intake of most vitamins by young people exceeded RNI levels. The only exception is in respect of vitamin A intake among 4–18 year olds which showed regional variations as well as variations in respect of socio-economic circumstances. Reference intake levels were least likely to be achieved by young people living in Scotland (82 per cent) and the Northern region (90 per cent) as well as those in poorer families or families of lower socio-economic status (Charts 4.3 and 4.4)

Separate analysis of the 1997 survey by Wynn and Wynn (2001) shows that there is greater variation in vitamin intake among individuals. Many young people fail to reach RNI levels and this increases with age, particularly among girls. On average over half of boys and girls fail to reach RNI levels of Vitamin A at all ages, while around half of girls and one-third of boys aged 11–18 do not reach RNI levels for Folate B9 and Riboflavin B2. Vitamin C intake levels are also low, with around one in five boys and one in four girls failing to reach RNI levels (Table 4.5).

The Wynns' further question the relevance of official recommended levels

Chart 4.3: Vitamin A intake as % of RNI by region

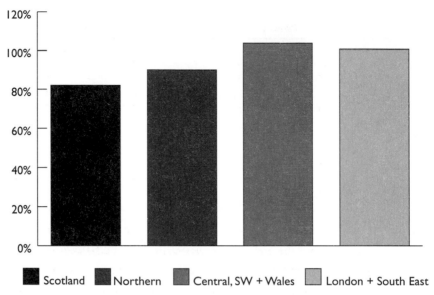

Source: Gregory and Lowe (2000), Table 8.42

Chart 4.4: Vitamin A intake as % RNI by socio-economic status

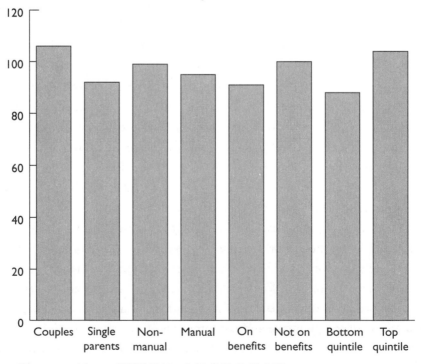

Source: Gregory and Lowe (2000), Tables 8.44, 8.46, 8.48, 8.50

Table 4.5: Percentage of children aged 4–18 failing to reach RNI levels for intake of vitamins

	Males (years)				Females (years)			
	4–6	7–10	11–14	15–18	4–6	7–10	11–14	15–18
Vitamin A	42	57	65	69	42	59	74	70
Folate B9	4	13	33	18	5	22	50	52
Riboflavin B2	10	12	25	28	7	21	40	40
Vitamin C	8	8	14	20	9	9	20	26
Pyridoxine B6	3	1	11	5	8	2	3	13
Thiamine B1	6	1	6	7	0	2	3	10
Niacin B3	2	0	4	0	2	2	2	5
Cobalamin B12	0	0	1	1	5	1	3	18

Source: Wynn and Wynn (2001)

which were set well over 10 years ago and have greatly differing rates for different age groups. For example, the Recommended Daily Intake of Vitamin A is only 75 per cent of that recommended for girls in France and the USA, and only 70 per cent of that recommended for boys (Wynn and Wynn, 2001). Vitamins are essential for normal growth and development at all ages, deficiencies therefore can impinge on a young person's health and well-being. In particular, Vitamin A is essential in respect of the cardiovascular and nervous system, the pancreas and insulin production, as well as cell proliferation of the brain. Moreover, there is continual research producing further evidence of the biological role of vitamin A. Deficiencies in vitamin A are associated with blindness, diabetes and neurological disorders as well as increasing the risk of cancer. Folate B9 is essential for the replication of cells, and deficiencies may result in congenital malformation and impaired fertility. It is therefore desirable that older boys and particularly girls have sufficient levels of folate in their diets. Following recent research in the USA, recommended folate intake levels in Britain for women who are planning pregnancy or are pregnant have been increased from the 1991 level of 200 mcg/d to 400 mcg/d (Wynn and Wynn, 2001).

As they do with vitamins, the Wynns argue against the relevance of British RNI levels for minerals, which are between half and two-thirds of those recommended in France and USA, and which are considerably lower for younger children than adolescents (Wynn and Wynn, 2001). Growth and development of young people is controlled by hormones, which are themselves dependent upon adequate energy intake and consumption of protein and minerals. It has already been shown that energy intake levels are below EAR in all circumstances (Table 4.3 and Charts 4.1 and 4.2). Protein intake on average exceeded RNI in

Table 4.6: Percentage of children aged 18 months to 18 years failing to reach RNI levels for intake of minerals.

	All <4 years	Males (years)				Females (years)			
		4–6	7–10	11–14	15–18	4–6	7–10	11–14	15–18
Calcium	11	10	19	79	68	15	29	79	76
Copper	36	38	33	35	50	52	49	60	78
Iodine	24	19	24	37	33	27	39	61	61
Iron	84	14	39	60	43	28	59	96	93
Magnesium	7	11	56	86	75	13	75	97	97
Potassium	3	5	43	88	85	5	46	97	99
Zinc	72	79	73	84	68	89	83	96	72

Sources: Gregory *et al.* (1995), Wynn and Wynn (2001)

both the 1992/93 and 1997 surveys (Gregory *et al.*, 1995, Table 6.2; Gregory and Lowe, 2000, Table 6.3). However, as with vitamins, many young people are failing to reach RNI levels of minerals, and this increases with age, particularly among girls. While between half and three-quarters of boys aged 11–18 are falling below RNI levels of mineral intake, this rises to between three-quarters and nearly all of older girls (Table 4.6).

Mineral intake on average is lower for boys and girls in poorer, lower socio-economic households. While boys in lower socio-economic households achieve RNI levels for mineral intake (Chart 4.5a), for girls intake is on average below RNI for calcium, magnesium, potassium, zinc and copper and is particularly low for iron (Chart 4.5b). Girls in Northern Ireland were reported to avoid milk and red meat because of a mistaken belief that it was fatty (HPA, 2001) and this has significant consequences on calcium and iron intake. Iron deficiency syndrome increases significantly among adolescent girls at the onset of sexual maturity, since they do not compensate for their increased loss of iron during menstruation (Holden and MacDonald, 2000).

Deficiencies in minerals can have important consequences on the present and future health of young people and are therefore important to growth and development at all ages. Iron stores in the body are influenced by long-term nutrition. Deficiencies, which are particularly common among adolescent females, can lead to anaemia and also functional impairments in relation to intellectual performance and behaviour (DoH, 1991; Holden and McDonald, 2000). Calcium is an important component of bone health: deficiencies, particularly among women, have been associated with increased risk of osteoporosis and fracture (Acheson, 1998). Magnesium, potassium and copper

Chart 4.5a: Mineral intake as % RNI by socio-economic circumstances, males 4–18 years

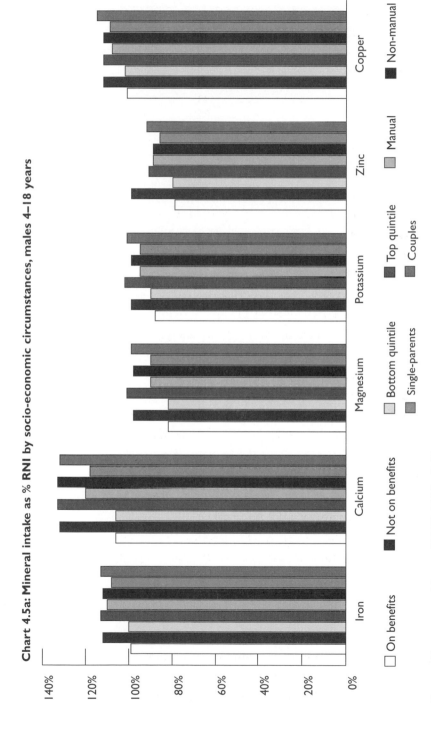

Source: **Gregory and Lowe (2000), Table 9.45**

Chart 4.5b: Mineral intake as % RNI by socio-economic circumstances, females 4–18 years

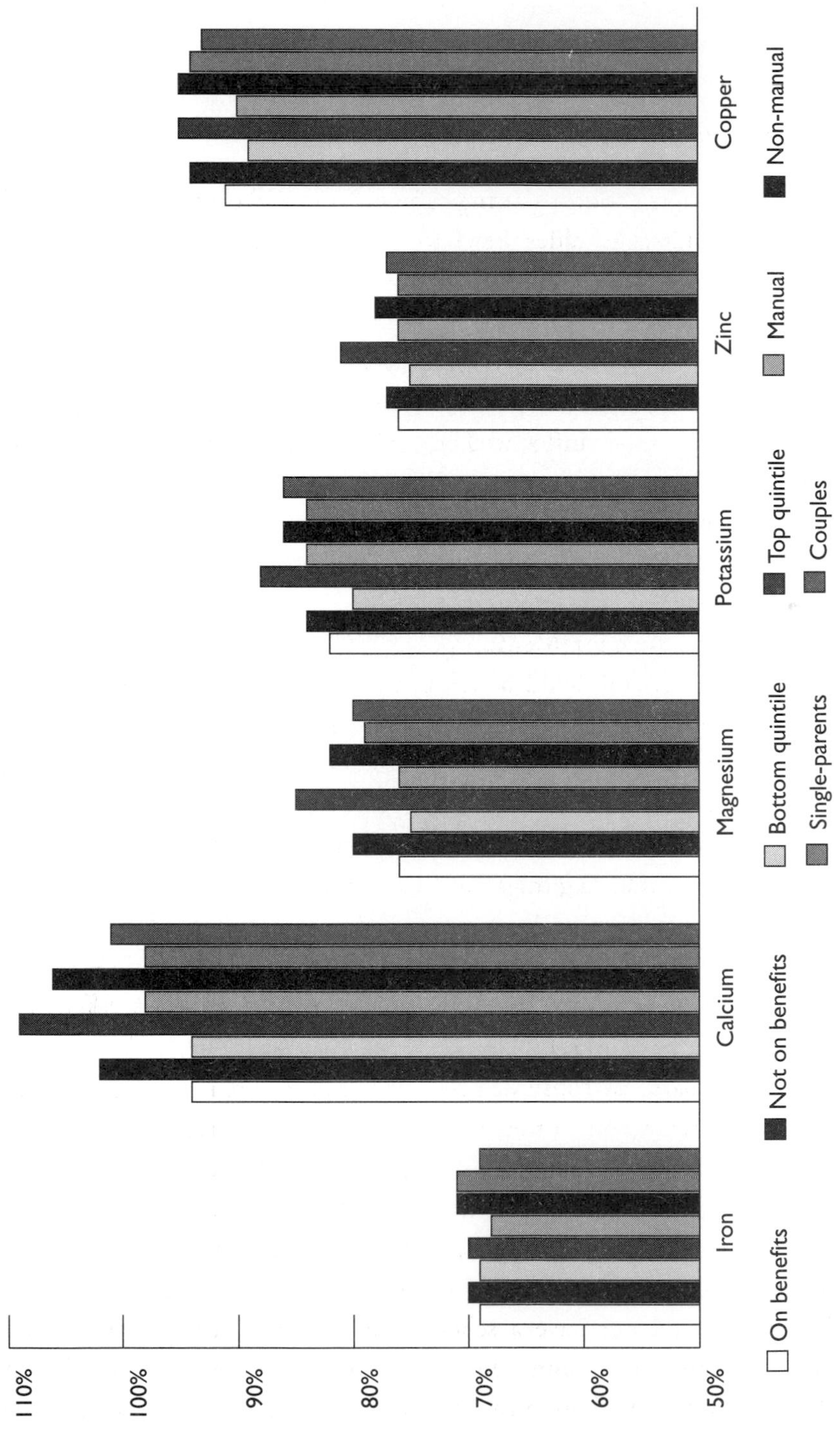

Source: Gregory and Lowe (2000), Table 9.45

deficiency can lead to progressive muscle weakness, skeletal fragility and mental depression and confusion, while low zinc intake is associated with restricted growth and deficiencies in skin tissue and the immune system (DoH, 1991).

Changes in dietary practices

Although younger children's eating habits are more likely to reflect those of their parents, as children get older they have greater opportunity for purchasing their own food (Dobson *et al.*, 1994; Wynn and Wynn, 2001). Young people's dietary habits are increasingly influenced by economic and lifestyles changes (Holden and MacDonald, 2000; Leather, 2000). Young people in poorer families are more likely to experience food poverty (Leather, 1997), while eating practices in general are increasingly influenced by the 'fast food' culture (Lynch *et al.*, 1997).

Changes in eating habits and less active lifestyles have been associated with the increase in obesity among school-aged children in the UK (National Audit Office, 2001b; see Chapter 16). Research shows a negative association between obesity and socio-economic status, with the risk of obesity increasing as socio-economic status declines (McMurray *et al.*, 2000; Reidpath *et al.*, in press). One of the reasons for this could be associated with poor eating behaviour among lower socio-economic status families leading to higher consumption of 'fast foods' (Lynch *et al.*, 1997). Compared with children from more affluent families, young people in low income families are more likely to be given what they like to eat in order to avoid waste and are less likely to be restricted in their access to unhealthy foods, resulting in greater consumption of their preferred foods such as chips, beans, burgers and fish fingers (Dobson *et al.*, 1994; Hupkens *et al.*, 1998). Cultural factors may also play a role in obesity, with some ethnic groups having a desire for a fuller body in contrast to the Western ideal of slimness (O'Dea and Caputi, 2001).

Foods prepared or consumed outside the home are making an increasingly important contribution to nutritional intake. 'Current trends have resulted in the traditional "proper cooked meal" being continually overshadowed by the rise in demand for prepared convenience and fast foods' (Brown *et al.*, 2000, p. 105). Such trends can be seen to be reflected in the nutritional value of a main source of food outside the home, namely school meals. The 1997 survey showed that children who did not have a school meal had significantly lower fat, fibre, protein, calcium and vitamin A intake than those who ate school lunch, and that children having free school meals obtained a higher proportion of daily energy and nutrients intake compared to those who paid for their meal (Gregory and Lowe, 2000, Table X3). Despite this, school meals failed to meet recommended provisions of access to healthy and unhealthy foods (Gregory and Lowe, 2000). The re-introduction of Minimum Nutrition Guidelines (Local Authority Caterers Association, 2000) and the National Fruit Scheme (DoH, 2001h) are two of a number of initiatives for improving children's health. Although the fruit scheme is meeting with some success, its implementation is restricted to children in England (DoH, 2001e). The impact of nutritional guidelines may also be limited where local education authorities are not required to ban individual foods, such as fast foods, or where school meals services are contracted out and provision of food is determined more by local market forces than by central government guidelines. These limitations therefore may have serious implications for the future nutritional health of young people in the UK.

Conclusion

The diets and nutrition intake of British school children have failed to improve over the past two decades. Young people still consume too much fat and sugar and not enough fruit and vegetables. They also fail to meet recommended levels of vitamin and mineral intake, and have experienced a reduction in energy intake. Poor diets and lack of nutrients can have a significant impact on physical and mental well-being. Deficiencies in vitamins and minerals can cause restricted skeletal and muscular growth and development and may also impair cognitive development leading to educational and behavioural difficulties. Low energy levels limit young people's engagement in physical activity, placing them at greater risk of obesity, cardiovascular diseases and high blood pressure.

International comparisons show that the diets of young people in the UK are among the worst in industrialised nations, and this is particularly so for Scotland. Socio-economic variations also exist, with young people from poorer households being at greatest risk of experiencing food poverty. Parental choice and budgetary decisions can reduce the variety and quality of food available in the home, and the influence of the 'fast food' culture outside the home acts as a disincentive for the provision of healthier food options in schools.

Government intervention is seeking to improve the diets of school children as part of a wider initiative to improve their health generally. In alleviating food poverty, consideration needs to be given to factors other than monitoring nutritional intake. Dietary behaviour is influenced by home, school and social environments. Family budget, parental preferences, access to food and social and cultural 'trends' all play an important role in young people's preferred eating pattern.

5 Children's Health

Bryony Beresford

Key statistics:
- The incidence of initial breastfeeding varies between the four countries, with higher rates in England and Wales compared to Scotland and Northern Ireland.
- Immunisation rates are high (~95 per cent) in all four countries though lower than the peak in the mid-1990s.
- Levels of parental and/or self-reported good health are high, with around 90 per cent of children reporting good or very good health.
- Factors such as social class and household income are associated with perceived health.
- In 2000, a quarter of boys (aged 2–15 years) and 18 per cent of girls had a longstanding illness.
- The presence of a longstanding illness is associated with socio-economic status. However, not all chronic conditions are associated with indicators of deprivation, for example diabetes.
- Estimates based on data available in 1998 suggest that at any one time at least 6,000 children in the UK are living at home but dependent on one or more items of medical technology to maintain health or sustain life.

Key trends:
- Compared to other age groups, the rate of increase in the prevalence of chronic ill health is greatest among children.
- There is an increasing prevalence of insulin dependent diabetes and asthma among children.
- For some chronic or life-limiting conditions, eg, cancers and cystic fibrosis, there have been significant improvements in survival or life expectancy rates.
- The number of children born to HIV-infected mothers is rising, but the proportion of children being infected by the virus is declining.
- The number of diagnoses of sexually transmitted infections in young people is increasing, particularly among females.

Key sources:
- OECD Health Data (2001)
- Infant Feeding Survey (2000)
- Health Survey for England (1997)
- Health in Scotland (2000)
- General Household Survey (1972–2000)
- Key Health Statistics from General Practice (1998)
- Office of National Statistics: cancer registrations
- AIDS/HIV Quarterly Surveillance Tables
- Communicable Disease Surveillance Centre: annual tables

Introduction

The health of children in the UK improved enormously over the last century. Contagious conditions such as polio and tuberculosis have all but been eradicated, and advances in medical science mean that the prognoses of previously fatal conditions are continually improving. At the same time 'new' child health issues have emerged. The 1990s saw increasing attention being paid to the irrefutable evidence on the inequalities in child health (Spencer, 2000); the impact of increasingly rapid advances within medicine and medical care is widespread; and there is a growing concern about the incidence of sexually transmitted infections among older adolescents.

This chapter seeks to provide an overview of what is known about children's health in the UK at the beginning of the 21st century. The subject of 'child health' is vast with ambiguous boundaries, and different health issues are pertinent at different ages across childhood. It is not possible to be comprehensive in the space available here. We have, however, endeavoured to present child health data on the key, or emerging, issues. The focus in this chapter is on physical health/ill health; separate chapters deal with other health-related issues such as mental health (Chapter 22), health-related behaviours (Chapters 12, 16 and 19) and diet (Chapter 4).

The chapter tackles the issue of child health from two perspectives: first, we present data on what is known overall about the health of children in the UK at the turn of the century and we examine the relationship between social, demographic and economic factors on children's experience of health or ill health. Here we look at indicators of infant health and then child and adolescent health more generally. The second part of the chapter focuses on specific health conditions chosen either because they represent examples of changes in children's health over the past 20 years or so, or because they are the emerging health issues which have the potential to become key health issues in the future.

Health and disability: definitions

The traditional (or medical) model of disability in which the presence of an impairment or illness is viewed as the cause of disability has been challenged over the last decade or so by an alternative model known as the social model of disability (eg, Oliver, 1990). This states that it is not an impairment or health condition, *per se*, that results in disability: rather it is environmental (for example, unsuitable housing, inaccessible public buildings and facilities) and social barriers (for example, individual and group attitudes) that disable individuals whose abilities differ from 'the norm'. Some of the health conditions discussed in this chapter are likely to result in the experience of disability – others will not. In addition, there are impairments which are labelled as disabilities (such as Downs syndrome, learning difficulties, autistic spectrum disorders and sensory impairments) which may, or may not, have (physical) health implications. These impairments or conditions do not fall within the scope of this chapter.

Sources of data

Data on health among children – both illness and 'well-ness' – is frustratingly limited, with considerable differences between the four countries of the UK on the extent to which children are represented in national data collection exercises. This is in striking contrast to the considerable amount of data on adult health which is routinely collected across all UK countries.

For example, the Welsh Health Survey 1998 collected *no* data on children and their health, and *Health Statistics Wales 2001* (published in March 2002), aside from data on dental health, offers only one table (Table 3.2: 'Patients visiting general practice by diagnosis in 1999') in which children are identified as a specific age group. In the case of other indicators of health/morbidity, the data concerns only adults or does not contain an age split. Except for that collected at a UK-wide level, we could find no population datasets on children's health in Northern Ireland. The Health and Social Well-being Survey conducted in 1997 and repeated in 2001 does not include children. It appears that the most recent data collected at a national level was the 1991 census in which parents were asked to report whether or not their child/ren had a chronic illness or disability. Once available, the 2001 census will provide some more up-to-date figures.

Inadequacies in child health data in Scotland are being addressed. Child health has been acknowledged as a priority area by the Scottish Executive and in 1999 the Child Health Information Team was established in order to act as a centralised team for information concerning the health of children in Scotland. The team initially focused on health data collected by pre-school health surveillance systems, but there are plans to co-ordinate and collate a wider range of data from a number of different sources. It will be important to track the work of the Child Health Information Team and its publications in any future reports.

In England, a key source of health data is the annual Health Survey for England. Along with the core set of questions, each year the survey focuses on a specific topic and/or population. Children and young people were the population focus in the 1997 survey, and are again the focus for the 2002 survey. The 2002 survey will also include specific questions on asthma, accidents, physical activity, eating habits and oral health. These conditions/areas will also be covered in the 2003 survey in which the proposed population focus is minority ethnic groups. This survey will clearly be an important source for any future reports, with the potential for some data comparisons over time.

In terms of cross-country data, the annual General Household Survey (covering England, Scotland and Wales) contains key, but limited, data; its particular value being the opportunity to explore the relationship between health indicators and socio-economic and demographic variables. The UK-wide General Practice Research Database, recently taken over by the Medicines Control Agency, is a potentially useful source. This database is the world's largest computerised database of anonymised clinical records from general practice, and a report of the database was produced in 1998. The Medicines Control Agency plans to provide greater access to the database for research purposes, and this is a source that might be used more fully in any future reports.

More specifically, the Institute of Child Health collects UK-wide data on the incidence of HIV and AIDS, and this is supplemented by data for older adolescents held by the Public Health Laboratory Service, which also collates data on sexually transmitted infections. Data on specific conditions may be collected at a local level for registers (for example, district diabetes registers). The extent to which these data can be collated to provide national data is limited for a number of reasons. For instance, some areas may not collect the data at all, or different diagnostic or severity criteria may be used. The same problem occurs when looking at data on the prevalence of physical impairments. Following an examination of child health information systems held by health authorities, Johnson and King (1999) concluded it was 'impossible to monitor trends in the prevalence rates of disabling disorders in childhood using child health information systems'. They called for greater collaboration between health authorities in order that the systems of collecting and recording local information could be made more compatible and thus enable collation of the data. For some conditions, specialist research groups, for example the UK Cystic Fibrosis Survey and EURODIAB (a European collaboration of research on diabetes), work together to collect national population data. Finally, the OECD provides access to annually updated datasets: a small minority of these are pertinent to child health.

Immunisations

Routine immunisation of infants has been shown to benefit the health of children and their communities where immunisation rates are high (eg, Nicoll *et al.*, 1989). Table 5.1 shows primary immunisation uptake rates for the four UK countries in 2000.

Scotland shows the highest immunisation uptake rates across UK countries. Northern Ireland is the second best performing country. England has the lowest uptake for all immunisations except for MMR which is lower in Wales.

OECD Health Data (2001) provide international comparative data on the proportion of children immunised against measles (Table 5.2). This table shows the considerable increases in immunisation rates in some countries. For example, immunisation rates in Italy increased from 50 per cent to 75 per cent during the 1990s. Other countries, such as Hungary, Slovakia, Sweden and Poland, have maintained consistently high immunisation rates over that period. Data for the

Table 5.1: Primary immunisation uptake rates, 2000

| | % coverage at 24 months | | | | | |
	Diphtheria 3	Tetanus 3	Pertussis 3	Polio 3	Hib 3	MMR
Scotland	97.5	97.5	96.8	97.5	97.3	92.8
England	94.6	94.6	93.7	94.6	94.2	87.6
Wales	96.1	96.2	94.1	96.2	95.9	87.2
Northern Ireland	96.6	96.6	95.6	96.5	96.7	91.9
UK	95.0	95.0	94.1	95.0	94.6	88.2

Source: Scottish Executive (2001e), p. 58.

Table 5.2: The proportion of children immunised against measles by 2 years old by country and year

Countries*	1991	Year 1995	1999
UK	**90.0**	**92.0**	**88.1**
Turkey	73.0	65.0	81.0
Sweden	95.0	96.0	96.3
Spain	85.0	90.0	95.0
Slovakia	98.0	99.0	99.3
Poland	97.0	96.0	97.1
Norway	94.0	92.0	88.0
Japan	71.4	93.0	96.5
Italy	50.0	50.0	75.0
Iceland	98.0	98.0	99.9
Hungary	100.0	100.0	100.0
Finland	97.0	98.0	98.0
Denmark	86.0	88.0	92.0
Czech Republic	98.0	96.0	95.0
Belgium	67.0	85.0	82.4

* The countries shown in this table are restricted to those where data was available for 1991, 1995 and 1999.

UK show lower immunisation rates at the end of the 1990s than at the beginning of the decade, with a peak in the mid-1990s.

Social inequalities in immunisation uptake are well documented (eg, Reading *et al.* 1994) and evidence from small-scale studies suggests that it is extremely difficult to improve, and maintain improvements, in uptake (Morgan and Evans, 1998). In terms of reducing social inequalities it is suggested that targeted interventions with deprived groups and young mothers, as opposed to overall uptake interventions, are needed (Reading *et al.*, 1994; Morgan and Evans, 1998). However, there is a lack of rigorous evaluation of different intervention approaches.

Figures published at the time of writing suggest that the widely reported concerns among parents and some medical practitioners about a possible association between the MMR vaccination (which includes the measles vaccination) and autism and bowel disorders are affecting immunisation rates, with the knock-on affect of outbreaks of measles being reported across the UK. This is something that will clearly need to be tracked, and any future report may wish to focus on the time-related changes in the incidence of communicable diseases such as measles, mumps and rubella.

Infant feeding

The health benefits of breastfeeding are well documented, and it is appropriate in this chapter on child health to report on infant feeding practices. An interim report on the Infant Feeding Survey 2000 (DoH, 2001d) provides up-to-date data on incidence of initial breastfeeding (that is, breastfed at birth – even if only on one occasion) in all four nations and offers comparisons with earlier Infant Feeding Surveys.

There have been statistically significant increases in the incidence of breastfeeding in the past 10 years (DoH, 2001d). Initial incidence of breast-feeding second babies, while increasing, remains lower than initial incidence of breastfeeding firstborns. The data, by country, are summarised in Table 5.3. Greater gains in initial incidence are found in Scotland and Northern Ireland than England and Wales. However, the actual incidence of initial breastfeeding in the former two countries is lower.

Analysis of the Infant Feeding Survey 2000 has found that incidence of initial breastfeeding increases with mother's age, with a particularly sharp increase being noted between mothers under 20 years and those aged 20–24 years. As in previous surveys, the 2000 survey found that mothers who left full-time education at 16 years were least likely to breastfeed, while those who continued their education beyond 18 years were most likely to do so. In all countries, mothers in Social Class I and II had the highest breastfeeding rates. However, in England and Wales, the greatest change in incidence of initial breastfeeding was among mothers in social class V (1995: 50 per cent; 2000: 62 per cent). In contrast, mothers in social class V in Scotland and Northern Ireland were the only social class group where incidence of initial breastfeeding fell.

Table 5.3: Initial incidence of breastfeeding by birth order and country, 1995–2000

Birth order	England and Wales 1995	England and Wales 2000	Scotland 1995	Scotland 2000	Northern Ireland 1995	Northern Ireland 2000	UK 1995	UK 2000
			Percentage who breastfed initially					
First birth	74	75	61	67	52	59	72	74
Second or later births	62	66	50	59	40	51	60	65
All births	68	70	55	63	45	54	66	69

Source: DoH (2001d)

Self-reported health

Given that much of the data reported here is drawn from datasets gained from large-scale survey work it is not surprising that there is virtually no data which is self-reported by children themselves. It therefore seems important to include in this report data from a survey that did not entirely rely on proxy informants. (It may be useful in any subsequent reports to offer an overview of the quite sizeable literature on children's reported health concerns – this is essentially qualitative data with some local population survey data.)

The annual 1997 Health Survey for England took the health of children and young people (aged 2–24 years) as its specific focus (Prescott-Clarke and Primatesta, 1998). Children aged 13 years and over completed the questionnaire themselves, while parents acted as proxy informants for younger children. Among other things the survey asked about self-assessed general health. There are no similar datasets for children living in Wales, Northern Ireland or Scotland, nor is there earlier data for comparison. There is no available international comparative data on perceived health among children, the lower age band for OECD data being 15–24 years.

Informants were asked to rate their health in general on a five-point scale ('very good' to 'very bad'). Among 2–17 year olds, almost all children (~90 per cent) rated their general health as either 'good' or 'very good', and there were no differences between boys and girls. This figure fell slightly among respondents in their late teens and early 20s (Table 5.4). Very few children rated their health as 'bad' or 'very bad'.

Chart 5.4: Self-rating of general health by age

	Age																	
	2	3	4	5	6	7	8	9	10	11	12	13	14	15	16	17	18	19
Girls: 'very good' or 'good'	91	91	90	92	91	92	93	93	94	93	93	90	87	89	87	86	85	85
Girls: 'very bad' or 'bad'	1	1	1	1	2	1	1	1	1	1	0	1	1	1	1	1	1	2
Boys: 'very good' or 'good'	89	87	89	89	91	94	91	95	93	94	89	88	90	91	91	92	86	88
Boys: 'very bad' or 'bad'	1	3	1	1	1	1	1	2	0	0	0	1	1	0	0	1	1	2

Factors associated with self-assessed general health

The best predictor of self-assessed good health was whether or not the child had a longstanding illness. Four factors were found to be associated with self-reported 'good' or 'very good' health:

- social class
- household income
- ethnic group
- presence of longstanding illness

For both boys and girls there were differences in the proportions reporting 'good' or 'very good' health by social class and household income (Table 5.5). Children in the top social class were more likely to report their health to be good or very good compared to children in the lowest social class. Similarly, a significantly greater proportion of children living in households with an income in the top 5 per cent of household incomes in England reported good or very good health compared to those children in households with the lowest 5 per cent of incomes.

Ethnicity was also associated with self-reported health. White informants were one-and-a-half times more likely to report having better health than Asian informants. More specifically, Pakistani and Bangladeshi boys were less likely to report 'good' or 'very good' health than boys in the general population.

Table 5.5: Association between self-assessed general health and social class and household income

	% reporting 'good'/'very good' health	
	Boys	Girls
Social class		
Class I	96	97
Class V	86	89
Household income		
Household with income in top 5%	95	94
Household with income in lowest 5%	87	89

Longstanding illness and limiting longstanding illness

Information on the prevalence of longstanding illness and, more specifically, limiting longstanding illness among children, has been routinely collected by the General Household Survey since the earlier 1970s. This is an annual multi-purpose survey collecting information about a range of topics from people living in private households in Great Britain (there is no comparable data for children living in Northern Ireland). Parents are asked whether they have a child with a longstanding illness or disability which has troubled them for some time. Those reporting that their child has a longstanding illness are asked whether it limits their activities in any way. Table 5.6 displays the trends in parent-reported longstanding illness and limiting longstanding illness among children.

What Table 5.6 shows is an increase in the prevalence of both parent-reported longstanding illness and parent-reported limiting longstanding illness over the past 30 years. The increases are greater for longstanding illness than limiting longstanding illness.

The child's age and sex affect whether the child is reported to have a longstanding illness. The increases in prevalence are more marked among children over 5 years, than among those aged 0–4 years. Indeed there is evidence of a

Table 5.6: Trends in parent-reported longstanding illness by sex and age, 1972–2000

	1972	1975	1981	1985	1991	1993	1995	1996	1998	2000
					Year data collected					
% reporting that their child had a longstanding illness										
Boys										
0–4	5	8	12	11	13	15	14	14	15	14
5–15	9	11	17	18	17	21	20	19	21	23
Girls										
0–4	3	6	7	9	10	12	11	13	15	13
5–15	6	9	13	13	15	16	17	16	19	18
% reporting that their child had a limiting longstanding illness										
Boys										
0–4	–	3	3	4	4	5	5	4	4	4
5–15	–	6	8	8	7	9	8	8	8	9
Girls										
0–4	–	2	3	3	3	3	3	4	5	5
5–15	–	4	6	6	5	8	8	8	8	8

Sources: Office for National Statistics (2002), The Stationery Office (2002)

Table 5.7: Rate per 1,000 reporting longstanding illnesses, by sex and age

Condition group (ICD)*	Age band (years)											
	2–3		4–6		7–9		10–12		13–15		16–19	
	m†	f†	m	f	m	f	m	f	m	f	m	f
Infectious disease	–	1	0	–	0	3	1	5	3	1	4	1
Neoplasms and benign growths	–	2	4	0	0	2	1	–	1	3	1	1
Endocrine and metabolic	2	1	6	2	2	5	7	6	2	10	4	14
Blood and related organs	2	–	5	3	0	1	4	1	5	3	1	3
Mental disorders	11	4	13	8	14	9	18	7	15	10	12	5
Nervous system	9	6	6	7	14	10	27	14	26	16	12	34
Eye complaints	3	7	12	15	13	19	11	11	13	8	14	9
Ear complaints	20	10	30	31	34	27	24	18	18	13	4	12
Heart and circulatory system	11	5	9	14	5	6	9	6	5	3	6	9
Respiratory system	141	100	164	122	133	113	165	134	165	137	126	130
Digestive system	13	9	14	7	7	6	6	12	9	10	8	13
Genito-urinary system	8	5	6	13	3	8	10	7	2	7	3	4
Skin complaints	73	45	51	40	38	39	37	48	25	38	17	32
Musculoskeletal system	8	8	10	7	15	7	14	20	45	36	42	35
Other complaints	1	–	1	0	4	2	2	4	2	–	2	3

* Illnesses were coded into broad categories which were then aggregated into groups which corresponded as far as possible to the Ninth Revision of the International Classification of Diseases (ICD)
† m = male, f = female
Source: Prescott-Clarke and Primatesta (1998), Chapter 2, Table 2.2.

plateauing of the rising trend among the 0–4 year olds. There are also sex differences in the prevalence of longstanding illness among children aged 5–15 years. In the year 2000, almost a quarter of boys (23 per cent) aged between 5 and 15 years were reported by their parents as having a longstanding illness; this figure falls to less than one in five (18 per cent) for girls of the same age.

Compared to data collected on other age groups using these same measures, it is children who have registered the greatest relative rise in the prevalence of reported chronic ill health over the past 25 years (Yuen and Office of Health Economics, 2001).

Data collected by the 1997 Health Survey for England provides similar findings in terms of the prevalence of longstanding illnesses among children. It found that a quarter of children aged between 2 and 15 years reported having a longstanding illness, with more boys reporting a longstanding illness (26 per cent) than girls

(22 per cent). In addition, one in 20 children reported having more than one longstanding illness. The Health Survey for England also usefully provides information about the prevalence of the different types of conditions (Table 5.7).

The most commonly reported group of conditions were those related to the respiratory system, followed by conditions of the skin and of the musculoskeletal system. The prevalence of conditions of the respiratory system was higher in boys (up to 15 years). The prevalence of musculoskeletal conditions increased with age among boys and girls. For conditions of the skin, there was a decrease in prevalence above 15 years of age – the decrease being more marked for boys.

Factors associated with rates of longstanding illness

Taking the data from the 2000 General Household Survey, among boys there is a clear association between rates of reported longstanding illness and socio-economic group (see Table 5.8) with an increase in prevalence with decreasing socio-economic status. While, this pattern is not replicated among girls, overall the prevalence rates of longstanding illnesses among girls in the highest socio-economic group are much lower than among girls in the lowest socio-economic group. In terms of limiting longstanding illness, the pattern is less strong for both boys and girls. However, for both sexes, the presence of limiting long-standing illness is higher in the lower socio-economic groups compared to the top socio-economic groups.

Table 5.8: Rates of longstanding and limited longstanding illness by sex and socio-economic group

	I	II	III	IV	V	VI	VII
Boys – longstanding	15	16	20	20	21	24	27
Girls – longstanding	18	15	11	16	19	18	27
Boys – limiting longstanding	5	5	9	6	9	10	12
Girls – limiting longstanding	4	6	5	7	8	8	9

I: Professional
II: Employers and managers
III: Intermediate non-manual
IV: Junior non-manual
V: Skilled manual & own account non-professional
VI: Semi-skilled manual and personal service
VII: Unskilled manual
Source: 2000 General Household Survey.

Predictors of longstanding illness

The 1997 Health Survey for England looked at factors predicting longstanding illness in children. Parental longstanding illness was the strongest predictor of longstanding illness among children. Ethnicity was the second most important predictor, with those of Asian origin least likely to report longstanding illness. The authors cautioned interpretation of this finding, citing research by Pilgrim *et al.* (1993) which indicates that differences in cultural definitions of longstanding illness may have caused this effect as opposed to a difference in real prevalence. Gender was the third strongest predictor, with boys 28 per cent more likely to report a longstanding illness than girls. Finally, children living with a parent who was a current smoker were 23 per cent more likely to report a longstanding illness than those with non-smoking parents.

Childhood chronic illnesses: detailed exemplars

In this section we focus on particular childhood chronic conditions. First we report data on the two most common chronic conditions where increases in prevalence are being reported: diabetes and asthma. The possible factors underlying these increases are discussed. Next, we look at examples of conditions where there have been significant changes in mortality rates: cancer and cystic fibrosis. Following this we present data on HIV/AIDS. Finally, we report on what is known about the outcomes of children who have had a chronic childhood illness.

Common chronic conditions with increasing prevalence: diabetes

Type 1 (or insulin dependent) diabetes is one of the more common chronic childhood conditions. Maintaining adherence to the treatment regimes required to control the diabetes is acknowledged as a problematic issue – especially among teenagers. Yet the consequences of poor adherence are significant – in terms of both current and future health. Insulin dependent diabetes is believed to be due to genetic predisposition coupled with exposure to 'environmental' risk factors, including perinatal infection and rapid growth rate in early life, though these have yet to be definitively identified. Data collected by the EURODIAB collaborative group show marked variations in the incidence of diabetes across

Table 5.9: Summary of prevalence of insulin treated diabetes per 1,000 patients, by age, sex and country

Country	Rate per 1,000 0–4 years Male	Female	5–15 years Male	Female	16–24 years Male	Female
England	0.2	0.3	1.5	1.7	3.2	3.2
Wales	0	0.3	1.2	2.5	3	5.5
Scotland		0.26			–	–

Sources: England and Wales: ONS (1998a) Table 6A8; Scotland: Rangasami *et al.*, (1997)

European countries (EURODIAB, 2000). Incidence rates are higher in northern and north-western areas compared to other areas of Europe. Across Europe the incidence of diabetes is increasing, particularly among the under-5s.

Equivalent prevalence data for the four UK countries has not been identified. Table 5.9 summarises the most recent available data on the prevalence of insulin treated diabetes among children.

Comparing prevalence data between England and Wales shows lower rates of prevalence for boys in Wales compared to boys in England across all age bands. The pattern for girls is the reverse, with increasingly higher prevalence rates of diabetes in Wales with increasing age (a trend which continues into young adulthood).

The Scottish Study Group for the Care of Young Diabetics hold a register of all diagnoses of type 1 diabetes in Scotland. Analysis of incidence data between 1984 and 1993 showed a rising incidence of type 1 diabetes in Scottish children (0.23 per 1,000 to 0.26 per 1,000) of about 2 per cent per year. Boys are more likely than girls to be diagnosed with diabetes. In common with EURODIAB, the Scottish Study Group suggested that changes in exposure to environmental factors underlie increasing incidence.

Data collected from general practices in England and Wales (ONS, 1998) was used to explore the impact of deprivation on prevalence. This analysis suggests that insulin dependent diabetes in childhood runs counter to the usual pattern, with higher prevalence among the least deprived groups compared to the most deprived groups (Table 5.10). It will be important to report the findings from the Scottish Diabetes Survey being carried out in March 2002 in our next report. Among other things, this survey will be exploring the association between type 1 diabetes and factors such as age and deprivation.

Table 5.10: Prevalence of insulin treated diabetes by age, sex and deprivation category, England and Wales

		Rate per 1,000					
		0–4 years		5–15 years		16–24 years	
Deprivation scale		Male	Female	Male	Female	Male	Female
Least deprived	1	0.2	0.4	1.8	2.8	4.5	4.4
	2	0.2	0.3	1.6	1.5	3.9	2.5
	3	0.3	0.2	1.6	1.9	3.2	3.1
	4	0.1	0.4	1.4	1.7	3.0	3.5
Most deprived	5	0.3	0.1	1.2	1.1	2.4	3.4

Source: ONS (1998a), Table 8A8

Common chronic conditions with increasing prevalence: asthma

Asthma is the most common chronic childhood illness and Britain has one of the highest prevalence rates of asthma in the world (Central Health Monitoring Unit, 1995). As in other countries its prevalence in Britain is rising, although the mechanisms underlying this are unclear, with features of the domestic and external environments and genetic pre-disposition being suggested as contributory factors.

Drawing on data collected for the General Practice Research Database, it appears that there was an increase in the prevalence of treated asthma among young adults (16–24 years) over the period 1994–1998. However, this was not the case with children less than 4 years of age, among whom a slight decrease occurred in 1998. Among children aged 5 to 15 years there is no clear trend (ONS 1998a; 2000d). Across all child age bands, boys have a higher prevalence of asthma than do girls. The age band with the highest prevalence of asthma is 5–15 years: in this group 13 per cent of boys and 10 per cent of girls were being

Table 5.11: Prevalence of treated asthma per 1,000 patients by age, sex and deprivation category

		Rate per 1,000					
		0–4 years		5–15 years		16–24 years	
Deprivation scale		Male	Female	Male	Female	Male	Female
Least deprived	1	78.0	43.4	129.2	98.6	74.1	90.5
	2	99.2	65.6	127.4	97.9	73.1	85.4
	3	106.2	69.1	133.1	110.0	73.2	87.2
	4	97.1	69.3	132.7	107.0	69.5	83.5
Most deprived	5	109.0	70.4	129.2	98.1	60.8	70.3

Source: ONS (1998a), Table 8A10

treated for asthma in 1998. By contrast, 10 per cent of boys and 6 per cent of girls in the 0–4 age band were being treated for asthma.

Table 5.11 reproduces general practice data on the prevalence of treated asthma by age, sex and deprivation category. Overall, among children up to 15 years, increased deprivation appears to be associated with the prevalence of treated asthma. The association is particularly marked among girls aged 0–4 years. This association appears to reverse among older teenagers and young people: in these groups the highest prevalence rates are among the least deprived. This may be being caused by the known relationship between deprivation and use of/contact with health professionals and by issues to do with the relationship between adherence to treatment regimes and deprivation indicators.

Data collected by general practices show that overall prevalence levels are higher in Wales than in England for boys up to 15 years of age, and for girls under 5 and over 16 years (Table 5.12).

Table 5.12: Prevalence of treated asthma per 1,000 patients, by age, sex and country, England and Wales

| | Rate per 1,000 | | | | | |
| | 0–4 years | | 5–15 years | | 16–24 years | |
Country	Male	Female	Male	Female	Male	Female
England	100	65	130	103	69	82
Wales	104	77	141	103	74	90

Source: ONS (1998a), Table 6A10, 69.

Chronic conditions with changes in mortality: cancers and cystic fibrosis

Only a small proportion of cancer registrations relate to children. For example, in 1997, less than 1 per cent of cancer registrations were for children less than 15 years in age (Quinn et al., 2000). The most common forms of cancer found in children are the leukaemias and brain/spinal cord tumours. Boys are more likely to contract cancer, with a greater incidence of leukaemias, brain and spinal cord tumours and lymphomas in boys than in girls. Overall, in England and Wales over the period 1971 to 1993 there was an increase in the incidence of cancer in boys and girls. It will be important to monitor new incidence data as it emerges.

Analysis of survival rates from childhood cancer across the 1970s and 1980s show an enormous improvement over that period (Coleman et al., 1999). For example, the 5-year survival rate for children diagnosed with leukaemia has doubled from 33 per cent to 69 per cent; and for brain tumours, survival rates have risen from 43 per cent to 58 per cent. Inclusion of children in national and international clinical trials of new treatments, and increased use of tertiary care have contributed to these improvements (Stiller, 1994). Levels of deprivation do not appear to be associated with survival rates in childhood cancer (Quinn and Babb, 2000).

Analysis of incidence data over the period 1968 to 1994 found the incidence of cystic fibrosis to be constant. The population of children (16 years and under) with cystic fibrosis in 1995 was estimated to be around 4,500, with one in 2,500 births being that of a child with cystic fibrosis (Dodge *et al.*, 1997). Cystic fibrosis is one of the chronic childhood conditions which have shown significant increases in life expectancy. Changes in clinical practice and advances in treatment regimes mean that more and more children with cystic fibrosis are surviving into adulthood. However, while there is a continuing decrease in childhood mortality, cystic fibrosis remains a life-limiting condition and there have only been small improvements in maximum life expectancy.

HIV and AIDS

Since recording began in 1982, over 1,100 children have been infected with the HIV virus, of these 310 have died. The most common source of exposure to HIV virus among children under 14 years is mother-to-infant transfer (Table 5.13). Among boys only, exposure to the virus through blood products for the treatment of conditions such as haemophilia accounts for over a third of cases of HIV infection in England, Wales and Northern Ireland, and almost half the infection cases in Scotland. Despite its relative rarity, the availability of recent UK data on HIV/AIDS are in marked contrast to some of the other health conditions we have covered in this chapter.

At the end of June 2001, the total number of recorded cases of AIDS in children (who were under 14 years of age when first diagnosed) was 482; of these, 200 children had died (PHLS, 2002).

Data on children born to HIV-infected mothers over the past 20 years suggests that, while the numbers of children being born to HIV-positive mothers are rising, there is a decline in the proportion of children infected by the virus (Table 5.14).

Thus in the period 1979 to 1983 all children born to an HIV-infected mother were infected with the virus. By early 1990s just over a half of children were infected. In contrast, figures for the period 1998–99 show that less than

Table 5.13: HIV infection* and deaths in children*** by exposure category and sex: cases reported to the end of June 2001#**

How children probably acquired the virus	England, Wales, N. Ireland			Scotland			Total ##	Deaths
	Male	Female	NS	Male	Female	NS		
Mother to infant	374	364	2	21	19	0	780	172
Blood factor (eg, for haemophilia)	264	0	0	21	0	0	285	123
Blood/tissue transfer (eg, transfusion)	19	16	3	2	2	0	42	14
Other/undetermined	15	7	2	1	0	0	25	1
Total	672	387	7	45	21	0	1,132	310

* Includes all children with AIDS, or with virus detected, or with HIV antibody at age 18 months or over
** Deaths in HIV-infected children without AIDS are included
*** Infected when aged 14 years or under
# The introduction of a new computer system at the Institute of Child Health has delayed the release of data for the second half of 2001
Includes 337 children who were aged 15 years or over at the end of July 2000 or at death (44 children infected through mother-to-infant transmission (1 died), 268 haemophilia patients (106 died), 18 blood recipients (4 died) and 6 in other/undetermined category
Source: PHLS (2002)

Table 5.14: Children born to HIV-infected mothers, year of birth by infection status and country of report, 1979–2001

Year of birth	Infected				Indeterminate*		Not infected		
	England, Wales Northern Ireland		Scotland		England, Wales, Northern Ireland	Scotland	England, Wales, Northern Ireland	Scotland	Total
	AIDS	Not AIDS	AIDS	Not AIDS					
79–83	9	6	1	0	0	0	0	0	16
84–85	20	12	6	4	2	2	4	11	61
86–87	24	19	4	3	11	3	14	35	113
88–89	45	27	3	1	13	4	26	26	145
90–91	64	61	1	3	26	3	51	22	231
92–93	74	56	1	3	37	3	77	12	263
94–95	60	55	1	2	40	4	88	19	269
96–97	56	57	3	1	44	4	151	12	328
98–99	37	35	2	1	82	2	261	13	433
00–01	18	6	0	0	271	10	139	7	451
Total	407	334	22	18	526	35	811	157	2,310

* Aged less than 18 months when last tested positive for HIV antibody without other evidence of HIV infection.
Source: PHLS (2002)

one in five children (17 per cent) born to an HIV-infected woman have tested positive to the virus (though it should be noted that it is not yet possible, for a number of reasons, to determine whether a further 19 per cent of this cohort are infected). The implication of this change in the pattern of infection between mother and infant is that, while fewer children are contracting the HIV virus, an increasing number of children are living in families where at least one family member has HIV or AIDS.

HIV/AIDS acquired through sexual intercourse among 15–19-year-olds

Young people aged between 15 and 19 years who become infected with the HIV virus through sexual intercourse form a very small proportion of the total number of individuals who become infected in this way. However, as Chart 5.1 shows, the number of young people becoming infected with HIV through sexual intercourse is rising dramatically – especially among females (PHLS Aids Centre & the Scottish Centre for Infection and Environmental Health, 2002).

Chart 5.1: HIV infected individuals aged 15–19 years, infections probably acquired through sexual intercourse, UK data

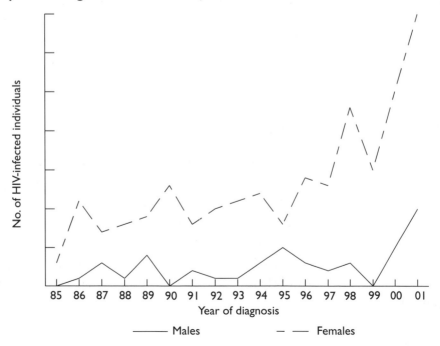

Surviving chronic childhood illness: psychosocial outcomes

There is a body of research looking at the psychosocial outcomes of surviving chronic physical illness in childhood. Gledhill *et al.* (2000) reviewed this evidence and drew the following conclusions. On measures of psychiatric outcome, there were no differences compared to healthy or general population controls. However, in terms of social outcomes (such as employment, educational attainment and the development of independence), survivors of a childhood chronic illness were more likely to experience difficulties than those who have not experienced childhood chronic illness. Survivors whose condition involved the brain or central nervous system and/or involved treatments which affected cognitive functioning, were at greatest risk of poor social outcomes. The processes underlying these observed associations are not fully understood. Other research has shown that the nature of the condition, quality of professional support, and family and individual psychological and social factors may all contribute to individual outcomes (for example, LaGreca *et al.*, 1992).

Finally, the authors note that the quality of paediatric care and psychosocial support will have a role to play in ensuring the most positive outcomes in adulthood for children with potentially life-limiting or life-threatening conditions. Other research has noted that responsibility for meeting this demand need not fall only on health professionals and parents, but also on schools and teachers (Lightfoot *et al.*, 1999). There is clearly a need for research on developing effective interventions to support children in achieving the best possible outcomes.

Sexually transmitted infections

Young people are vulnerable to acquiring sexually transmitted infections (STIs) as they are more likely to have a higher number of sexual partners and to change these partners more frequently than older age groups. In line with other age groups since 1995, the trend in the total number of diagnoses of STIs in young people is rising (PHLS *et al.*, 2000). This follows a plateauing of, or even decline in, numbers of many STIs in the late 1980s and early 1990s which was thought to reflect changes in sexual behaviour brought about in response to the HIV epidemic.

Table 5.15: New episodes of selected diagnoses by age and sex, England and Wales,* 1995–2000

Diagnosis	(age, years)	1995		1996		1997		1998		1999		2000**	
		male	female	male	female	male	female	male	female	male	female	male	female
Infectious syphilis	<16	1	0	1	0	2	0	0	0	0	0	0	0
(1° and 2°)	16–9	2	2	4	3	1	3	5	3	5	12	4	7
Gonorrhoea	<16	42	128	29	136	47	142	37	158	44	168	58	224
(uncomplicated)	16–19	690	1025	915	1411	1064	1462	1009	1509	1392	1854	1854	2350
Genital chlamydia	<16	45	396	40	466	50	522	52	584	77	714	69	808
(uncomplicated)	16–19	1184	4917	1434	5868	1873	7530	2423	8618	2997	10398	3702	12055
Genital herpes	<16	12	124	10	119	12	106	11	96	4	115	14	125
(first attack)	16–19	280	1637	272	1672	266	1818	323	1849	354	1894	402	1996
Genital warts	<16	90	481	88	499	101	469	94	457	100	477	95	450
(first attack)	16–19	1853	6845	2086	7714	2520	8381	2878	8700	3170	8644	3294	8631

* Data for Scotland and Northern Ireland are not yet available.
** 2000 figures are provisional

Table 5.15 shows the number of new episodes of certain STIs among under-16s and 16–19 year olds in England and Wales (PHLS *et al.*, 2000). Overall, it is clear that females are more likely to be diagnosed with an STI than males. Among young people under 16 years of age, there is an ongoing increase in diagnoses of gonorrhoea among males and females, and of genital chlamydia among girls. Similar patterns are found among the 16–19-year-old age group, though with a greater number of cases. Diagnoses of genital herpes and genital warts in males and females within this age group have also increased over the past five years. In reporting these data, the Public Health Laboratory Service noted that during 2000 almost 40 per cent of diagnoses of gonorrhoea and 34 per cent of chlamydial infections were in those aged 16–19 years. It is hypothesised that a lack of skills and confidence to negotiated safer sex renders young women particularly vulnerable to STIs (Hillier *et al.*, 1998).

Technologically dependent children

The impact of medical and technological advances on child health is most notable in two groups. First, advances which relate to the management of prematurity and congenital defects; and, secondly, advances in the treatment of conditions such as cancer and cystic fibrosis. In addition, the early discharge of medically frail babies and the increased practice of community-based paediatric care means there are increasing numbers of children living at home with complex health care needs or who are 'technologically dependent' (Kirk, 1998). Children who are technologically dependent 'need both a medical device to compensate for the loss of a vital bodily function and substantial and ongoing nursing care to avert death or further disability' (Wagner *et al.*, 1988). The types of technologies included in the term 'technologically dependent' include: mechanical ventilation, parenteral nutrition, intravenous drug therapies, peritoneal dialysis, haemodialysis, oxygen therapy, tracheostomy tube, enteral feeding, cardio-respiratory monitoring, urostomy, colostomy, ileostomy and urethral catheter.

Clearly, technologically dependent children are not a population independent of those already described in this chapter. Rather, some children who are chronically ill and/or have life-limiting or life-threatening conditions will be technologically dependent. What is significant about this group is their presence in the community, and the fact that the possible impacts of technological dependency on child and family functioning are yet to be identified, or even acknowledged.

In 1998 the Department of Health commissioned a piece of work to assess the number of technologically dependent children in the UK (Glendinning *et al.*, 1999). The researchers drew attention to the lack of comprehensive or long-term information on the numbers of technologically dependent children living in the community. However, an attempt was made to estimate the number of technologically dependent children in the UK using data from a number of sources. They estimated that it is likely that there were at least 6,000 technologically dependent children. Of these, '2,500 would be receiving artificial feeding, 1,000 with tracheostomies, over 1,000 on intravenous infusions, 150 on peritoneal dialysis, over 1,000 on oxygen and 93 on long-term ventilation at home' (Glendinning *et al.*, 1999, p. 17). Given the continued improvements in survival rates of technologically dependent children, the cumulative total will increase year by year and will need to be monitored.

Conclusions

A number of themes emerge from this discussion of the evidence on the current status of children's health in the UK. There are clearly a number of areas of child health which trend data suggest are a cause of concern. These include the increase in the number of children reporting a longstanding illness. We have looked in detail at the increases in the prevalence of asthma and diabetes and have highlighted the difficulties scientists are facing in identifying the factors contributing to these increases. Other populations are also increasing: survivors of chronic illnesses and previously life-limiting illnesses, children dependent on medical technology and cases of children with sexually transmitted infections. Set against this, the great majority of children in Great Britain (we have no comparable data for Northern Ireland) report, or are reported to be, feeling healthy. However, the impact of deprivation is clear here, with the most deprived children being least likely to report good health.

Throughout the chapter we have highlighted things 'to watch out for': this might be the future availability of a new dataset, or the suggestion that current figures or events indicate the emergence of a new, and perhaps unexpected, child health issue. The dramatic fall, in some areas, of the take-up of the MMR vaccine is a good example.

Care was taken at the beginning of this chapter to highlight the gaps and overall paucity of data on some areas of child health. This includes data at a national and 'four country' level on health or well-ness, ill health, chronic conditions and physical impairments. While there is some evidence of cross country differences on measures of child health, data enabling a detailed exploration of differences *within* countries is either not collected, or is not easily accessed by external researchers. In addition, the limitations of the data collected make it difficult, if not impossible, to unpick or understand the processes underlying any observed differences. Yet without this understanding it is impossible to devise appropriate and effective interventions.

In any case, it is important not to lose sight of the fact that children will continue to be born with physical impairments and children will continue to fall ill or have accidents which compromise their health. Multi-disciplinary research which improves our very limited understanding of how to best promote and protect the short- and long-term outcomes for these children and their families is a priority.

Finally, while there is some small-scale quantitative work on the health concerns of older children/teenagers, no national data is collected nor have attempts been made to collect such data from younger children. Given the call for greater participation by children in service development (Lansdown, 2000: DoH, 2001g), this seems to be a significant omission in what is known, at national levels, about child health. It may be helpful for any future report to include a brief review of the burgeoning body of qualitative research evidence in this area.

6 Unintentional Injuries

Karen Croucher

Key facts:
- Unintentional injuries remain the leading cause of death for children and young people in the UK, as in all industrialised nations.
- The major cause of unintentional injury related to mortality and morbidity is traffic accidents. The highest number of deaths and injuries are among child pedestrians.
- Drowning, falls, thermal injuries and poisoning are the other main causes of fatal and non-fatal unintentional injuries.
- A strong relationship between social class and/or levels of area deprivation and deaths related to unintentional injury has been demonstrated in the UK, although the evidence to link injury-related morbidity and social class is less consistent.

Key trends:
- Child injury death rates have fallen dramatically in the last three decades.

Key sources:
- UNICEF
- Registrar Generals for England and Wales, Scotland and Northern Ireland

---

Introduction

The focus of this chapter is on the nature and extent of unintentional injuries and deaths related to unintentional injury in childhood, using data drawn from a number of different sources. While recognising that it may be controversial, where possible the use of the word 'accident' has been avoided, as it implies an event which is unavoidable, unpredictable and not preventable, when in fact many so-called 'accidental' injuries and deaths might well have been avoided and prevented if individuals, parents, agencies and sometimes children themselves had taken different actions (Davis and Pless, 2001). There is a vast literature on injury prevention (see for example, NHS Centre for Reviews and Dissemination, 1996) which is not considered here. Similarly there is no room for a discussion on risk, children's and parents' perceptions of risk or the desirability of allowing children to take risks and develop risk management skills (see for example, Scott et al., 2000). Nor is there a discussion of the changing physical and social landscapes of children's lives in the 21st century (see for example, O'Brien, 1998).

International perspective

'In the world's richest nations, more than 20,000 children will die from injuries in the next twelve months' UNICEF (2001a)

Although child injury death rates in industrialised countries have fallen dramatically in recent decades, injuries remain the leading cause of death in children aged 1–14 years in all the world's richest nations. The first standardised league table of child deaths by injury (unintentional and intentional) in the OECD nations, published by UNICEF (2001a), shows that between 1991 and 1995 the UK had the second lowest child death by injury rate with an annualised rate of 6.1 deaths per 100,000 for children aged 1–14. Sweden had the lowest child death by injury rate (5.2 per 100,000 children) and Korea the highest (25.6 per 100,000 children). The number of deaths due to injury reflects an even larger number of non-fatal injuries, trauma and disability. It has been estimated that for every one death among children aged 0-14 years, there are 160 hospital admissions, and 2,000 accident and emergency department visits. Childhood injuries account for approximately 30 per cent of the total burden of disease among the industrialised world's children (UNICEF, 2001a). The child injury death rate continues to decline, but not as swiftly as other causes of child death. Consequently, in industrialised nations during the last 25 years the proportion of all child deaths accounted for by injuries has risen from 25 per cent to 37 per cent (UNICEF, 2001a).

The leading cause of injury-related deaths in all the OECD countries is transport accidents. Such 'accidents' accounted for 41 per cent of all injury-related child death between 1991 and 1995. The other main causes of injury-related child deaths are: intentional harm (accounting for 14 per cent of child injury deaths between 1991 and 1995), drowning (15 per cent), fire (7 per cent), falls (4 per cent), poisoning (2 per cent), firearms accidents (1 per cent) and other unintentional injuries such as medical accidents and death by choking (14 per cent).

UK perspective: sources of data

In the UK, data relating to injury-related child deaths can be derived from a number of sources including: Registrar Generals for England and Wales, Scotland, and Northern Ireland (mortality statistics); the Department of Transport, Local Government and the Regions (on road accidents in England and Wales); the Home Office (on residential fires); and the Scottish Executive and Welsh Assembly. There are also a number of data sources on non-fatal accidents, including the General Household Survey, the Home Accident/Leisure Accident Surveillance Schemes, the recently commissioned Health Survey for England, as well as school and GP records and hospital admission rates. However, no one source provides comprehensive evidence on unintentional injury-related child morbidity rates (Quilgars, 2001b). Different agencies code, collate and present data in different ways, and publish data at different times, thus comparisons are not easily made between different parts of the UK.

Data on unintentional injuries and deaths related to unintentional injury in the UK are relatively accessible. They are often collated on an annual basis, albeit by a number of different agencies. However, they are rarely, if ever, combined with data on social class. The relationship between social class and unintentional injuries and injury-related deaths has tended to be investigated by one-off studies. Quilgars (2001b) noted that since the early 1980s, few studies have investigated the class gradient of child injury mortality. She could only identify two studies which considered the relationship between poverty and child deaths related to unintentional injury: a study reported by Roberts and Power (1996) and a study reported by Morrison *et al.* (1999). Both studies consider death rates over time in geographical areas against measures of social deprivation in the local population. A further study (Sharples *et al.*, 1990) investigated child fatalities from head injuries. Similarly, Quilgars notes that, although there is a large body of work on childhood morbidity caused by unintentional injuries, very few studies address the issue of social class differentials. Those that have addressed this issue do not demonstrate a particularly consistent relationship between poverty and morbidity related to unintentional injury. This may be in part due to the difficulties in determining the underlying exposure to risk experienced by individuals from different socio-economic backgrounds, and the difficulties in separating the effect of the home environment from the effect of the wider area where people live (White *et al.*, 2000).

Child mortality and morbidity

Unintentional injury became the leading cause of child mortality in the 1950s and remains the single largest cause of death for all children over the age of 1 year in the UK. Child mortality due to unintentional injury has declined in the last three decades, with mortality rates for children aged 1–9 years halving over the period 1970 to 1990, although the decline has been less pronounced for older children (Jarvis *et al.*, 1995). Due to the smaller populations in Scotland and Northern Ireland, the death rates are subject to greater variation; however, the trend continues downwards. The decline in fatalities has not been as steep as for other causes of death, such as whooping cough, TB and measles (see Chapter 3), which has led to unintentional injury accounting for an increasing proportion of all child deaths. It is also important to understand that the decline in fatalities does not necessarily reflect a decrease in the number or severity of injuries, but may well be a reflection of improved health technologies and services.

In 1999 in England and Wales, 426 children aged 14 and under died as a result of unintentional injury or poisoning (ONS, 2000); in 1999 in Northern Ireland 21 children died as a result of unintentional injury or poisoning (NISRA, 2000a); in Scotland 47 children died as a result of accidents and adverse events (General Registrar Office for Scotland, 2000). In the same period more than 2 million children attended hospital accident and emergency departments (CAPT, 2000a). It is difficult to estimate the numbers of children whose injuries resulted in long-term or permanent disability. One study estimated that about 3 per cent of children under the age of 15 admitted to hospital following an accident have a permanent disability as a consequence. However, other data suggest that the percentage of children with permanent disability following accidents which resulted in hospital admission might be as high as 9 per cent (Roberts, 1996). It is very likely that, apart from accidents that require hospital admissions, many more children suffer minor injuries which are treated by general practitioners or in the home. In 1995 it was estimated that the direct costs of childhood injury to the NHS was £200 million annually (Jarvis *et al.*, 1995).

Leading causes of unintentional death and injury in the UK

There are several main causes of death and unintentional injury to children. As in all industrialised countries, traffic accidents are the most common cause of injury-related child death in the UK. Outside the home, apart from traffic accidents, drowning and falls are the most likely cause of child deaths related to unintentional injury (Roberts, 1996). Fatal injuries sustained in the home are most likely to be as the result of thermal injuries (burns and scalds), following by suffocating, drowning, falls and poisoning. Although these are the most common causes of death across the industrialised world, there are variations in the death rates in different countries for different types of injury.

In comparison with the 15 most populous OECD countries, the UK appears to have some of the lowest death rates per 100,000 children for almost all of the major injury-related causes of death (transport accidents, drowning and falls) for the period 1991–1995. The exception, however, is the death rate from thermal injuries, reported as 0.66 per 100,000 children. Only the USA, Korea, Canada, and Australia were reported to have higher rates (UNICEF, 2001a).

Road accidents

In the UK, as in all industrialised nations, road accident fatalities remain the single largest cause of all accidental deaths in the child population (Table 6.1). Apart from fatalities, thousands of children are injured every year (Table 6.2). It has been estimated that one in three children involved in a road accident suffers

Table 6.1: Road deaths as a percentage of all accidental deaths in Great Britain, 1999

Road accident deaths as percentage of all accidental deaths

Ages	Male	Female	All
0-4 years*	20	26	23
5–9 years	61	68	63
10–14 years	55	67	59
15–19 years	70	78	72
All ages	35	17	27

* NB: In some cases 0 may have been coded when the age of casualty was not reported.
Source: DETR *et al.* (2000)

Table 6.2: Child road deaths and casualties in Great Britain by age, road user type and severity of injury, 1999

Ages	1999				1981–85 averages			
	0–4*	5–7	8–11	12–15	0–4*	5–7	8–11	12–15
Pedestrians								
Killed	11	22	32	42	70	86	93	101
KSI**	455	677	1,165	1,160	975	1,535	2,334	2,304
All severities	1,999	3,082	5,873	5,873	3,331	5,369	8,503	8,389
Pedal cyclists								
Killed	2	5	11	18	2	8	30	58
KSI**	21	137	302	490	31	236	733	1,450
All severities	118	935	2,552	3,685	150	1,010	3,295	6,996
Car passengers								
Killed	21	7	10	32	28	15	18	32
KSI**	226	153	236	417	335	229	362	615
All severities	3,227	2,802	4,394	4,700	2,605	1,785	2,716	3,361
All road users								
Killed	34	34	54	99	102	109	144	208
KSI**	718	977	1,757	2,247	1,380	2,027	3,501	4,773
All severities	5,804	7,100	13,546	15,601	6,587	8,410	15,065	20,272

* NB: In some cases 0 may have been coded when the age of casualty was not reported
** KSI = killed or seriously injured
Source: DETR et al. (2000)

from post-traumatic stress disorder (Stallard *et al.*, 1998). Of all child road users, the highest number of deaths and injuries are among pedestrians. Scotland and Northern Ireland suffer higher child pedestrian casualty rates than do England and Wales (White *et al.*, 2000).

To the figures for Great Britain, figures for Northern Ireland must be added. The Royal Ulster Constabulary reports that 20 children were killed on roads between April 1999 and March 2000; a further 201 were seriously injured, and a further 1,546 sustained minor injuries.

Of all road users of all ages, children between the ages of 5 and 15, and particularly children between the ages of 12 and 15, have the highest rates of all types of injury and serious injury compared to rates in the general population as a whole.

For years, the Scottish child road casualty rates per head of population have been higher than those in England and Wales for fatal and serious injuries, although there is little difference between rates for all types of injuries. Using averages for 1995–99, Scottish rates for fatal injuries were 35 per cent higher than in England and Wales, and 39 per cent higher for fatal and serious injuries.

Table 6.3: Road death and injury rates per 100,000 population by age bands and road user type, Great Britain, 1999

	Age band (years) 0-4*	5-7	8-11	12-15	All ages
Pedestrians					
Killed	0.3	1.0	1.0	1.4	1.5
KSI**	13.0	30.0	38.0	40.0	17.0
All severities	57.0	137.0	194.0	202.0	74.0
Pedal Cyclists					
Killed	0	0.2	0.4	0.6	0.3
KSI**	0.6	6.1	10.0	17.0	5.5
All severities	3.4	42.0	84.0	127.0	40.0
Car passengers					
Killed	0.6	0.3	0.3	1.1	1.0
KSI**	6.4	6.8	8.0	14.0	13.0
All severities	92.0	125.0	144.0	162.0	127.0
All road users					
Killed	1.0	1.5	1.8	3.4	5.9
KSI**	20.0	44.0	58.0	77.0	74.0
All severities	166.0	316.0	444.0	537.0	554.0

* NB: In some cases 0 may have been coded when the age of casualty was not reported.
** KSI = killed or seriously injured
Source: DETR et al. (2000)

This represents a slight worsening in Scotland's fatal and serious figures relative to England and Wales. When examined, the figures show that child pedestrian casualty rates in Scotland in particular are higher than in England and Wales, with double the fatality rate, and a 51 per cent higher rate for fatal and serious pedestrian casualties. The casualty rates for child pedal cyclists casualties were lower across all categories in Scotland compared to England and Wales (Scottish Executive, 1999).

Table 6.4: Child road deaths and injury rates, Scotland, England and Wales

Rates per 1,000	Scotland			England and Wales		
	Fatal	Fatal and severe	All severities	Fatal	Fatal and and severe	All severities
1999	0.02	0.62	3.17	0.02	0.47	3.63
Average 1995–99	0.03	0.75	3.58	0.02	0.54	3.76

Source: Scottish Executive (1999)

The numbers of children killed and injured in road accidents in the UK are falling. Comparing 1999 with 1981–85 averages, child deaths on the roads have fallen by more than 70 per cent, serious injuries by more than 50 per cent and all types of injury by 18 per cent. However, these figures need to be considered in light of changing travel patterns, with fewer and fewer children undertaking journeys by foot and by bicycle. The downward trends in fatal and serious casualties have not been the same for all age groups, for all social classes or for both sexes. The greatest reduction in fatalities has been among the under-5s, and the smallest among 12–15 year olds. Reductions in casualties among boys are slightly less than among girls (CAPT, 2000b). The decline in fatality rates has been much less for children in the manual social classes and the risk of death for child pedestrians appears to be highly class-related. Children in the lowest socio-economic groups are over four times more likely to be killed as pedestrians than their counterparts in the highest socio-economic groups (White *et al.*, 2000).

Thermal injuries

The majority of deaths caused by thermal injuries (burns and scalds) result from house fires, with a small number being associated with severe scalds, often from bath water. Apart from fatalities, serious thermal injuries often require extensive (and painful) treatment over many years, and leave lasting scars and psychological damage.

House fires exhibit the greatest socio-economic gradient of any cause of injury-related death. The risk of house fires is strongly related to the type of housing and is greatest in the poorest housing – houses in poor repair, temporary accommodation, and houses in multiple occupancy. Children in social class V are 16 times more likely to be killed by fire or flames than those in social class I (Roberts and Power, 1996). The trend in fatalities from house fires is downwards, and is thought to be due in part to the increasing number of homes with smoke alarms installed. Table 6.5 shows the number of children killed or injured by fire in the UK in 1999.

Around 4,675 children under 18 are admitted as inpatients each year to accident and emergency departments or specialist burn units as a result of burn and scald accidents in the home. Pre-school children are most at risk, accounting for 75 per cent of all serious injuries. Some 3,500 children in this age group require admission to hospital every year, and many require plastic surgery. There are three main causes of these injuries: scalding drinks, scalding baths and kettles.

Table 6.5: Casualties from fire, by age and sex, 1999, UK

Age	Total	Rate per million population	Males	Rate per million population	Females	Rate per million population
Fatal						
0–4	6	8	4	11	2	6
1–4	24	8	13	9	11	8
5–10	7	1	3	1	11	8
11–16	10	2	6	3	4	2
Non fatal						
0–4	157	222	77	212	79	229
1–4	816	280	447	299	364	256
5–10	731	156	427	178	301	132
11–16	856	189	460	198	396	179

Source: Watson et al. (2000)

On average two very young children a year die as a result of being scalded in the bath (DTI, 1999). More than 26,000 pre-school children suffer minor or less serious burns every year (DTI, 1999).

Falls

Very few falls prove fatal. Using data from the Home Accidents Death Database and the Home Accidents Surveillance System, it has been estimated that pre-school children are involved in approximately 230,000 falls per year (DTI, 1999). The average child has an almost 25 per cent chance of being taken to hospital as the result of a fall at home before reaching the age of 5. Children between the ages of 5 and 14 are involved in 145,000 falls per year. One in every 40 children in this age group visits hospital each year because of a fall at home. Children in social class V are 10 times more likely than those in the highest social class to die as a result of a fall at home (Roberts and Pless, 1995). This disturbing inequality in risk has to be seen against the very small number of deaths resulting from falls, and the annual death rate from falls (see Tables 6.6 and 6.7 below).

Asphyxiation

Using data from the Home Accidents Death Database and the Home Accidents Surveillance System, it has been estimated that about 34 children in the 0–4 age

Table 6.6: Annual number of falls

Age	Trivial	Minor	Serious	Total	Fatal
0–4	46,000 (20%)	157,000 (68%)	28,000 (12%)	231,000	6
5–9	9,000 (10%)	66,000 (73%)	16,000 (18%)	91,000	1
10–14	4,000 (7%)	41,000 (76%)	9,000 (17%)	54,000	1

Source: DTI (1999)

Table 6.7: Annual fall rates per 10,000 per year

Age	Trivial	Minor	Serious	Total	Fatal cases per 10 m population per year
0–4	110	384	70	564	14
5–9	23	174	25	222	3
10–14	11	115	25	151	3

Source: DTI (1999)

group and 17 children in the 5–14 age group die every year as a result of asphyxiation. Such incidents include drowning in the bath, garden ponds, swimming pools and lakes, postural asphyxiation (in which the victim falls or lies in such a way as to constrict breathing) and constriction of the neck (for example, when a child has become tangled in a harness or dressing gown cord). Most of these incidents take place within the home or garden. Drowning is the third largest cause of unintentional death in the home in the under-5s (DTI, 2000).

Poisonings

Most cases of poisonings (adults and children) involve children under 5 years old and there are about 30,000 incidents every year. Household chemicals and medicines are the most common causes of poisoning in young children. The overall rate of poisonings decreases up until the age of 9 years old, and then shows an increase in the 10–14 age band. Poisoning in older children is largely due to alcohol, which accounts for about 41 per cent of cases in the 10–14 age band: there are about 1,400 cases of alcohol poisoning every year.

Variation in types and numbers of injuries by age, sex, social class, and ethnicity

Children under 15 undergo rapid developmental change. At different stages in this development they are differentially exposed to different types of activities and environmental hazards. Young children and toddlers are more likely to be injured in the home environment, reflecting the proportion of their time spent in the home. As children get older, they are more likely to get injured in external environments – at school, in the playground, during sporting activities and on the roads.

At every age, boys are more likely to die from unintentional injuries than girls. This pattern is seen across the industrialised nations. The difference between the sexes is greatest in older age groups. However, even in pre-school children, boys are more likely to die from unintentional injuries. Differences between boys and girls in attitudes to risk and risk taking behaviours, and the greater likelihood of boys participating in more dangerous activities or sports, may explain the differences in injury rates between the sexes.

Quilgars (2001b) examined the unintentional injury rates for children over the last 20 years and presents a detailed consideration of social class gradients and discussion of the causes of differences in childhood unintentional injury rates. She concluded that a strong relationship between social class and/or levels of area deprivation and deaths related to unintentional injury has been demonstrated in the UK, although the evidence to link injury-related morbidity and social class is less consistent. The decline in children's injury-related death rates over time has been less for children in the manual social classes than for children in the non-manual classes – consequently socio-economic differentials in mortality have increased. Between 1979 and 1983 the injury-related death rate for children in social class V was 3.5 times that of children in social class 1. However, between 1989 and 1992 the injury-related death rate for children in social class V was five times that of children in social class 1 (White *et al.*, 2000).

A number of studies have found that children in poverty, particularly young children and children of lone parents, are at greater risk of non-fatal unintentional injuries. Children of single parents have injury rates twice those of two parent families (Roberts and Pless, 1995) and their risk of pedestrian injury is 50 per cent higher. There are various possible explanations for this apparent increase in risk, some related to the immediate home and family environment, and others to area factors and greater exposure to hazardous environments. Lack of access to a car is associated with doubling the risk of injury as a pedestrian; lack of a car is most likely among the poorest households and single parents have particularly low rates of car use (White *et al.*, 2000). The number of roads children cross is a key determinant of risk of pedestrian injury; children in the lowest income quarter of the population cross 50 per cent more roads than children in the highest income quarter (White *et al.*, 2000). This may be because they are more likely to live in urban areas or because they do not have alternative means of travel. Children in homes without play areas are five times more at risk of pedestrian injury than children in homes with play areas. Poor quality housing is an important risk factor, particularly for younger children who are more likely to be injured in the home. Accidents to children under 5 years old in the home are strongly associated with overcrowding and type of tenure (White *et al.*, 2000). Similarly the risk of house fires is associated with the poorest housing conditions. Use of smoke alarms is lowest among low income groups and among those in rented accommodation (Roberts, 1996).

There is little in the literature relating to the ethnic origins of children who suffer injuries, and it is unclear whether there are any differences in injury rates, types and severity of injuries or fatalities suffered among children from different ethnic and cultural backgrounds. Data on ethnic origin are not routinely collected in mortality and morbidity statistics. Studies of traffic accidents rates have, however, found significant differences in accident risk rates based on ethnicity (White *et al.*, 2000). A recent literature review concludes that in almost all countries where data are available children of minority ethnic backgrounds are at increased risk of pedestrian injury relative to the norms for the host county as a whole (DTLR, 2001).

Conclusion

In the UK, as in all industrialised nations, unintentional injury remains the biggest single cause of death among children and young people. Between 1991 and 1995 the UK had the second lowest child death by injury rate among the OECD nations with an annualised rate of 6.1 deaths per 100,000 for children aged 1–14. In the UK child mortality due to unintentional injury has declined in the last three decades; with mortality rates for children aged 1–9 years halving over the period 1970 to 1990, although the decline has been less pronounced for older children.

As in all industrialised countries, traffic accidents are the most common cause of injury-related child death in the UK. Outside the home, apart from traffic accidents, drowning and falls are the most likely cause of child deaths related to unintentional injury. Fatal injuries sustained in the home are most likely to be as the result of thermal injuries (burns and scalds), followed by suffocating, drowning, falls and poisoning.

A strong relationship between social class and/or levels of area deprivation and deaths related to unintentional injury has been demonstrated in the UK, although the evidence to link injury-related morbidity and social class is less consistent. Data linking unintentional injuries with social class are rare, and are usually drawn from single studies rather than data collected on an annual basis. A number of studies have found that children in poverty, particularly young children and children of lone parents, are at greater risk of non-fatal unintentional injuries. There are various possible explanations for this apparent increase in risk, some related to the immediate home and family environment and others to area factors and greater exposure to hazardous environments.

7 Maltreatment of Children

Carol-Ann Hooper

Key statistics:

- A survey of young people born between 1974 and 1980 (Cawson *et al.*, 2000) found the following rates of maltreatment in childhood:

  eg, physical abuse (serious, by parents or carers) – 7 per cent

  eg, physical neglect: serious absence of care – 6 per cent

  eg, serious absence of supervision – 5 per cent

  eg, sexual abuse – 16 per cent

  eg, emotional maltreatment – 6 per cent

  [definitions given in text]

Key trends:

- There is some evidence of a decline in the frequency of physical punishment of children between the 1960s and the 1990s.
- There is insufficient evidence to establish trends in any other form of maltreatment.

Key sources:

- Cawson *et al.* (2000), *Child maltreatment in the UK*, NSPCC, London
- There are no government statistics which show the extent of child maltreatment. Statistics on child protection registrations refer only to those children for whom an inter-agency protection plan is held by child protection agencies.

Introduction

Definitions of child maltreatment (or child abuse and neglect) are variable and contested. Under the broadest definitions, some of the issues covered elsewhere in this report, such as poverty (Chapter 1) and homelessness (Chapter 14), would be included. This chapter takes a narrower focus, and covers fatal child abuse, physical punishment and abuse, physical neglect, sexual abuse and emotional maltreatment (including exposure to domestic violence between parents). The chapter reviews what is known about the extent and patterns of child maltreatment in the UK.

Sources of data

There are no government statistics which show the number of children who have experienced maltreatment. Research has shown that only a small minority of incidents of abuse are reported to any agency. The Bristol ALSPAC study (a prospective cohort study of children born in 1991/92 and their parents) found that only 6.6 per cent of cases of 'physical cruelty' and 3.9 per cent of cases of 'emotional cruelty' (as reported by parents) were known to child protection agencies (Sidebotham et al., 2000). Similar findings have been reported for sexual abuse – only 5 per cent of incidents reported in a survey of young adults' own childhood experiences (Kelly et al., 1991) and in a similar study by Cawson et al. (2000) hardly any were known to any statutory agency. To be included in government data on child protection registrations, a case must not only be reported to child protection agencies but must also be one in which a case conference is held and an inter-agency child protection plan developed. Where data on referrals are available, they suggest that only around a quarter of cases referred for child protection inquiries are later registered – 26 per cent in Scotland in 1999/2000 (Scottish Executive, 2001b). Registered children include some who have not been maltreated (but who are thought at risk) and exclude many who have been maltreated, where for example the abusive parent has later left the household. Trends in registration are affected by public and professional awareness and reporting, by the categories for registration defined by government guidance and by developments in professional knowledge, all of which have changed over time. Moreover, there is considerable local variation in registration rates, which has been found to be associated with a wide range of factors, both socio-demographic and operational (Gibbons et al., 1995). Some of these factors (eg, a high unemployment rate) may reflect different levels of maltreatment, others (eg, different thresholds for intervention and regular updating of the register) have more to do with local policy and practice. As the Department of Health has noted, local authorities may reduce their registration rate by addressing operational factors, but 'changing the rate will not necessarily improve the situation of abused children or the service they are offered' (DoH, 1995a, p. 31).

The data on child protection registrations are generated as part of the child abuse management system and are not intended as a record of levels of maltreatment. They do, however, tell us something about trends in child protection intervention, and data are given below under the section on comparisons between the four countries of the UK. Criminal justice statistics are not used in this chapter (with the exception of homicide statistics). They have some similar limitations to child protection registration data in that few cases of child maltreatment are reported, and among those that are, the attrition rate is high and variable both between areas and between forms of abuse. Cases drop out of the system for a wide range of reasons other than whether maltreatment is thought to have taken place (Social Services Inspectorate, 1994; Davies *et al.*, 1995; Crown Prosecution Service, 1998). Criminal justice statistics are no indication of the extent of maltreatment. Moreover, it is not even possible to identify all offences against children in criminal justice statistics, since while some offences are specific to children (eg, infanticide), others (eg, rape) are not and statistics are not always broken down by age.

To establish the extent and patterns of child maltreatment it is necessary to turn to research. Research on the extent of child abuse takes two forms. Incidence studies focus on the number of cases reported per year (in which abuse may have occurred that year and/or earlier). Prevalence studies examine the proportion of the population affected, using surveys of adults (or sometimes children) to ask about their childhood experiences (or sometimes their parenting). Incidence studies, especially those which collect reports not just from social services but from all agencies which may come to know of or suspect abuse, including health, social services, police and voluntary organisations (eg, Royal Belfast Hospital, 1990), have their uses for the planning of services. It is only prevalence studies, however, which attempt to address the extent of abuse in children's lives without the limitations of reporting bias. This chapter therefore draws extensively on prevalence research. It is difficult to establish trends in this way, partly because studies are not carried out frequently enough and partly because methodology often varies between studies so that findings are not strictly comparable. However, it is only through this research that a realistic assessment of the extent of maltreatment in children's lives, and hence of its possible relevance to other indicators of children's well-being, eg, mental health (see Chapter 22), homelessness (see Chapter 14) and suicide (see Chapter 20), can be made. In any future reports, more attention would need to be focused on trends in the child protection system, but, to establish a baseline, child maltreatment itself is the focus in this report.

The most comprehensive and methodologically sophisticated prevalence study in the UK is now Cawson *et al.*'s *Child Maltreatment in the UK* (2000). In this, a random probability sample of 2,689 18–24-year-olds were interviewed (using computer-assisted personal interviewing to increase privacy) to explore both their views on acceptable treatment of children and their experience of family life, abuse, bullying and discrimination. Prevalence rates for a wide range of behaviours with the potential for harm were gathered and summary rates calculated at three or four levels for each form of abuse, using definitions which reflect both the professional knowledge base and the views of the young people themselves on unacceptable treatment. The respondents were born between 1974 and 1980 and the sample was defined both to give a picture of recent childhoods and to gather data before the cumulative effects of later events confounded the impacts or memory was lost. The findings are likely to be an underestimate. This is partly because the sample excluded young people who were either homeless or in institutional settings (among whom there are likely to be higher rates of abuse). In addition, events in early childhood are unlikely to be remembered and young people who are still living with their parents (as 56 per cent of this sample were) may also be less likely to have regained memories of abuse (from early or later childhood) to which they have lost access through dissociation, amnesia or repression. Nevertheless, it is overall the best data available and findings are displayed in boxes in the relevant sections of this chapter (with the definitions to which prevalence rates apply). Commentary on the findings in the light of other research (taking into account sample, methodology and interpretation of the data) is given in the text.

The extent of maltreatment

Fatal child abuse

The number of children who die from maltreatment each year is difficult to establish precisely. A commonly cited estimate of 'one to two children die from maltreatment each week' is supported by official statistics. These have a number of limitations, however. First, homicide statistics are broken down by age of victim and by relationship of victim to principal suspect, but not by both together. Secondly, Wilczynski (1997) has calculated that the true incidence of deaths to which maltreatment has contributed is 3–7 times higher than that recorded in official statistics on child homicide. Some deaths classified as by accident or natural cause involve maltreatment or negligence, as Squires and Busuttil (1995) have shown in relation to child fatalities through house fires (see also Chapter 6). Other deaths are misclassified – 10–20 per cent of deaths attributed to Sudden Infant Death Syndrome have been estimated to involve maltreatment (Wilczynski, 1997). In other cases, the child's body may not be found or identified, or the evidence may not be sufficient to prove homicide. Given the limited reliability of homicide figures and the small base numbers, great caution is necessary in interpreting trends over time. An apparent decline from the 1970s to the 1980s identified by Pritchard (1992) has since been attributed largely to changes in the classification system (Lindsey and Trocme, 1994). On the basis of official statistics, however, infant and child homicide rates seem to have remained fairly stable during the 1980s and 1990s, at least in England and Wales.

Although for adults Scotland has a significantly higher homicide rate than England and Wales, Soothill *et al.* (1999) found that for children aged 14 or below the rate (proportional to the population) was broadly similar over the period 1985 to 1994. In both contexts, the rate is highest for children under 1 year of age.

Northern Ireland has the highest homicide rate overall of the UK countries

Table 7.1: Child homicides in England and Wales

Years	Age under 1	Over 1 and under 16	0–15 total	By parent
1980–84	125	273	398	289
1985–89	138	268	406	313
1990–94	130	243	373	281
1995–2000*	153	254	407	288
2000/01**	50	48	98	82

* In 1997 the period for which figures are recorded changed from the calendar year to the financial year. Home Office statistics give the figures for both 1997 and 1997/98 but the degree of double-counting which aggregating both would entail has been estimated to produce the figures for this period. The period itself is not strictly comparable with the earlier periods as it covers five and a quarter years.
** The figures for 2000/01 are provisional – in over half the cases court proceedings were still pending at the time of publication.
Source: Home Office, Criminal Statistics England and Wales, 1990, 2000

Table 7.2: Child homicides in Scotland

Years	Age under 1	Over 1 and under 16	0–15 total	By parent
1990–94	17	26	43	35
1995–99*	10	40	50	26
2000	6	4	10	8

*These figures include the 17 children killed in Dunblane in
1996.
Source: Scottish Executive, Statistical Bulletin CJ/2001/9,
Homicide in Scotland 2000

(and indeed of the EU member countries for the years 1997 to 1999) but it is not known how far this applies to children (Barclay *et al.*, 2001). Only very limited data was available from the Northern Ireland Police Service, indicating that there had been 16 victims of homicide under the age of 17 in the period April 1998 to March 2001. One reason for the higher homicide rate, however, is clearly the political situation in Northern Ireland, and 257 children below the age of 18 were killed in troubles-related deaths between 1969 and 1998 (Smyth, 1998).

Physical punishment and abuse

A certain level of physical violence to children is extremely widespread. While in 10 countries (Sweden, Finland, Norway, Austria, Cyprus, Denmark, Latvia, Croatia, Germany and Israel), children are now protected by law from all corporal punishment, and Scotland is considering a partial ban, in the rest of the UK hitting a child can still be defended in court by a parent as 'reasonable chastisement'. The case for change has been made on the basis of justice, evidence of effectiveness (Leach, 1999) and prevention of physical abuse (which often starts with punishment), but this kind of 'normalised' violence is not generally regarded as maltreatment. As part of the context of maltreatment, it is worth noting that the vast majority of children are still smacked at some point. There is some evidence of a decline in frequency between the 1960s and the 1990s (Newson and Newson, 1989; Smith *et al.*, 1995). Creighton and Russell's (1995) survey of 1,032 adults aged 18–45 in England, Wales and Scotland strikes a cautionary note about focusing on this trend in isolation, however. While the youngest age group recalled the least physical punishment, they reported more of every other type of disciplinary measure, including being shouted or roared at constantly or frequently. Some non-physical forms of discipline, such as isolation (eg, sending/locking a child in their room), silence (not speaking to a child), verbal threats of a beating, making a child miss a meal or embarrassing/humiliating a child were regarded as less accceptable than smacking with an open hand by Cawson *et al.*'s (2000) respondents.

Studies of physical punishment have also uncovered behaviour which would clearly be defined as abuse. Of the parents in the Newsons' study, 22 per cent had used an implement to hit their children by the time they were aged 7, and 9 per cent were still hit with implements at age 11 (Newson and Newson, 1989). Cawson *et al.*'s (2000) findings are given below. The 'serious' category refers to those who experienced violent treatment from their parents either regularly, or which caused injury or had physical effects lasting to the next day or longer. The 'intermediate' category refers to less serious incidents which occurred regularly or serious incidents which occurred occasionally but caused no serious injury. Taking both these categories together, the findings of other UK studies are fairly similar (Smith *et al.*, 1995; Creighton and Russell, 1995), with the exception of the ALSPAC study. That showed a much lower rate, which is probably a reflection both of the short lifespan of the children so far and the methodology used (which involved only one question each about physical and emotional 'cruelty', rather than more descriptive questions about specific behaviours).

Physical abuse

Definition based on experiences of: being hit with an implement or fist, kicked hard or shaken, thrown or knocked down, beaten up (hit again and again), grabbed round the neck and choked, burned or scalded on purpose or threatened with a knife or gun.

Rates:

At least one of the behaviours specified above:

25 per cent (78 per cent at home, 15 per cent at school)

Physical abuse by parents or carers:

serious – 7 per cent

intermediate – 14 per cent

cause for concern – 3 per cent.

(Cawson *et al.*, 2000)

Physical neglect

The term neglect covers a wide range of behaviour broadly characterised by omission or absence of parental care. Definition is problematic partly because it inevitably involves assumptions about what standards of care should be expected of parents, and raises questions over whether universal standards are appropriate for parenting in varied socio-economic and cultural contexts. Cawson *et al.*'s (2000) findings are given below. While the 'serious' categories were used for exceptionally low levels of care and supervision known to carry a high risk of harm, the 'intermediate' categories cover a broad range of experience with lesser and more variable risks.

Physical neglect

Definition on two dimensions:

- absence of physical care and nurturing: includes lack of health care, feeding, clean clothes, medical and dental care, children being left to look after themselves (parents away or with drug/alcohol problems)
- failure to safeguard through appropriate supervision: a series of indicators about the ages at which children left unsupervised in particular circumstances and for how long.

Rates:

Absence of care:
some absence of care (total) – 18 per cent
    serious – 6 per cent
    intermediate – 9 per cent
    cause for concern – 2 per cent
Absence of supervision:
less than adequate supervision (total) – 20 per cent
    serious – 5 per cent
    intermediate – 12 per cent
    cause for concern – 3 per cent
(Cawson *et al.*, 2000)

Sexual abuse

What makes sexual activity involving children abuse, aside from the use of coercion, is their inability to give informed consent in relationships of unequal power. Definitions in research vary here as elsewhere. One area in which definitions differ is in the type of activity included: a distinction is often made between abuse involving physical contact, such as actual or attempted penetration, touching or forced masturbation, and 'non-contact abuse', such as flashing or voyeurism. There are also differences in the cut-off point adopted for 'childhood' and the age difference across which it is assumed that informed consent is not possible. Kelly *et al.* (1991) made differences of definition explicit by calculating nine prevalence rates in their study of 16–21 year olds. The rates they arrived at ranged from 59 per cent of women and 27 per cent of men who reported at least one sexually intrusive experience before the age of 18, to 5 per cent of women and 2 per cent of men who reported some form of penetration or coerced/forced masturbation (the narrowest definition). Cawson *et al.*'s (2000) are given below, and are broadly comparable with Creighton and Russell's (1995) findings.

Sexual abuse
Definition based on sexual experiences if i) the other person was a parent or carer, ii) they were against the person's wishes, or iii) they were felt to be consensual but involved a person other than the parent who was 5 years older when the child was 12 or under.

Rates:
Sexual abuse – 16 per cent (21 per cent girls, 11 per cent boys)
Excluding non-contact abuse – 11 per cent (16 per cent girls, 7 per cent boys)
Including 13–15-year-olds who had had sexual experiences regarded as consensual with someone at least 5 years older – 20 per cent
(Cawson *et al.*, 2000)

Unlike other forms of abuse, only a small minority of incidents of sexual abuse are committed by parents (largely fathers/stepfathers). Brothers and stepbrothers seem to be equally if not more implicated (Kelly *et al.*, 1991; Cawson *et al.*, 2000). Other known people account for far more incidents either than family members or strangers. In fact, much of what falls under the category of sexual abuse occurs with peers, especially during adolescence, and may be better seen as 'date rape' or (school or other) peer group sexual harassment.

Both Kelly *et al.* (1991) and Cawson *et al.* (2000) found that 1 per cent of respondents reported sexual abuse by parents (virtually all fathers/stepfathers). This is a considerably lower figure than the 4.5 per cent of Russell's (1984) US random sample who reported sexual abuse by fathers (biological, step, adoptive or foster). Different samples and contexts make it premature, however, to conclude that this is indicative of a positive trend. Significant cohort effects have been found within US studies, however. No evidence has been found to support the idea of an increase in child sexual abuse following the 'sexual revolution' of the 1960s. However, higher rates of abuse have been found among women born 1936–45 who experienced the disruption of war and its aftermath, including fathers who left then returned after a long absence (see 'Family structure and process', below) (Russell, 1984; Finkelhor *et al.*, 1990).

Emotional maltreatment

Emotional maltreatment is increasingly seen as underpinning all forms of abuse, and often the most important influence on the impact of physical and sexual abuse. Even more than other forms of abuse, it comes in many guises since there are not only many ways to cause children emotional distress but different ways to hurt specific children in specific contexts. Cawson *et al.*'s (2000) rates based on an aggregate score for all forms of emotional maltreatment are given below, and are broadly comparable with the findings of Smith *et al.* (1995) and Sidebotham *et al.* (2000). However, far higher rates were found for at least one of the dimensions of abuse. A striking 34 per cent reported some form of 'terrorising', the most common experience. Both Ghate and Daniels (1997) and Doyle (1997) report significantly higher rates of emotional abuse than Cawson *et al.*'s overall rate, and it may be that the cut-off point adopted in Cawson *et al.*'s study is too conservative.

Emotional maltreatment

Definition based on seven dimensions:

- psychological control and domination
- psycho/physical control and domination (eg, mouth being washed out with soap, being locked in cupboard or room)

- humiliation/degradation
- withdrawal (absence of affection or exclusion from family activities)
- antipathy (active dislike or hostility)
- terrorising
- proxy attacks (including domestic violence between parents as well as attacks on pets and treasured possessions)

Scoring system used and cut-off point adopted representing adverse experiences on at least four dimensions.

Rates:

Emotional maltreatment – 6 per cent (8 per cent girls, 4 per cent boys) (a further 6 per cent came close to this level)

(Cawson *et al.*, 2000)

Significantly fewer children were found to have witnessed violence between their carers by Cawson *et al.* (2000) than by Creighton and Russell (1995), although 26 per cent had still experienced this at some time, and for 5 per cent it was constant or frequent. It may be that this indicates a positive trend, and one that might be expected given the increased economic independence of women and awareness of domestic violence among the police and public. Once again, however, caution is necessary in interpreting such trends. The British Crime Survey data suggest that rates of domestic violence have been declining since 1993, but still remain higher than in the 1980s (although people may also have become more willing to reveal such experiences to interviewers) (Mirrlees-Black, 1999).

Patterns of maltreatment

Poverty and social class

Research both in the UK and elsewhere has consistently suggested that physical abuse and neglect are more prevalent among lower socio-economic groups, while sexual and emotional abuse occur fairly evenly across classes. Cawson *et al.*'s (2000) study is particularly useful in confirming this as it addresses all forms of abuse and is not confined to reported cases (where reporting/intervention bias may play a part in the over-representation of lower socio-economic groups). The effect of class was most marked for serious physical abuse and serious absence of care (neglect), while slight effects were found for intermediate absence of care, absence of supervision and sexual abuse, and none for intermediate physical abuse or emotional abuse. It is worth noting both these trends and that all forms of serious abuse occurred across classes (Cawson *et al.*, 2000). It is possible that class effects are slightly exaggerated since class was assessed more by present than past situation, and socio-economic status may be affected by childhood abuse as well as vice versa. The effects of abuse on brain development (Maclean, 2000) and cognitive ability (Leach, 1999) are beginning to be recognised, and reported maltreatment has been found associated with reduced school attendance and performance (Sullivan and Knutson, 2000). Those abused at home may also be more vulnerable both to being bullied and to bullying others at school (Creighton and Russell, 1995) and hence perhaps to truancy and/or exclusion. The effects of abuse on school performance and later work are complex and variable, however, (Sanford, 1991) and the different extent of class effects between different forms of abuse suggests that the association between poverty and an increased risk of physical abuse and neglect is real.

Other UK research addressing the association between poverty and maltreatment has been confined to reported cases. Here too, however, the strongest relationship has been found with neglect, a smaller relationship with physical abuse and a much weaker relationship (if any) with sexual or emotional abuse. Gillham *et al.* (1998), who explored the relationship between poverty and maltreatment by focusing on area rather than individual characteristics, found some association with all indicators but the strongest association with male unemployment, especially in relation to physical abuse. In a study of all families on child and family social work caseloads, Sheppard (1997) found high levels of abuse (especially multiple forms of abuse) associated with high levels of maternal depression, and both associated with social deprivation and a range of other problems including domestic violence, marital problems and social isolation.

Gender

Children's gender affects their vulnerability to abuse in different ways for different forms. All UK prevalence studies (and most in other countries) have found girls significantly more vulnerable to sexual abuse than boys – the risk is usually around 1.5–3 times as high for girls. For other forms of abuse the differences tend to be slighter although the Cawson *et al.*'s (2000) study also found girls twice as likely to be emotionally abused as boys. Some dimensions of emotional abuse were more gender differentiated than others, however – in particular girls were twice as likely to report antipathy from a parent. Boys appear overall to be more vulnerable to physical abuse, although Cawson *et al.* (2000) found girls more vulnerable to serious physical abuse. Girls were also found slightly more vulnerable to serious absence of care, although again boys were more vulnerable to absence of care overall. With regard to supervision, girls were more likely to have been expected regularly to care for younger siblings, but boys were more likely to have been left without supervision themselves.

While all forms of abuse are committed by both men and women, the responsibility for abuse is also gendered, to different extents for different forms. The vast majority of sexual abuse is committed by men. Research on both domestic violence and physical abuse of children suggests that men are also more prone to physical violence, once time spent with children is taken into account, although the number of cases of physical abuse attributed to mothers and fathers is fairly similar (Nobes and Smith, 2000). Neglect and emotional abuse are often not attributed to a particular parent in research, although in practice neglect is referred to predominantly in relation to women simply because women carry primary responsibility for children's care. Some gender differences emerged in Cawson *et al.*'s (2000) study in patterns of emotional abuse – most strikingly, significantly more respondents (both boys and girls) reported being 'sometimes really afraid' of their father/stepfathers than of mothers/stepmothers (20 per cent compared with 7 per cent) (Cawson *et al.*, 2000). Creighton and Russell (1995) also found higher levels of fear of fathers than of mothers, and that more children felt close to their mothers than to their fathers.

Race

While it is well established that black children (especially those of mixed parentage) are over-represented in the care system (see Chapter 8), UK research has not shown any significant race differences in the prevalence of abuse. There are some forms of abuse to which black children are particularly vulnerable, however. Many experience racial abuse and harassment within the community directly and/or witness such attacks against others including their family members and friends. Black children in predominantly white families or families with one white parent may also suffer racial abuse or racially motivated abuse, and/or witness racism directed against others, within their own families. Black children in care may have similar experiences within children's home settings (Race Equality Unit, 1996).

Disability

Disability (both some physical impairments and learning disabilities) can be the consequence of abuse. There is also strong evidence that disabled children are at greater risk of all forms of abuse, although some disabilities increase vulnerability more than others (Sullivan and Knutson, 2000). Research on this issue, mostly in the US, has so far relied on incidence studies based on cases known to professionals. Since it is possible that disabled children's greater involvement with a number of service providers increases the likelihood of abuse being detected (though equally both professional misinformation and the nature of some disabilities may impede it) it would be helpful also to address disability in prevalence studies.

Age

Babies are most vulnerable to fatal child abuse. Physical punishment peaks a bit later, then declines. Age trends are more difficult to assess in relation to sexual abuse since early abuse is less likely to be remembered, though some argue there are two peaks, the first around 6 years, the second around 13 years (Rees and Stein, 1999). Emotional abuse seems to be fairly constant, or perhaps to increase with age (Rees and Stein, 1999). Neglect cannot be considered in this way as definitions are necessarily age-related.

The abuse of adolescents is beginning to be recognised as a problem meriting further research in the UK, with somewhat different patterns and dynamics from the abuse of younger children. It is clear from research with runaways/ homeless young people that physical, sexual and emotional abuse in the home are all significant problems for this age group (Hendessi, 1992; Safe on the Streets Research Team, 1999). US research suggests that the abuse of adolescents is less concentrated in lower socio-economic groups, occurs significantly more in reconstituted families than in others, and may reflect both the life-stages of parents and adolescents and the changing power dynamics between them (Rees and Stein, 1999). Gelles and Straus (1988) found teenagers as likely as children under 3 years old to be the targets of physical violence from parents. The abuse of adolescents by peers outside the family also merits attention, particularly the experience of adolescent girls as they begin to explore sexual relationships. Very high rates of stalking ('persistent and unwanted attention') have been reported by young women aged 16–19 (Budd and Mattinson, 2000). The highest rates of domestic violence are also reported by young women, though this peaks a little later, between 20–24 (Mirrlees-Black, 1999).

Family structure and process

Both lone parent families and stepfamilies have been found significantly over-represented among registered cases, but this may be at least partly the result of reporting bias and recording practices (Andrews, 1994). The most reliable evidence (both from the UK and USA) suggests that these family forms do carry some increased risk. Growing concern about the association between domestic violence and child abuse, however, suggests that it is as important to consider family relationships as family structure.

Severe physical abuse has been found more common in lone parent families (lone father families more than lone mother families) (Gelles and Straus, 1988). Poverty, the stress of sole responsibility for children, higher rates of mental illness, alcohol and drug problems, may all contribute to violence in lone parent households. Nobes and Smith (1997), however, argue that violence in two-parent families is often underestimated because of the tendency for researchers to interview only one parent. Children in two-parent households may be vulnerable to more violence since both parents tend to use fairly similar levels.

The evidence regarding stepfamilies is mixed. Young people who live with a step-parent are significantly more likely than others to run away from home, and the quality of family relationships, including maltreatment, are common influences on running away (Safe on the Streets Research Team, 1999). Adults who lived in stepfamilies as children have been found more vulnerable both to constant criticism (Ghate and Daniels, 1997) and in the USA to sexual abuse, by stepfathers and other men (Russell, 1984). Cawson *et al.* (2000), however, report that very few respondents were physically, sexually or emotionally abused by step-parents.

The overlap between domestic violence (most of which, though not all, occurs in two-parent families) and physical abuse of children is now estimated to be about 30–60 per cent, and domestic violence appears to increase risk of all forms of abuse (Creighton and Russell, 1995; Mullender, 2000; McGuigan and Pratt, 2001).

Vulnerability to child sexual abuse involves rather different dynamics than other forms because the majority of perpetrators are not parents. No family factors have been found to have particularly strong predictive power, but an unhappy family life has been found the strongest predictor of child sexual abuse (Finkelhor *et al.*, 1990).

Comparisons between the countries of the UK

There is little evidence to suggest significantly higher or lower rates of any of the forms of maltreatment discussed in this chapter between England, Wales, Scotland and Northern Ireland, although children in Northern Ireland clearly face greater exposure to community violence. Cawson *et al.* (2000) drew their sample from across the UK, but the samples from Wales, Scotland and Northern Ireland are too small to conduct much meaningful comparative analysis. No significant differences have emerged so far, although analysis is continuing (Pat Cawson, personal communication, 2001). Comparable surveys conducted earlier by ISPCC for the whole of Ireland and NSPCC for England, Wales and Scotland (Creighton and Russell, 1995) do suggest some significantly different patterns and responses in Ireland, although overall rates were the same for sexual abuse. They were very close for physical punishment (slightly higher in Ireland, 86 per cent compared with 81 per cent reported some experience). Differences were found in the form of punishment used, in the context in which it occurred (Irish children were more likely to be physically punished in school), in attitudes to punishment and in patterns of sexual abuse (more neighbours and teachers of religious subjects were involved in sexual abuse in Ireland). Most importantly perhaps, fewer people in Ireland said they would tell authorities (police/social workers) if they suspected physical abuse in a neighbouring family (more would tell respected local figures).

The last finding highlights probably the main significance of the political situation in Northern Ireland for child maltreatment. Childline (1998) reports too that callers from Northern Ireland are less likely already to have told an authority figure of their abuse and are considerably more reluctant to allow counsellors to refer them to other helping agencies than callers from other parts of the UK. For children who experience the same forms of maltreatment as children throughout the UK, the effect of 'the Troubles' as a backdrop may be to intensify their fears of seeking help, either because of the involvement of members of paramilitary organisations and the possibility of reprisals or because of the more contested legitimacy of the state (Garrett, 1999; Geraghty, 1999).

Levels and patterns of child protection registration in each country are given in the table overleaf. The apparently lower rate of registration in Scotland may be a reflection of the lower age threshold used. The drop in the registration rate in England in 2000/01 is probably because most local authorities are now excluding temporary registrations (which had often been double-counted in previous years) (DoH, 2001a). In England and Scotland registrations for neglect and emotional abuse have been rising and those for physical and sexual abuse falling over the last few years. This is most likely a response to the research reviewed in *Child Protection: Messages from Research* (DoH, 1995a) and also to a concurrent concern in the professional and research communities at the 'neglect of neglect'. *Child Protection: Messages from Research*, which has been widely publicised since it was issued, argued for less focus on specific incidents of abuse and more attention to the overall family environment. The pattern in Wales is fairly similar, although less clear in relation to emotional abuse. In Northern Ireland, data is only available for three years but suggests a rather different pattern, with registrations for physical abuse increasing and those for emotional abuse decreasing. It is impossible to say whether these differences reflect variations in actual maltreatment or in the practices of agencies.

International comparisons

It is clear from the growing body of research across the world that child maltreatment is a global problem (Kempe Children's Center, 1998; Schwartz-Kenney *et al.*, 2001). However, differences of definition and methodology in research, and the impact of changing public and professional awareness and different approaches to reporting and recording on the level of recorded cases, make comparison difficult. Cross-national comparisons have been attempted in relation to infant and child homicide, since the definitional problem is less here and data are at least widely available from the World Health Organization, if not wholly reliable. A league table of child deaths by injury in rich nations shows the UK with the fifth lowest rate of death from intentional injury of 15 listed countries for the years 1991–95 (UNICEF, 2001a). In other such studies covering longer periods of time, a number of southern European countries (Italy, Spain, Greece, Portugal) and others (Netherlands, Norway, Ireland) have consistently lower rates than England and Wales, while the USA and Japan in particular have consistently higher rates across age groups. Income inequality and male unemployment have not been found

Table 7.3: Number of children on child protection register, and rate per 1,000 children under 18

Date	England	Wales	Scotland*	Northern Ireland
31/3/97	32,400 (2.9)	n/a	2,280 (2.3)	n/a
31/3/98	31,600 (2.8)	2,450 (3.7)	2,303 (2.3)	n/a (3.0)
31/3/99	31,900 (2.8)	2,670 (4.0)	2,361 (2.3)	n/a
31/3/00	30,300 (2.7)	2,416 (3.6)	2,050 (2.0)	1,483 (3.2)
31/3/01	26,800 (2.4)	2,126 (3.2)	n/a	n/a

*For Scotland, the rate given in brackets is per 1,000 children under 16
Sources: DoH (2001a), Scottish Executive (2001b), Social Services Inspectorate (2001), Welsh Assembly (1999/2000/2001)

Table 7.4: Percentage of registrations 2000/01 in each category of abuse

Category of abuse	England	Wales	Scotland*	Northern Ireland*
Physical abuse	30%	30%	38%	34%
Sexual abuse	16%	15%	15%	18%
Emotional abuse	17%	15%	12%	14%
Neglect	46%	50%	39%	47%

Note: Some children are registered under more than one category, hence totals may be over 100 per cent
* Figures for Scotland and Northern Ireland are for 1999–2000, the latest figures available.
Sources: DoH (2001a), Scottish Executive (2001b), Social Services Inspectorate (2001), Welsh Assembly (1999/2000/2001)

significantly associated with child homicide rates in such studies. High female labour force participation, where it is accompanied by low status of women (as indicated by participation rates in higher education) and low investment in welfare spending have been found to be significantly associated with higher child homicide rates. So too have high divorce rates and a culture of violence (as indicated by eg, reported rape rates) (Fiala and LaFree, 1988; Briggs and Cutright, 1994). The findings on women's labour force participation are consistent with Gelles's (1987) US research which found that mothers' employment overall was not associated with increased risks of violence to children, but that a lack of choice over whether to work and a sense of having excess responsibility for domestic activities alongside paid work were associated with more violence. While it would not be surprising if children suffer where women (as their primary carers) are particularly overburdened and oppressed and/or where stable relationships are difficult to maintain, too much weight should not be placed on comparative analyses given the concerns about child homicide data discussed above.

Conclusions

While the impacts of child maltreatment are variable and by no means determined, there is consistent evidence that it both undermines children's well-being in childhood and increases vulnerability to a wide range of problems in later life. These include mental health problems, low self-esteem and difficulties with interpersonal relationships including parenting (Duncan *et al.*, 1996; Fergusson *et al.*, 1996; Bifulco and Moran, 1998). The evidence presented in this chapter shows that child maltreatment is also a far more widespread problem than is indicated by data on cases reported to agencies. Too much reliance should not be placed on official statistics, therefore, when considering the relevance of child maltreatment to children's well-being. Moreover there are dangers in drawing conclusions from trends in such data without a full understanding of the processes affecting them. The fall in the re-registration rate used as an indicator in the government's *Opportunity for All* reports (see Chapter 1) could be accounted for by successful work when children are first registered, by changes in practice regarding deregistration and/or by changes in the threshold for registration.

It would be useful if all countries recorded data on referrals and investigations as well as registrations, to enable a fuller picture of the operation of the child protection systems across the UK. Such data will remain limited to reported cases, however, and the issue of child maltreatment needs also to be brought into the mainstream of research on children's well-being, with due attention to the development of appropriate methodology for this issue. The ALSPAC study, for example, presents a good opportunity to follow the example of Fergusson *et al.* (1996) in New Zealand, and use a survey of the young people at age 18 (if not before) to gather data on their experiences of abuse retrospectively and explore its relationship to other aspects of their lives studied prospectively. More research is also needed on the abuse of adolescents (both within and outside the family), the involvement of children in prostitution, the vulnerability of disabled children to abuse and the exposure of children to racism and community violence. Trends in relation to any form of abuse are so far difficult to assess, although Cawson *et al.*'s (2000) plan to repeat their survey every 10 years should make this possible in the long term.

8 Looked After Children

Ian Sinclair and Ian Gibbs

Key statistics:
- Around four in 1,000 children are looked after away from home by the state in the UK.
- Most are with foster carers, but others are placed for adoption, with relatives or in residential care.
- Those entering the system do so for reasons connected with poverty, family dysfunction or their own behaviour.

Key trends:
- Over the past 20 years the proportion of children entering the system for reasons connected with abuse has risen rapidly while the proportion entering for other reasons has fallen.
- The result is that fewer children enter the care system but they stay for longer. Outcomes are poor and costs are high.
- The challenge is to provide high-quality stable care that gives a good upbringing to vulnerable children without diverting an undue proportion of resources from preventive work.

Key sources:
- Department of Health (England), Welsh Assembly, Scottish Executive and the Northern Ireland Statistics and Research Agency
- Academic research

Introduction

At the turn of the century around 75,000 children and young people under the age of 18 were in the UK care system and looked after by the state. Some were 'voluntarily accommodated' because they or their parents had asked for this. Others were in 'care' because the courts had ordered it. This chapter covers all these 'looked after' children (a term we shall now use for children and young people). It does not cover private fostering or boarding education.

In official policy, the care system appears as an unfortunate necessity. Scandals and escalating costs have undermined confidence in it. Its critics see it as cutting children off from their families, stigmatising them and failing to give them secure long-term placements, a sense of identity or the skills to make their way in life. The aim, therefore, is to reduce the size of the system and the lengths of time children spend in it, while improving its quality and outcomes. An important part of this effort concerns the introduction of a form of National Quality Assurance characterised by Standards, Care Councils and Performance Indicators.

This chapter is relevant to the feasibility and achievement of these aims. We will look at:
- the number of looked after children
- where looked after children are placed
- which children are looked after and why
- the length of looked after placements
- variations between local authorities
- various changes over time
- the cost of looked after a child
- outcomes of the looked after system.

Children in the care system commonly complain they are viewed as the odd ones out, objects of pity or sources of trouble. Some research (e.g., Rowe *et al.*, 1989) has included their good qualities, but most concentrates on their problems and misfortunes, a tradition we inevitably reflect.

The number of looked after children

Table 8.1 gives the numbers of children looked after in the UK. Children placed for an agreed series of short breaks are excluded. The numbers can be used to calculate the rates of children looked after per 1,000 under the age of 18. Table 8.2 shows that the rate in Scotland (10) is much higher than in Northern Ireland (5.3), England (5.1) or Wales (4.9). Scotland counts as looked after children who are at home on supervision orders, who would not be counted as looked after in the rest of the UK. A more valid yardstick for comparison may therefore be the rate of children who are looked after and not placed with parents. On this

Table 8.1: Children looked after by country, by placement, 31 March 2000

	England No.	%	Wales No.	%	Scotland No.	%	N. Ireland No.	%	UK No.	%
Foster placements	37,900	65	2,691	75	3,058	27	1,611	66	45,260	60
Children's homes – local authority, voluntary, private										
	6,300	11	234	6	723	6	285	12	7,542	10
Placed with parents or family*										
	6,500	11	364	10	6,368	56	472	20	13,704	18
Placed for adoption**										
	3,100	5	138	4	123	1	–	–	3,361	5
Lodgings, living independently, other community										
	1,200	2	58	2	176	1	–	–	1,434	2
Schools and associated homes and hostels										
	1,100	1	24	1	629	6	–	–	1,729	2
Other accommodation***										
	1,900	3	65	2	233	2	54	2	2,276	3
Totals	58,000		3,574		11,310		2,422		75,306	

* In England, Wales and N. Ireland these figures refer to children placed on a care order with adults who have parental responsibility for them. In Scotland they include children on supervision orders.
** Not included in the returns in N. Ireland.
*** Includes Youth Treatment Centres, Young Offenders Institutions and various other categories in England and secure and other residential accommodation in Scotland.
Percentages may not add up to 100 due to rounding
Sources: DoH (2001c), Welsh Assembly (2001c), Scottish Executive (2001c), NISRA (2000b)

measure Northern Ireland has the lowest rate (around 4.2), Scotland and Wales the next lowest (4.4), and England the highest (4.5).

The rates are still not strictly comparable since children placed with relatives in Scotland would mainly be on supervision orders and not fostered. If we count

Table 8.2: Children looked after per 1,000 population aged under 18, selected years 1978–2000

	England	Wales	Scotland	Northern Ireland
1978	7.6	6.6	11.7	3.9
1983	7.0	6.2	11.8	5.1
1988	5.9	5.2	–	5.8
1993	4.6	4.6	–	4.4
1998	4.9	4.9	–	5.0
2000	5.1	4.9	10.0	5.3

Sources: Central Statistical Office (1981), ONS (2000c, 2000e)

such children as 'placed with parents or family', the rate of children looked after away from home drops again for England and Wales to around 3.9. The Northern Ireland statistics do not count children fostered with relatives as a separate category so a similar calculation cannot be done for them (DoH, 2001c; Welsh Assembly, 2001c; Scottish Executive, 2001c; NISRA, 2000b).

Where looked after children are placed

A quarter of children in the UK are in 'informal placements' with their parents, in lodgings or residential employment, with potential adopters, or (in Scotland) with relatives and friends. For reasons already explained, Scotland has a much higher proportion (59 per cent) of informal placements than England (14 per cent) and Wales (14 per cent). Northern Ireland does not provide separate figures on those in lodgings or with future adopters. Informal placements probably account for around 20 per cent of its total.

Most informal placements are with parents (England 60 per cent, Scotland 80 per cent, Wales 69 per cent). The difference reflects a greater use in England of adoption out of care. Only 123 Scottish children are with possible adopters as against 3,100 children placed for adoption in England. To put the figures in perspective, England has, in comparison with Scotland, 12 times as many foster children but 25 times as many placed for adoption (DoH, 2001c; Scottish Executive, 2001c).

Foster care accounts for 80 per cent of 'formal placements'. Placements with relatives and friends account in England and Wales for about a sixth of all foster placements (16 per cent) – a calculation that cannot be made for Scotland and Northern Ireland. The proportion of 'formal placements' with 'stranger' foster carers is very similar in Scotland, Wales and England, suggesting a similar overall use (DoH, 2001c; Welsh Assembly, 2001c; Scottish Executive, 2001c; NISRA, 2000b).

The remaining formal placements are in some form of residential care. In England around two-thirds of the residential places are in children's homes, around one in ten in boarding schools and the remainder in a wide variety of other accommodation (eg, mother and baby homes). On 31 March 2001, 377 children were in secure accommodation (including 17 in Wales) (DoH, 2002). In comparison with England, Scotland appears to make more use of boarding schools, and less use of children's homes and 'other accommodation'.

Most, but not all, formal placements are provided by the statutory sector.

According to figures collected by the Chartered Institute of Public Finance and Accountancy (CIPFA) the growing independent sector (composed of agencies other than local authorities which provide care services either on a 'profit' or on a 'not for profit' basis) accounts for around 10 per cent of the total time spent in foster care in Great Britain (CIPFA, 2001). 'Snapshot' figures suggest that a quarter of the places in English children's homes, and a sixth of those in Northern Ireland and Wales, are provided by the independent sector. This also accounts for 29 per cent of the establishments used in Scotland, but nearly half (48 per cent) of its residential placements at any one time.

Which children are looked after and why

The kinds of difficulties experienced by children entering the care system vary with their age and reasons for entry. A variety of studies (Berridge, 1985; Farmer and Parker, 1991; Millham *et al.*, 1986; Packman *et al.*, 1986; Packman and Hall, 1998; Sinclair and Gibbs, 1998; Vernon and Fruin, 1986) have suggested broad distinctions between children entering because of family misfortune or disadvantage, family dysfunction (eg, excessive drinking or abuse) and child behaviour.

Children from poor and disadvantaged families are much more likely to enter the care system (Bebbington and Miles, 1989; St Claire and Osborn, 1987). The risk of doing so increases if:

- the family is on social security benefits, is impoverished in terms of possessions (washing machines etc.) and facilities, lives in poor or overcrowded housing and is either large or headed by a lone parent
- the child is of 'mixed race' and does not live with both birth parents
- the children's families are troubled.

Between a third and a half of the children come from families where marital/partner relationships, if any, are discordant and often marked by violence. Their parents quite often have chronic ill health and minorities have a history of alcohol and drug misuse and psychiatric problems. Many parents experienced abuse in childhood and were themselves in care. In later life, relationships with their own children are likely to be seriously disturbed. There may be a longstanding pattern of resolving these difficulties by permanent or temporary separation of the warring parties. The parents are often out of touch with their own parents or extended family (sometimes because of moves) or on bad terms with them; friends, if any, do not often give practical help so that there is a greater reliance on public services (Bullock *et al.*, 1993; Fisher *et al.*, 1986; Millham *et al.*, 1986; Packman *et al.*, 1986; Packman and Hall, 1998; Schaffer and Schaffer, 1968; Sinclair *et al.*, 1995; Wedge and Mantle, 1991).

These difficulties are reflected in the children's health and behaviour. Recent re-analysis of a major study carried out in the mid-1980s suggested that 27 per cent of children in care were 'disabled'. In this 'disabled group' half of those aged 5–15 were said to have problems of behaviour only, and around a quarter more had problems combining learning difficulties and behaviour. The rate of disabled children in the care system was high and remained so even if those with behavioural difficulties were excluded (Gordon *et al.*, 2000). The Children in Need data (DoH, 2001f) gives less prominence to behavioural problems in defining disability, but still identifies around 14 per cent of the children in the care system as disabled.

Looked after children are also much more likely than their contemporaries to show symptoms of disturbance (Koprowska and Stein, 2000). A study in Oxfordshire (McCann *et al.*, 1996) suggested that two-thirds had some form of psychiatric disorder, whereas the figure for the comparison group was 15 per cent. Diagnoses of conduct disorder, over-anxious disorder and major depressive disorder were each made for around a quarter of the group. None of these diagnoses were made for more than 3 per cent of the comparison group.

The length of looked after placements

In England at least, most stays in care are short. Studies in the 1980s found that 50 per cent or more of the children left within six months of arrival and the majority of these did so within six weeks. After six months the chance of return home fell rapidly. Those who remained beyond this period constituted an increasing proportion of the total. They were on average older, more likely to be white, and more often admitted compulsorily and for reasons other than the situational difficulties of their families (Bullock *et al.*, 1993; Packman *et al.*, 1986; Rowe *et al.*, 1989; Vernon and Fruin, 1986).

English statistics for the year 2000 suggest a similar picture (DoH, 2001c). Just over a third of those who had left the care system over the previous year had had a period of care of less than eight weeks. Just over half had left within six months. Voluntary arrangements predominated. Two-thirds of these 'leavers' had been accommodated on a voluntary basis, as opposed to a quarter who had been either on a full care order (14 per cent) or an interim one (11 per cent). Periods in care were strongly related to legal status. Only 1 per cent of those leavers who had been on a full care order and 33 per cent of those on an interim one had left within six months. By contrast, two-thirds (65 per cent) of leavers voluntarily accommodated had left within this period.

The 'snapshot' picture of those in care at any one time was very different. Nearly half of those looked after (49 per cent) were on a full care order. A further 14 per cent were on an interim one. Only a third were voluntarily accommodated. Lengths of stay were long. Only 16 per cent had been in the care system for less than six months. Four in ten had been there for over three years. One in 20 had been looked after for over ten years. Northern Ireland statistics for 2000, the only comparable source, suggest even longer stays (NISRA, 2000b). Over half (54 per cent) of the children had been looked after for three years or more. A staggering 19 per cent had been looked after for over ten years.

Variations between local authorities

There are wide variations in the rates of children looked after in different authorities. For example, on 31 March 2001 Rutland looked after one child per thousand under the age of 18, Islington 14, East Renfrewshire 4 and Glasgow City 19. The use of care and the cost of children's services is higher in disadvantaged local authorities and districts. High use goes with high proportions of lone parents, high housing density, poor housing, and high proportions of minority ethnic and transient populations. Other explanations may include the attitudes of key individuals, an authority's willingness to spend on social services, professional thresholds for the use of care, the availability of alternative provisions, adoption policies, discharge policies, preventive measures and local court policies (Bebbington and Miles, 1989; Carr Hill *et al.*, 1997; Cliffe with Berridge, 1991; Davies *et al.*, 1972; Packman, 1968, Rowe *et al.*, 1989).

Authorities also vary in the way they deal with looked after children. On 31 March 2001 English local authorities showed the following ranges:
- using care orders for between 31 per cent and 84 per cent of their looked after children
- using children's homes for between 1 per cent and 23 per cent
- placement with parents for between 2 per cent and 32 per cent
- placement for adoption from between none and 35 per cent.

Fifty-eight per cent of the children ceasing to be looked after in Haringey, but only 1 per cent of those in Waltham Forest, were said to have been looked after for 5 years or more (DoH, 2001c). Independent foster care provision was concentrated in a small number of authorities – notably Cornwall and Lambeth (CIPFA, 2001). Northern Irish Health and Social Services boards have proportions of children looked after for over ten years which vary from 11 per cent to 27 per cent (NISRA, 2000b).

Changes over time

Rates

The rates of children in the care system have fallen over the past 20 years (see Table 8.2). This decline was halted in 1994 and 1995. Recently there has been a slight rise.

Scotland and Northern Ireland provide two apparent exceptions to these trends. In Scotland the fall has been less than elsewhere. This has to do with the greater number of children supervised at home – a number which has declined only slightly. Between 1977 and 1999 the numbers in residential care or 'stranger' foster care halved, falling from 9,942 to 4,939 (Scottish Executive, 2001c). Northern Ireland had an apparently low rate in 1978 (Central Statistical Office, 1981). This was at least partly explained by its exclusion of children in training schools, who would have been included in the other statistics.

Reasons for admission

One explanation for the fall in rates has been a change in reasons for admission. In England between 1982 and 1991 there was a sharp drop in the numbers entering the care system for reasons to do with 'family misfortune' – homelessness, short- or long-term parental illness, hospital confinement, the absence of parents (including 'abandonment'), imprisonment of parents and 'illegitimacy'. Over the same period the number of children officially in care in England because they were guilty of an offence or were not receiving full-time education fell from roughly 15,600 to 1,700 (DoH, 1992a). A variety of factors may explain these and earlier reductions. Lengths of stay in maternity wards and psychiatric hospitals shortened. Home helps were used to prevent receptions into care because of parental illness. Housing departments took responsibility for dealing with homeless families. The *Children and Young Person's Act 1969* discouraged the use of care as a response to delinquency and school refusal. The police made greater use of cautioning. The changes anticipated the *Children Act 1989*, which confirmed them.

In contrast to these reductions the numbers of children admitted under orders concerned with abuse and neglect, the presence of adults convicted of offences against children or as wards of court (a device often used to control dangerous situations) did not fall between 1981 and 1991 (DoH, 1992). The increase in the proportion of abused and neglected children has continued. Between 1993 and 2000 the numbers entering for reasons attributed to abuse and neglect rose from 3,800 to 8,600 (DoH, 2001b).

Such children tend to stay in care longer than others and thus constitute a high percentage of those looked after at any one point in time. The Children in Need survey suggested that 55 per cent of children in the English care system are looked after because of concerns about abuse and neglect (DoH, 2001f). One study (Sinclair *et al.*, 2000) found that in around two-thirds of a large sample of foster children social workers thought there was strong evidence of prior abuse and neglect. In a further quarter there was said to be some evidence.

A contrasting trend is provided by the increasing numbers of unaccompanied children seeking asylum. Expenditure figures from CIPFA suggest that the impact of these children is likely to be substantial, but limited to Greater London and a handful of other authorities (CIPFA, 2001). Elsewhere in England the 'unfortunate' and the delinquent are largely no longer in the system. The remainder are abused and neglected children whose return home may be difficult to arrange with safety.

Types of placement

The reluctance to look after children simply on the grounds of delinquency has contributed to the decline of residential care. Other reasons include the high costs of residential care and professional doubts about it. Between1979 and 2000 the number of children in English community/children's homes fell from 30,000 to 6,000 and the number in residential care in Scotland from 6,647 to 2,088. Between 1980 and 1999 the number of children in children's homes in Wales fell from 1,329 to 170. The remaining residential establishments are, on average, much smaller and – in part as a consequence of this – much more highly staffed. Almost certainly they cope with a more difficult population (Berridge and Brodie, 1998).

Over a similar period the numbers in foster care have not fallen. In England in 1979 there were around 34,000 children in foster care. There are now around 38,000. The proportion of looked after children in foster care has approximately doubled (DoH, 1980 and 2001b).

Lengths of stay

Over time there have been shifts in average lengths of stay. In the mid-1970s lengths of stay in the care system increased in response to anxiety about child abuse. Reductions in care numbers in the 1980s reflected decreasing lengths of stay as well as fewer admissions. The recent increase in the numbers looked after in England reflects an increase in the lengths of stay of children in the system and is highest for the youngest age groups where anxiety about abuse is likely to be most intense. The numbers of children who are looked after on a compulsory basis is also up by 25 per cent since 1996. The numbers of children voluntarily accommodated has fallen slightly (DoH, 2001b).

Two factors cut across the trend towards longer stays in care. First, there has been a growth in the use of 'an agreed series of short stays'. These provide a service to families with disabled children (in about six out of ten cases) or in difficulty. In England the number of children making such stays has increased from 10,600 in 1996) to 12,200 in 2000. Most UK statistics are meant to exclude these children (in England just over 1,000 at any one point time) thus increasing the apparent average length of stay. Second, there has been an increased emphasis in England on adoption out of care (42 per cent up from 1,900 in 1996 to 2,700 in 2000). This represents a small proportion of children looked after over a year (5 per cent). However, the children adopted are young (two-thirds are under five years old) and would otherwise probably stay a long time in the care system. Over time, the impact on the volume of care and on average lengths of stay should be considerable.

The cost of looking after a child

CIPFA collects annual expenditure statistics on 'Children and Families' of social services departments (England and Wales) and social work departments (Scotland). The figures cover Great Britain (although a small minority of departments do not make returns) and the most recent ones allocate 75 per cent of 3.2 billion pounds gross expenditure to identifiable services (foster care, residential care, day nurseries and so on). The remaining 25 per cent is spent on 'cost of purchasing' and 'care management' and has to be apportioned between services. After this apportionment, estimates of the proportion of social services expenditure on children in the care system in England (fostering, residential care and secure provision) vary from 57 per cent (Carr Hill *et al.*, 1997) through 62 per cent (from Children in Need data) to 64 per cent (from local authority treasurers) (DoH, 2001f).

A small proportion of children take up a high proportion of expenditure. In 1996 a child cost around £1,200 per week in an English children's home, £275 in foster care and around £66 when officially looked after elsewhere (Carr Hill *et al.*, 1997). These figures ignore factors such as the child's age and difficulty, which increase the expected cost of residential care. Nevertheless, the concentration of costs on a few individuals is striking. At any one time social services departments in England have an estimated 400,000 children in need on their books (DoH, 2001b). Of these, the 15 per cent who are looked after take upwards of 60 per cent of expenditure. Less than 2 per cent of the 400,000 are in children's homes, which account for around a third of expenditure (Carr Hill *et al.*, 1997). In children's homes a small minority (probably around 15 per cent) stay more than six months and take up half the places (Sinclair and Gibbs, 1998).

Costs have varied over time and continue to vary between authorities. Over the 1980s rapidly increasing staff ratios drove up the costs of residential care. Both the unit and total costs of the care system have further increased since 1993 – a finding that makes allowance for inflation (DoH, 2001f). Unit costs vary widely between authorities. Some of this variation can be explained by the characteristics of the authority. For example, competition between authorities, and perhaps the cost of living, drives up the unit cost of fostering in London. Other variation is less easy to explain. Why, for example, is the cost per fostering week in Liverpool (£137) so much lower than that in Birmingham (£261)? Some variation may be explained by higher standards. This is not always true. One study found that large variations in staff hours (the major 'driver' of costs in residential care) were quite unrelated to large variations in quality of care (Sinclair and Gibbs, 1998).

Outcomes of the looked after system

The outcomes of the looked after system are generally seen as poor. These difficulties are not necessarily 'caused' by the system. More probably they reflect a chain of cause and effects, including genetic mechanisms, with one bad or good experience making another more likely (Quinton and Rutter, 1988). Utting (1997), quoting the Social Services Inspectorate, summarises the outcomes as follows:

- more than 75 per cent of care leavers have no academic qualifications of any kind
- more than 50 per cent of young people leaving care after 16 years old are unemployed
- 17 per cent of young women leaving care are pregnant or already mothers
- 10 per cent of 16–17-year-old claimants of DSS severe hardship payments have been in care
- 23 per cent of adult prisoners and 38 per cent of young prisoners have been in care
- 30 per cent of single young homeless people have been in care.

There is now a general emphasis on the importance of educational outcomes for care leavers (see, for example, Scottish Executive, 2001f). So far only England provides national statistics on these outcomes. These show that the proportion of children leaving care at 16 or over with no educational qualifications falls with the length of time they have spent there. Between 80 and 90 per cent of those in the system for less than six months have no qualifications. The comparable figures for those there from six months to up to two years is 65 per cent to 75 per cent. Over that time the percentage falls to around 63 per cent.

Figures are also collected on the frequency of children's moves in the care system (a predictor of subsequent welfare – Biehal et al., 1995). The proportion of children with three or more placements is currently just under a fifth (18 per cent). This percentage has been falling, possibly because fewer children are being admitted to the care system. By contrast the proportion of long-stay children (four years over) who have been in the same placement for the last four years has remained constant at around 50 per cent.

Such findings do not in themselves justify criticism of the care system. Studies which do not control for the difficulty of the children or which only count those in prison or homeless, ignoring others, provide no evidence on its effects. Some follow-up studies have controlled for background and provided community comparison groups. These have not shown that care adversely affects behaviour, adjustment or education (Aldgate *et al.,* 1992; Colton and Heath, 1994; Essen *et al.,* 1976; Mapstone, 1969; St Claire and Osborn, 1987). Some children (eg, those failing to thrive) do better in certain respects if left in the care system than if returned home (Hensey *et al.,* 1983; King and Taitz, 1985). Return to a 'disharmonious' or otherwise 'unsatisfactory home' may encourage pregnancy (Quinton and Rutter, 1988) or delinquency (Sinclair, 1975). Children who have long stable careers in foster care can do well. Indeed the longer children have been in the care system, the less likely they seem to be to get into trouble (Minty, 1987).

Conclusion

The prevailing philosophy of care emphasises prevention, diversion and return home. Its success is seen in the large drop in children looked after because their families are in situational difficulties or they themselves are delinquent.

Despite these changes, prevention is not wanted by all parents and children and is not always effective. Many birth parents accept care for their child with relief and most children either compare care favourably with what went before, or have mixed feelings about it (Fisher *et al.,* 1986; Packman *et al.,* 1986; Rowe *et al.,* 1984; Sinclair and Gibbs, 1998). American evidence suggests that structured intervention with birth families can work. However, the effects tend to wear off and be less pronounced where the problems are most serious (Rutter *et al.,* 1999). Even in highly resourced American projects, re-abuse rates are high (Gough, 1993) and a heavy American emphasis on prevention has proved quite compatible with large increases in the care population (Dore and Alexander 1996).

In the UK, for the foreseeable future a sizeable care system seems here to stay. A high proportion of its clientele will have been abused and they are likely to stay longer in the care system. Policy for them is likely to emphasise:

- adoption
- long-stay fostering
- educational outcomes
- stability and staying after 18.

These emphases are already apparent. The challenges that arise include:

- variations in approach at a local level
- the high costs of a small proportion of children
- the apparently poor outcomes, particularly in children's homes
- the risks of breakdown in foster care
- the problems of coping with very difficult children in foster care
- difficulties over contact between children and abusive birth families
- the small proportion of children staying after reaching the age of 18.

Against these problems should be set the resilience of many children and the dedication, warmth and skill of many of the carers. It is above all on the quality of these frontline carers that the quality of the system depends.

9 Young People Leaving Care and Young People Who Go Missing

Mike Stein and Gwyther Rees

Key statistics:

- In England, Scotland and Wales the majority of young people leave care at 16 and 17 years of age. Only in Northern Ireland did over half leave at 18.
- One in nine young people run away overnight before the age of 16. There are an estimated 129,000 running away incidents per year in the UK.

Key trends:

- There has been a fall in the numbers of young people aged 16 to 18 leaving care.
- There is currently no trend data available on the issue of going missing or running away in the UK.

Key sources:

- Official statistics on young people leaving care in the four countries of the UK
- Still Running: Young People on the Streets in the UK

Introduction

This chapter reviews the official data and research evidence in relation to two groups of highly vulnerable young people: care leavers and young people who go missing. In addition to their vulnerability, the main connection between these two groups is between *living in* substitute care and going missing from care. There is no UK data or research which has explored the links between *leaving care* and going missing from care or home. In light of this, the chapter is presented in two distinct parts. First, we will begin by focusing upon young people, aged 16–18, who move from care to live independently in the community. Second, we will explore what we know about young people under the age of 16 who go missing from home and care. The weaknesses of the data sources, of which there are many, will be highlighted in the conclusion.

Young people leaving care

Official data: numbers and characteristics of young people who leave care

UK data

During the year ending 31 March 2000 (the latest year for comparable data for all four countries of the UK) 6,800 young people aged 16–18 and over left care in England; 1,057 aged 16–18 left care in Scotland; 106 aged 18 (no data on 16–17-year-olds) left care in Wales; and 178 aged 16–18 left care in Northern Ireland (see Table 9.1).

In England and Scotland a majority of these young people left at 16 and 17. Only in Northern Ireland did over half leave at 18. In England and Scotland a greater percentage of young men than young women, aged 16–18, left care, but in Northern Ireland over half were young women.

Regional data

The latest regional data (year ending 31 March 2001) for the four UK countries shows considerable variation in terms of numbers of care leavers, their final placements and their length of time in care. The highest and lowest numbers for areas within each country is outlined below (see Table 9.2).

Table 9.1: Numbers and characteristics of young people leaving care in the UK, year ending 31 March 2000

Country	Left care at 16 & 17		Left care at 18		Per cent	Per cent	Total
England	4,000	(58%)	2,880	(42%)	56.0	44.0	6,880
Northern Ireland	62	(34%)	116	(65%)	46.6	53.4	178
Scotland	929	(88%)	128	(12%)	60.5	39.5	1,057
Wales	No data		106		No data	No data	106

Sources: DoH (2001b), Scottish Executive (2001i), Social Services Inspectorate Wales (2001).

Table 9.2: Regional variations in the UK, young people leaving care aged 16–18, year ending 31 March 2000

Jurisdiction	Most young people		Least young people	
England – Inner London	Lewisham	82	Camden	38
England – Outer London	Waltham Forest	108	Kingston upon Thames	17
England – Metropolitan Districts	Birmingham	162	Tameside	18
England – Shire Counties	Kent	*272	Bedfordshire	30
England – Unitary Authorities	Bristol	65	Rutland	2
Northern Ireland	Foyle HSS Trust	45	Causeway HSS Trust	4
Scotland	Glasgow	161	Orkney Islands	1
Wales**	Cardiff	14	Merthyr Tydfil	0

* Includes unaccompanied young asylum seekers
** Data on 18-year-olds only
Sources: DoH (2001b), Scottish Executive (2001i), Social Services Inspectorate Wales (2001).

Trends

In the three UK countries for which data is available there has been a fall in the numbers of young people aged 16–18 and over who ceased to be looked after or who were looked after (see Table 9.3).

A longer-term trend in all four countries has been the increase in the numbers of young people leaving care from foster care placements and a decline in the proportion leaving care from children's homes.

In England, between 1993/94 and 1998/99, the proportion of care leavers (of all 16–18-year-olds and over) aged 16–17 rose from 51 per cent to 67 per cent, but in 1999/2000 fell back to 59 per cent. The latest data for England shows that since 1988 there has been a fall in the number of young people aged 16–17 leaving care and an increase in the number of those aged 18 and over (DoH, 2001b).

Also, data for England only shows that between 1996 and 2000, there was an increase in the percentage of young people whose final care period was more

Table 9.3: Young people, aged 16–18 and over, ceased to be looked after, or looked after, years ending 1997 and 2000

Jurisdiction	1997	2000
England (ceased to be looked after)	8,300	6,880
Northern Ireland (ceased to be looked after)	248	178
Scotland (ceased to be looked after)	No data	1,057
Wales (looked after)	376	273

than two years (from 46 per cent to 53 per cent) and an increase in the percentage of young men leaving care, from 53 per cent to 56 per cent and a decline in young women from 47 per cent to 44 per cent.

Research findings and performance evidence data

Leaving home, leaving care and homelessness

As the official data reveals, with the exception of Northern Ireland (confirmed by Pinkerton and McCrea in their 1999 research), most young people legally leave care at 16 and 17 years of age (see Table 9.1). Research completed since 1992 adds to this data. It shows that young people leave care to live independently at a much earlier age than other young people leave home. An English survey of 183 young people showed that two-thirds of young people left care before they were 18 and just under a third did so at just 16. This contrasts starkly with 87 per cent of 16–18-year-olds who were still living at home (Biehal *et al.*, 1992). In a 2001 Scottish survey of 107 young people, nearly three-quarters of those who legally left care did so at 15 (21 per cent) or 16 (52 per cent) years of age, in contrast to a modal age of 22 for males and 20 for females identified in an earlier Scottish study (Dixon and Stein, 2002).

Although no official data is collected on homelessness among care leavers, research studies have shown that they are over-represented among the young homeless population. A two-year follow-up study of young people leaving care suggests that over half of the young people will make two or more moves and just over 20 per cent will become homeless at some stage (Biehal *et al.*, 1995).

Comparative research drawing on data from England, Northern Ireland and Ireland showed that 15 per cent of young people in England, 20 per cent in Northern Ireland and 16 per cent in Ireland, experience homelessness at some point within six months after leaving care (Stein *et al.*, 2000). In the 2001 Scottish survey of 107 young people, 61 per cent of them had moved three or more times, and 40 per cent reported having been homeless since leaving care (Dixon and Stein, 2002). Estimates based upon young homeless people living in hostels suggest between 30 per cent and 59 per cent have been in care at some time in their lives (Randall, 1988, 1989).

Performance evidence data: In England only, care leavers' accommodation is measured under the evaluation of the Quality Protects programme. The latest data shows that 26 per cent were not known to be in suitable accommodation, 74 per cent were known to have suitable accommodation, based upon young people who left care between September 1998 and September 1999. The indicator is planned to improve to 88.5 per cent by March 2002. Also, English councils reported that on 30 September 1999, they were still in touch with nearly 70 per cent of the young people who had left care in the previous 12 months. They had lost touch with more than 30 per cent of care leavers in the course of a year. No comparable data was available from the other UK countries.

Education

Educational disadvantage casts a long shadow. Young people leaving care have lower levels of educational attainment and participation rates than young people in the general population. In the English survey of 183 young people, two-thirds had no qualifications at all, only 15 per cent had a GCSE (A-C grade) or its equivalent, and 0.5 per cent an A level pass. For the equivalent year, nationally, 38 per cent, and locally, 30 per cent, attained five or more GCSE passes at A-C grade. As regards A level, 25 per cent of boys and 29 per cent of girls attained at least one pass (Biehal *et al.*, 1992). In the Scottish survey almost two-thirds of young people had no standard grade qualifications compared to the national average of 7 per cent, and most had experience of truancy (83 per cent) and exclusion (71 per cent) (Dixon and Stein, 2002).

Analysis of data from the UK-wide National Child Development Study comparing 12,128 young people who had never been in care with 372 who had experienced care revealed that 43 per cent of the 23-year-olds who had been in care had no qualifications, compared with only 16 per cent of their peers who had never been in care (Cheung and Heath, 1994). (The Child Development Study was a longitudinal study of children born between 3 and 9 March 1958, designed to be nationally representative of all children in Great Britain; the secondary analysis by Cheung and Heath analyses the data at a UK-wide level.)

Performance evidence data: In England, the percentage of young people leaving care aged 16 and over with at least one GCSE or GNVQ, is one of the key Performance Assessment indicators. It monitors progress towards the government's National Priorities Guidance target, which is to:

- improve the educational attainment of children looked after by increasing to at least 50 per cent by 2001 the proportion of children leaving care at 16 or later with a GCSE or GNVQ qualification; and to 75 per cent by 2003.

- increase to 15 per cent in 2003/04 the proportion of children leaving care aged 16 and over with 5 GCSEs at grade A* to C.

At March 1998, only 40 per cent had gained at least one GCSE or GNVQ, and 60 per cent left with no qualifications. By the year ending 31 March 2000, the situation was worse, with less than 30 per cent achieving at least one qualification and 70.6 per cent leaving with no qualifications. Only 4 per cent left with at least five GCSEs grade A*-C. An analysis of the 2000 data shows that positive educational outcomes are linked to longer care duration, foster care (and those foster placements located within the authority did better than those outside the area) and gender – girls did better than boys (DoH, 2001b).

The latest data for England showed that 37 per cent had reached the target of at least one GCSE or GNVQ in 2000/01, an improvement on 2000, although this progress has not been made in all regions. Also, this contrasts dramatically with the 94 per cent of 16-year-olds in the general population who achieve this target.

Wales is also collecting data on the percentage of young people leaving care aged 16 and over with at least one GCSE grade A to G or GNVQ as an objective under the Children First programme, and has set a national target of 50 per cent. Due to substantially incomplete data returns for the years ending 2000 and 2001 it is not possible to arrive at a reliable comparable percentage for Wales. For those authorities which returned data, the percentage ranged between 11 per cent and 91 per cent for 2000 and 3 per cent and 78 per cent (excluding one authority with one successful young person returning 100 per cent).

There is no comparable data for Northern Ireland and Scotland.

Employment and careers

Care leavers are more likely to be unemployed than other young people aged 16–19 in the population at large. In a 1995 survey and follow-up study 36.5 per cent and 50 per cent respectively were unemployed compared to a mean of 19 per cent for other young people (Biehal et al., 1995). Nearly two-thirds of young people surveyed in the 2001 Scottish research had poor employment outcomes (Dixon and Stein, 2002).

Analysis of the National Child Development Study UK data revealed that young people who had been in care were much more likely to be unemployed or be in unskilled or semi-skilled manual work, and were less likely to be in managerial work than their peers who had never been in care (Cheung and

Heath, 1994). Analysis of the same data also revealed that unqualified young people who had been in care were more disadvantaged in employment opportunities than unqualified young people who had never been in care.

A survey of leaving care projects working with 2,905 young people showed that just 11 per cent of the total sample were working full time, 27.5 per cent were participating in youth training, further or higher education, 4 per cent were in part-time work and 51 per cent were unemployed – two-and-a-half times the unemployment rate for young people in this age range (Broad, 1998).

Comparative research showed that 66 per cent of care leavers in England and 50 per cent in Northern Ireland and Ireland left school with no qualifications at all. Most of those young people who had qualifications had low achievement levels and left school at the minimum school leaving age in their respective areas (Stein *et al.*, 2000).

Performance evidence data: In England and Wales, information on the percentage of young people who were looked after on 1 April aged 16 who were engaged in education, training or employment at the age of 19, is provided as part of the evaluation of the Performance Assessment Framework under Quality Protects and Children First respectively.

The latest provisional data for England, collected from local authority Management Action Plans, suggests a figure for this indicator of 41.3 per cent at 31 March 2000, or 57.8 per cent unemployed (based upon less than 50 per cent return).

The latest data for Wales suggests a figure for this indicator of 36 per cent at 31 March 2000 and 50.2 per cent at 31 March 2001.

The latest English data on the related Quality Protects interim indicator tracks the educational status of the young people who were looked after on 31 August 1999 aged 16 or more and who subsequently left care. The proportion of this group who were engaged in education or training or who were employed at 30 September 2000 was 50.4 per cent (just under 50 per cent unemployed).

There is no comparable data for Northern Ireland and Scotland.

Poverty

The impact of poor educational and employment outcomes leaves many care leavers ill prepared for an increasingly competitive youth labour market. The pattern for many of these young people was periods of unemployment punctuated by training schemes and short-term employment. A consistent finding from the UK studies completed since the mid-1970s has been that the vast majority of care leavers live at or near the poverty line at some time (see Stein, 1997; Broad, 1998; Dixon and Stein, 2002; Pinkerton and McCrea, 1999).

There is no official data of care leavers living in poverty. However, the English and Welsh government performance indicators for those not in education, employment or training would suggest a baseline for the year 2000 of just under 50 per cent for those dependent upon some form of financial assistance.

Young parenthood

There is no official data collected on young parents leaving care. Two English research studies reveal that young women leaving care aged 16–18 are more likely to be young mothers than other young women of that age group. They show that between 25 and 50 per cent of young women aged 16–19 were young parents compared to 5 per cent in the general population. Also, just over half of the young parents reported that their pregnancies were unplanned (Garnett, 1992; Biehal et al., 1992, 1995). For young parents who are supported, parenthood may bring some benefits – a renewal of family links and improved relationships as well as furthering an adult 'non care' status (Hutson, 1997).

Differences between black and white young people

Very few studies have been able to make significant comparisons between black and white young people or have been solely of black young people leaving care. The largest group of black young people being looked after and leaving care are young people of mixed heritage (Bebbington and Miles, 1989; Biehal et al., 1995; Rowe et al., 1989). As a group, black young people enter care earlier and stay longer than white young people. Research has also highlighted identity problems derived from a lack of contact with family and community as well as direct and indirect discrimination after leaving care (Ince, 1998).

After leaving care black young people had similar employment and housing careers, but were slightly more likely to make better educational progress than white young people. Most black young people had experienced racist harassment and abuse and some mixed heritage young people felt they were not accepted by black or white people (Barn, 1993; Barn et al., 1997; Biehal et al., 1995).

Young disabled people

There is no official data on young disabled people leaving care (although the first Children in Need census has provided data on looked after young people) and there has been very little research into the experiences of young disabled people leaving care (DoH, 2001b; Rabiee *et al.*, 2001). Data on 131 young disabled people showed that there was a lack of planning, inadequate information and poor consultation with them. Their transitions from care could be abrupt or delayed by restricted housing and employment options and inadequate support after leaving care (Rabiee *et al.*, 2001).

Research studies show that approximately 13 per cent of young people leaving care have special needs, including emotional and behavioural problems, learning difficulties, a physical disability or mental health problems. Compared to other young people leaving care, this group of young people have fewer educational qualifications, are more likely to be unemployed and are more likely to be homeless (Biehal *et al.*, 1995).

Young people with mental health problems

There is no official data on the mental health of young people after leaving care. Analysis of UK data from the National Child Development Study (not separately analysed for each UK country), comparing the mental health of care leavers with other young adults, indicates a higher risk of depression at age 23 and 33, a higher incidence of psychiatric and personality disorders and greater levels of emotional and behavioural problems (Cheung and Buchanan, 1997).

In a study of care leavers, 17 per cent had a long-term mental illness, including depression, eating disorders and phobias, females being greatly over-represented. In the same study, just over a third had deliberately self-harmed, two-thirds had thought about taking their own lives and 40 per cent had tried to between the age of 15–18, at the time of leaving care (Saunders and Broad, 1997).

Evidence from other countries

Research from both Europe and the United States reveals similar findings in respect of the poor outcomes of care leavers in comparison to other young people (see Stein, 1997 for a discussion).

Young people who go missing

This section will look at the issue of young people under the age of 16 going missing in the UK. This is an issue which has received increasing recognition over the last decade, and a number of research studies have been published.

Estimates of prevalence and incidence

It is important immediately to draw a distinction between different definitions of missing children and young people. There is a division between incidents of young people 'going missing' which are reported by parents and carers to the police, and incidents of 'running away' or 'being forced to leave' which have been reported by young people themselves via research studies.

Early UK research into the issue of missing children focused primarily on official missing person reports. Newman (1989) carried out a survey of police authorities in England and Wales. On the basis of the sample of responses it was estimated that there were 98,000 missing person incidents involving young people under the age of 18 each year. A similar study of four police authorities in England and Scotland (Abrahams and Mungall, 1992) estimated that around 43,000 young persons under the age of 18 went missing each year in England and Scotland and that there were 102,000 missing person incidents per year.

These early research studies established the widespread prevalence of children and young people going missing in the UK. However, the reliance on official reports of incidence does present difficulties. First, there is an over-reporting of young people going missing from substitute care (particularly children's homes). Standardised and fairly widespread procedures mean that a young person might be reported because they are late returning to a children's home. Conversely, there is no legal requirement for parents to report their child missing and there is therefore likely to be significant under-reporting of young people going missing from the family home. Newman (1989) suggested that only half of such incidents are reported to the police. Moreover, the inclusion of 16- and 17-year-olds in the statistics is problematic in that young people of this age can, in effect, leave home without parental permission.

An alternative source of data has been surveys of young people. Rees (1993) conducted a survey of 1,200 young people in schools and children's homes in Leeds. This research estimated that around one in seven young people ran away and stayed away for at least one night before the age of 16. A much larger survey of 13,000 young people in 25 areas in the UK was carried out in 1999 (Safe on the Streets Research Team, 1999). This survey found that 10 per cent of a sample of young people (primarily aged 14–15) had run away overnight. Taking into account the age distribution of this sample it was estimated that the proportion of young people running away overnight before the age of 16 was one in nine. On this basis around 77,000 young people under 16 run away for the first time each year in the UK and there are around 129,000 runaway incidents per year.

This latter study represents the most reliable evidence on young people going missing to have so far been gathered in the UK. The information from this study, plus findings from a Department of Health-funded study of young people going missing from the care system (Wade *et al.*, 1998) will be used as the basis for the UK evidence presented below. All findings, except where otherwise indicated, are from Safe on the Streets Research Team (1999). Unless explicitly stated, all running away rates quoted relate to running away incidents involving being away from home for at least one night. All statistics from the Safe on the Streets research refer to reported rates of running away in the survey sample made up primarily of 14–15-year-olds. As explained above, actual rates of running away before the age of 16 will be higher by a margin of 1 per cent or more due to the age distribution of the sample.

As the different studies mentioned above have used different definitions of going missing/running away, there is currently no trend data available on going missing in the UK.

Variations in running away rates between countries and areas of the UK

The Safe on the Streets research was able to compare rates of running away in the different countries of the UK and also rates between geographical areas with different economic and geographical characteristics.

Table 9.4 shows the reported rates of running away in the four countries of

Table 9.4: Reported rates of running away by country

Country	Number of young people surveyed	Per cent running away overnight
England	8,164	10
Northern Ireland	1,310	9
Scotland	1,802	10
Wales	1,214	8.5

the UK. While there is some variation in these rates, these were not found to be statistically significant.

Similarly, comparing areas on the basis of population density and indicators of economic prosperity, the research found no significant variation in running away rates.

Running away rates amongst different groups

There were, however, significant variations in running away rates between young people on the basis of their characteristics (see Safe on the Streets Research Team (1999) and Table 9.5).

Not surprisingly, the likelihood of running away increases with age. As detailed in *Still Running* (Safe on the Streets Research Team, 1999), the peak age for first running away is 13 years old, and over half of young runaways first run away at the ages of 13 to 15. However, around a quarter first run away before the age of 11 and these young people are the most likely to go on to run away repeatedly (Rees and Smeaton, 2001)

Females are significantly more likely to run away than males. On the other hand, male runaways tend to start younger and run away more often.

There are significant differences in running away rates among young people in different ethnic groups. Rates of running away are around 10.5 per cent for

Table 9.5: Rates of running away for young people by gender, ethnicity, family form and experience of substitute care

	Percentage
Gender	
Female	11.5
Male	8.5
Ethnicity	
Black-African/Caribbean	7.5
Indian/Pakistani/Bangladeshi	5.5
White	10.5
Family form	
Stepfamily	22
Lone parent family	14
Two parent family	7
Experience of substitute care	
Currently in substitute care	45
Have lived in substitute care	30

white young people, 7.5 per cent for young people of African-Caribbean origin, and 5.5. per cent for young people of Indian/Pakistani/Bangladeshi origin.

There are highly significant differences in running away rates among young people living in different types of family. Around 22 per cent of young people living in stepfamilies at the age of 15 have run away, compared to 14 per cent of those living in lone parent families and 7 per cent of those living in two-parent families (Rees and Rutherford, 2001). This pattern cannot be explained by differences in economic prosperity among the family types. In fact, evidence of a direct link between poverty (using indicators based on free school meals and number of adults in the family with paid jobs) and running away is very limited. Multivariate analysis reveals that the impact of poverty on likelihood of running away is quite small and that factors such as family type and quality of family relationships are far more significant.

There is a very strong link between running away and experience of living in substitute care. In the Safe on the Streets Research Team (1999) survey sample around 45 per cent of young people who currently lived in residential or foster care, and 30 per cent of those who had ever lived in care, had run away. Wade *et al.* (1998) found proportions of young people going missing from children's homes within a 12-month period ranging from 25 per cent to 71 per cent across four local authorities. These findings, together with high proportions of police missing person reports in relation to young people from children's homes (see earlier discussion), are open to misinterpretation. It must be remembered that young people in substitute care are a very small minority of the population of young people. It is estimated that between 5 and 10 per cent of young people who run away are currently living in substitute care. Additionally, a substantial proportion (probably around half) of these young people started running away before living in care (Rees, 1993; Wade *et al.*, 1998). On the other hand, young people who run away from care are more likely to do so repeatedly.

The issue of running away among some significant minority sub-groups of the population has not yet been fully explored. So far, there is no UK research on the link between running away and issues of sexuality for young people. In relation to disabilities, among the main survey sample in the Safe on the Streets Research Team study young people who defined themselves as having learning difficulties were significantly more likely than average to have run away, with a running away rate of 16 per cent. Among a small supplementary sample of 67 young people in six special needs schools there was a running away rate of 33 per cent, although this sample is too small to draw definitive conclusions. There has been no substantial research into the issue of running away among young people with physical disabilities.

Reasons for running away

Broadly speaking, research has shown that running away is primarily a response to problems experienced by young people within the family home. The most common immediate triggers for running away are conflict, physical abuse, emotional abuse and neglect. But there are usually also other underlying reasons, as suggested by the evidence on quality of family relationships above (see Chart 9.1). Personal problems and problems at school are also a factor in a minority of cases, but these are usually in conjunction with problems within the family.

For young people in substitute care, running away can be a response to quality of care issues. However, a number of other factors are also at play. These include a desire not to be living in care at all, a wish to be with family or friends, bullying by other young people and peer pressure to run away. Additionally, Wade et al. (1998) emphasise that 'histories of abuse, rejection and neglect' before moving into care are a key factor in understanding young people going missing from care.

Experiences of being away

Young people report positive aspects of the experience of being away from home. It provides an opportunity to reflect, a relief from pressure and an escape. It is also clear that running away carries risks for young people. Around a quarter of young runaways sleep rough, and around one in seven report having been sexually or physically assaulted while away. Survival options for young people under 16 are very limited. Runaways often resort to stealing, begging and other illegitimate means of survival. There is also evidence of a link between running away and sexual exploitation (Melrose et al., 1999).

Links between running away and other issues

The Safe on the Streets Research Team (1999) found significant links between running away and a number of other issues in young people's lives.

In terms of family relationships, young runaways are significantly more likely than other young people to report physical abuse, differential treatment of

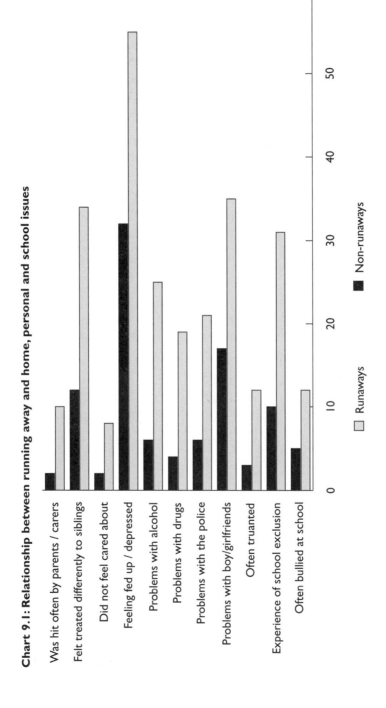

Chart 9.1: Relationship between running away and home, personal and school issues

Source: Compiled from information from Safe on the Streets Research Team (1999)

siblings and feelings of not being cared about or understood. At school, young runaways are significantly more likely to be bullied, to truant and to be excluded. In their personal lives, young runaways report high rates of offending, depression, and problems with alcohol and drugs.

As with young people leaving care, there is also some UK evidence of a link between running away under the age of 16 and youth homelessness after the age of 16 (Craig and Hodson, 1998; Centrepoint, 1998).

Evidence from other countries

The main source of international evidence on running away is the US, where a substantial body of literature has accumulated over the last 30 years. Rates of running away in the US are comparable to those in the UK. It is estimated that one in seven young people in the US run away by the age of 18 (National Runaway Switchboard, 2001). Patterns of running away and links with other issues also appear to be broadly in line with the UK findings (see the comprehensive study by Brennan *et al.,* 1978).

A notable aspect of the US research has been an exploration of the longer-term impacts of running away. Young people who go missing are, for example, significantly more likely than average to become homeless as a young adult (Simons and Whitbeck, 1991) and to have an early pregnancy (Greene and Ringwalt, 1998). It also seems that running away may be transmitted from one generation to another. Young people who have a parent who ran away have a higher than average likelihood of running away themselves (Plass and Hotalling, 1995).

Conclusion

In relation to young people leaving care there are three main weaknesses of the existing data sources. First, there is very little directly comparable data available in the four UK countries in terms of both year and category. Second, the amount of official data on care leavers is very limited in contrast to the more robust data on looked after children under 16 years of age. Third, and on a more positive note, performance measurement data has recently been published in England and Wales, and is being developed in Scotland and Northern Ireland. The partial account provided by the official data is complemented by the findings from research studies, but these are also limited in terms of directly comparable data –

due to differences in time, sample size and location. The overall picture is therefore constructed from a range of sources and where there are differences these have been detailed in the text.

In terms of going missing, the survey carried out by Safe on the Streets Research Team (1999) has provided a reliable broad overview of the incidence of running away in the UK, and some of the factors associated with it. However, there are a number of specific gaps and under-explored areas in current UK knowledge. There is a need for more detailed research to improve our under-standing of the issue of running away for particular sub-groups, including young people from minority ethnic backgrounds, disabled young people and lesbian, gay and bisexual young people. Furthermore, while many links have been established between running away and other issues, little is yet known about the nature and direction of these links. There is a need for research which investigates the chronology of the emergence of various issues such as running away, problems at school, offending, drug and alcohol problems and the relationships between them. Further, there is a need for further research to investigate the longer-term links between running away under the age of 16 and issues such as youth homelessness after the age of 16.

Finally, there is a notable lack of official data on the issue of going missing in the four UK countries. As discussed earlier, there are serious drawbacks regarding reports of young people going missing made by parents and carers to the police as a reliable indicator. There is evidence of both under- and over-reporting and there is likely to be variation between areas which is attributable to differences in reporting and recording procedures rather than due to substantive differences in actual rates of going missing. One solution to these problems is for official data to be based on self-reporting of going missing by young people.

10 Children as Carers

Sally Baldwin and Michael Hirst

Key statistics:

- Currently, up to 50,000 young people in the UK are heavily involved in caring for a family member who is chronically ill or severely disabled.
- 4 per cent of young people can expect to care regularly for a family member at some time during their childhood.

Key trends:

- Official recognition of the needs and circumstances of young carers has grown rapidly since the early 1990s.
- The number of support projects for young carers has grown nationally from 37 in 1995 to almost 150 in 2001.

Key sources:

- The 1995 survey of young carers aged 8–17 years and their families in Great Britain, carried out by the Office for National Statistics
- Surveys of children and young people in contact with young carers support projects, carried out during the 1990s by the Young Carers Research Group, University of Loughborough

---

Introduction

Most children are involved to some extent in the running of their households. When a member of their family is ill, some children take responsibility for their care and for household tasks for a short period. Such work can be useful preparation for the responsibilities of adult life. In recent years, however, it has been recognised that a significant number of children are more heavily involved in caring for relatives for longer periods. Evidence is beginning to accumulate on the potentially adverse effects of such caring, both on children's immediate quality of life and psychological well-being and, in the longer term, on their educational attainment and transition to adult life and employment.

Caring by children remains a difficult issue to study, partly because it raises difficult ethical questions. Both parents and children are involved; possible links to child protection proceedings inevitably raises fears that families may be broken up and children taken into care. It is also made difficult by the fact that 'we know very little about what contribution *any* children in *any* family make to the domestic smooth running of the household. Some children may be heavily involved for reasons such as gender, family size, tradition or expectation which have nothing to do with the presence or absence of a disabled or older person in the household. Assumptions that children who are involved in caring activities are thus *necessarily* more involved than their contemporaries cannot be upheld.' (Drewett *et al.*, 1999).

A wealth of qualitative research from all parts of the UK provides valuable evidence on the experiences of young carers, though with relatively little coverage of children from minority ethnic communities. By comparison, there is a dearth of representative data at the national level, and from the devolved administrations, on the volume, pattern and timing of caring among children and young people.[1]

It is difficult, then, to establish precisely the prevalence of young carers or the impact of caring on their lives. Estimates vary considerably, depending on how they are identified, the definition of what constitutes caring beyond what children normally do and the age at which children are included in studies. Even so, a substantial amount of evidence has accumulated since the early 1990s. In the remainder of this chapter, we summarise the main findings of this research, looking first at the numbers and characteristics of young carers.

How many young carers?

The most robust figures are based on a survey conducted in England, Scotland and Wales by the Office for National Statistics (ONS). Only children over 8 years old 'carrying out significant caring tasks and assuming a level of responsibility for another person which would usually be taken by an adult' were included (Walker, 1996, p. 3). According to this definition, 0.46 per cent of young people aged 8–17 years are carers. Given the usual margin of error in such surveys, the actual figure could lie between 0.27 per cent and 0.72 per cent (95 per cent confidence interval).

Applying these prevalence rates to the mid-1995 population, estimates for 8–17-year-olds in the UK gives the number of young carers shown in Table 10.1.

---

[1] The 2001 population census will for the first time provide national data on the number and characteristics of young carers, including the amount of time they devote to their caring activities. These data were not available at the time of preparing this chapter.

Table 10.1: Estimated number of young carers

	England	Scotland	Wales	Northern Ireland	UK
Low	16,300	1,700	1,000	700	19,700
Middle	27,700	3,000	1,700	1,200	33,600
High	43,400	4,600	2,700	1,900	52,600
All young people aged 8–17 years*	6,031,900	642,100	374,000	263,300	7,311,300

* *Sources*: ONS (1996), Registrar General for Scotland (1996), NISRA (1996)

Experts in the field of young carers suggest that the true figures are likely to be towards the higher estimate:

- The ONS definition excludes many children whose lives are significantly affected by caring (Becker *et al.*, 2000).
- Local studies have found children under 8 years old providing care for siblings, parents, or other relatives.
- Non-response to the survey, including the widely reported fear that children identified as carers may become involved in child protection proceedings, is likely to have reduced the estimates. According to Walker's calculations (1996, p. 6), non-response could add 7,500 to the UK mid-estimate shown above.
- The prevalence of disability among adults in Scotland, Wales and Northern Ireland is higher than in England and might give rise to greater proportions of young carers in those countries (Grundy *et al.*, 1999; McCoy and Smith, 1992). Using different definitions and survey procedures to those employed in the ONS study, the 1999 Scottish Household Survey estimates that there are over 6,000 children under age 16 providing informal care (Scottish Executive, 2001g).
- Over 50,000 adults with substantial care needs live in households containing children, although it is recognised that many will play only a limited role in providing care (Parker and Olsen, 1995).
- Our analysis of the British Household Panel Survey (BHPS) indicates that 2.9 per cent of young people aged 16–17 identify themselves as caring for someone in their own household. Applying *half* that rate to the 8–17 age group gives 106,700 young carers in the UK during the mid-1990s, or between 75,300 and 146,200.

Moreover, the ONS survey provides no more than a snapshot picture, yet individuals move in and out of a caring role over time. A survey of young adults aged 18–24 found that 4 per cent had 'regularly' cared for a family member who was ill or disabled *at some time* during their childhood (Cawson *et al.*, 2000).

In summary, then, we might be safe in saying that up to 50,000 young people are heavily involved in some caring activity at any one time. We *cannot* conclude that they are the only young carers whose lives are significantly affected by their caring responsibilities. That will depend on their individual circumstances and the support available.

Characteristics of young carers and the people they look after

From their UK-wide survey of 2,303 young people in touch with young carer support groups, Dearden and Becker (1998) found that:

- 86 per cent of young carers are of compulsory school age, ie, under 16 years
- although children can become involved in care-giving at any age, most young carers are between 11 and 15 years, with an average age of 12 years
- girls are more likely than boys to be involved in caring
- 14 per cent of young carers are from black and minority ethnic groups
- one in ten young carers are caring for more than one person.

Children and young people are involved in caring for grandparents, siblings or other relatives. However, parents are the commonest group of care recipients, and young carers are more likely to be caring for mothers than fathers.

Young carers look after people with a range of physical, mental or sensory impairments, although physical health problems predominate. In the survey by Dearden and Becker (1998):

- 63 per cent were caring for someone with physical illness or impairment – multiple sclerosis was the most commonly occurring condition
- 29 per cent were caring for someone with mental health problems, including schizophrenia and depression, and alcohol and drug misuse
- 14 per cent were caring for someone with learning disabilities
- 4 per cent were caring for someone with a sensory impairment

Similar figures are found in the authors' study of young carers in transition to adulthood (Dearden and Becker, 2000). However, nearly half the children in the study by Mahon and Higgins (1995) were caring for parents with mental health problems. The distinction between looking after parents with mental health problems, as against physical or sensory impairments, is important and warrants further study.

What does caring involve?

Young carers' responsibilities vary with the condition of the person they look after, their household circumstances and the amount of support available from other family members or external sources. The findings from two surveys of young people in touch with young carer support groups in the UK show that caring tasks range from household duties (eg, cooking and cleaning) to intimate personal care (eg, washing and using the toilet) (Table 10.2). In this table, 'Other responsibilities' includes managing benefits or interpreting for parents whose preferred language is not English. The increase in emotional support between 1995 and 1997 indicates a growing recognition that this is part of the caring role.

A study of young carers in transition to adulthood found similar proportions involved in domestic and general care, but a higher proportion of the older age group were involved in providing intimate, personal care (Dearden and Becker, 2000). These young carers found this very difficult, particularly where cross-gender caring was involved.

These tasks mirror those carried out by adult carers (Rowlands, 1998). However, Mahon and Higgins (1995) argue that there are particular elements of young carers' responsibilities that have a bearing on their experience of childhood:

Table 10.2: Caring activities

| | Percentage* | |
Caring activity	1995	1997
Housework (shopping, making meals)	65	72
General care (help with medicines, lifting, etc.)	61	57
Emotional support and supervision	25	43
Intimate, personal care (toileting, bathing, etc.)	23	21
Care of siblings	11	7
Other responsibilities	10	29
Base (=100 per cent)	640	2,303

*Percentages sum to more than 100 because some young people performed tasks in two or more of the areas listed
Source: Dearden and Becker (1995 and 1998)

- looking after siblings
- reversal of roles and responsibilities between the parent and themselves
- emotional labour or feeling responsible for a parent or relative.

How much time do young carers spend on caring activities?

It is difficult to gauge how much time young carers devote to looking after relatives. This is partly because some tasks are carried out concurrently with others. It is also is difficult to establish how much of what they do goes beyond what any child their age would do.

Evidence from the 1994 BHPS shows that 18 per cent of 11–15-year-olds living with a disabled parent devote three hours or more per week to household chores. The comparable proportion for those with parents who are not disabled is 12 per cent.

The ONS survey provides more detail on the time devoted to caring by young people with 'significant' caring responsibilities (Walker, 1996). In this in-depth study of 14 households containing young carers, only two families estimated that the young carer spent less than 14 hours a week providing care. Nine reported that the young person spent more than 20 hours a week, two spending some 32 hours. Most were said to spend more time at the weekend. None had particular days when they were not involved in caring.

Impact and outcomes

A large number of descriptive studies have identified ways in which caring for a chronically ill or severely impaired relative can affect young people's lives. Summarising this literature, Becker (1995) identifies the following 'recurrent problems':

- impaired educational development – more than one in four young carers experience educational difficulties or miss school because of their caring responsibilities
- isolation from peer group and extended family, and limited opportunities for developing friendships
- lack of time for usual childhood and leisure activities
- guilt and resentment caused by conflict between the caring role and the child's own needs

- feeling that nobody is there for them, or understands their experience
- fear of what professionals might do if the family's circumstances are known
- lack of recognition, praise or respect for their contribution
- feeling stigmatised, particularly where parents have mental health problems, misuse drugs or alcohol or have AIDS/HIV
- limited horizons and aspirations for the future.

Walker's (1996) study also confirms that some young carers feel their responsibilities as a burden and experience psychological stress.

Dearden and Becker's (2000) study of young carers' transition to adulthood focuses on their ability to achieve adult goals and ambitions. It identifies adverse effects on their:

- educational attainment and qualifications
- employment and training opportunities
- income levels
- ability to leave home.

Similar findings on the longer-term impact of caring are reported in a study of 25 *former* young carers. Around half or more reported continuing effects on their physical and mental health, education and employment (Frank *et al.*, 1999). However, there is evidence that caring for a close relative need not only have negative effects on children's lives. A number of studies point to ways in which caring can have positive effects and help young carers to acquire skills that are useful later in life. These include maturity, ability to take responsibility and make decisions, and a range of personal and practical skills.

Material well-being

Few studies have focused on the financial circumstances of young carers' families. Those that have identify low income and financial hardship as common problems. There are three main reasons:

- Family incomes are reduced when a parent is unable to work or incurs additional costs because of disability. The relationship between poverty and disability is well established (Matthews and Truscott, 1990) and most young carers' families will be poor.
- A disproportionate number of young carers live in households headed by

only one, disabled, adult – usually their mother – increasing the likelihood of poverty and social exclusion.

- Caring responsibilities can limit young people's ability to get a regular, spare-time job and earn their own money.

All the families in the ONS study were receiving some type of benefit; half felt in need of financial help and many did not understand the benefits system (Walker, 1996).

Dearden and Becker (2000) provide further evidence of family poverty and multiple deprivation of households in which the young carers lived:

- Half the families were headed by a lone parent.
- Of two-parent families, only a third contained anyone in paid work, mainly in manual occupations.
- None of the parents who were ill or disabled was in paid work.
- Most parents had previously been in manual occupations.
- Virtually all families lived on benefit income.
- Almost two-thirds lived in council or housing association rented accommodation.

Experience of financial hardship and social exclusion was common in this study of young carers aged 16–17 (Dearden and Becker, 2000). Few had earnings; only one or two received any benefit income in their own right. The remainder were completely dependent on parents who were financially stressed themselves. The young people reported difficulties in affording enough (much less healthy) food most weeks and were often excluded from the normal activities of their peer group.

Dearden and Becker (2000) raise a more fundamental concern: in the absence of education maintenance allowances and well-paid jobs (which their poorer educational qualifications rule out), continuing to care may be seen by families and young people alike as a sensible decision. That option, however, is likely to disadvantage their longer-term chances of competing in the labour market.

Support for young carers

Research indicates that adverse impacts on young people's lives can be reduced by support received from relatives and friends, and from statutory and voluntary services. Evidence from recent research suggests that such support has increased, but remains patchy. In some cases, support from informal sources plays an important role; in others, the child acts as the primary carer with virtually no support from other family members. Support from statutory and voluntary services, whether directly to the disabled person, to the household generally or to the young carer, also varies considerably.

Support to young carers from minority ethnic communities seems likely to be particularly patchy, though very little research has been carried out on this issue. A study by Shah and Hatton (1999), the first to look at the needs and experiences of young carers from South Asian communities, found that support was poor and based on inaccurate stereotypical assumptions about the capacity of extended families to provide care. The report of this study includes recommendations for how best to work with and support young carers from Asian communities.

In Dearden and Becker's (1998) survey:
- Half the families received support from social workers, although the proportion receiving other forms of support was small.
- A quarter of the families received no support at all.
- Only 11 per cent had been assessed under any legislation, and only 5 per cent under the 1995 Carers Act – much smaller proportions than was the case with families of adult carers.

By comparison, 'very few' of the families in the ONS study were receiving help from any voluntary or statutory services, some had been refused help and none had regular visits from a social worker (Walker, 1996, p. 11).

Help aimed directly at relieving young carers' situation within their families is often limited. They mostly want the kinds of support that enable them to continue their involvement in the caring relationship without too great a sacrifice. This requires information, practical help, substitute care to let them have time off or to go away for a short spell, financial support and equipment such as mobile phones to help them keep in touch. Some young carers would also welcome psychological support – someone to talk to from time to time (DoH, 1995b).

Young carers projects have been developed to meet some of these needs and are highly valued by the young people and their families (Aldridge and Becker, 1998). As well as providing information, counselling, advocacy and befriending services, these projects provide opportunities for young carers to enjoy themselves and meet other young people in similar circumstances (Becker et al., 2000).
- Since 1992, when two pilot projects were established in Merseyside, the

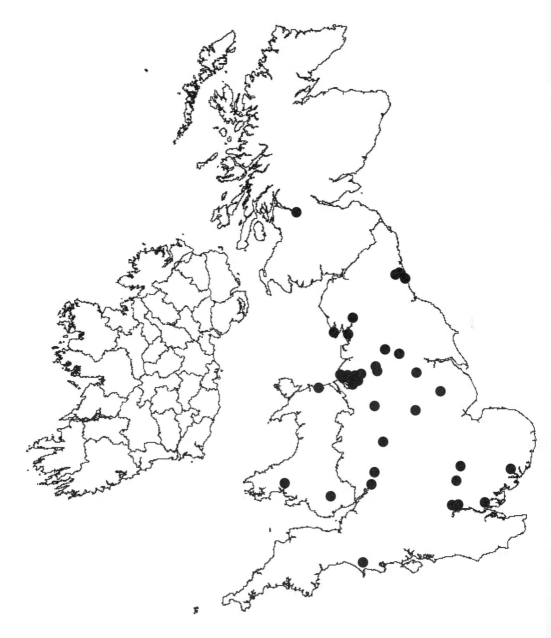

Figure 10.1a: Number of young carers projects in 1995
Compiled from information supplied by Professor Saul Becker

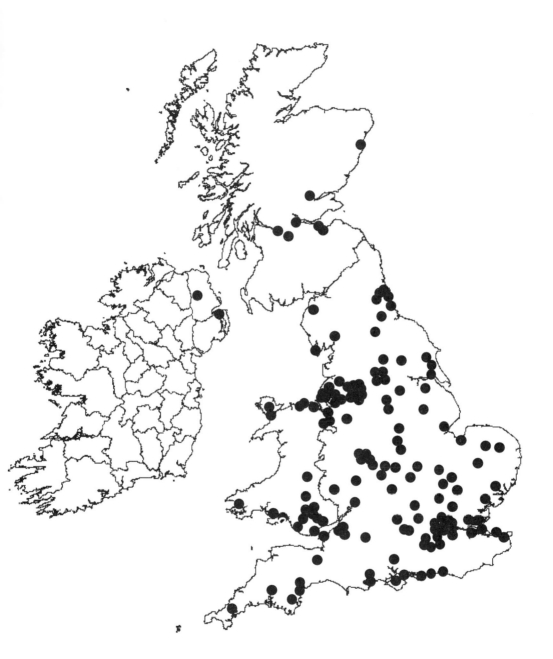

Figure 10.1b: Number of young carers projects in 2001
Compiled from information supplied by Professor Saul Becker

number of young carers projects has grown rapidly – to 37 in 1995, just over 100 in 1998, and almost 150 in 2001 (Figure 10.1).

- Each project caters for between 70 and 100 young people, perhaps more in metropolitan areas. This suggests that between 10,000 and 15,000 young carers benefit from the support services they provide.
- Without these projects, it is estimated that up to a quarter of these young people would have no outside support at all (Dearden and Becker, 1998).

There will be many young carers who do not have access to such projects. On current estimates they cater for no more than one in three of the 50,000 young people who might be heavily involved in providing care. More-over, their scope is limited. They are not responsible for assessing young carers' and their families' needs – nor, in general, for arranging, providing and co-ordinating services. Responsibility for these functions lies with local authorities.

Sensitive assessment of young carers' needs is an important route to increased support. However, research has identified two dilemmas service providers must resolve in providing the right kind of support:

- A danger that increasing support to young carers may lock them inappro-priately into the role of carer. A better approach to reducing young carers' risk of social exclusion is by providing more support to parents who are disabled – particularly in their role *as parents* (Dearden and Becker, 2000; Social Services Inspectorate, 1995, 1996).
- Young carers can also be locked into their caring role by service support that is experienced as intrusive, inappropriate and inconvenient – or for which local authorities charge a significant price. For these reasons, many families reject the services that are offered and choose to rely on their own resources – which include care provided by their own children.

International perspectives

There is a lack of reliable and comparable data from countries outside the UK on children's involvement in caring, its impact on their lives and any support available. The only cross-national study so far conducted focused on four European countries: Great Britain, France, Germany and Sweden (Becker, 1995). This study, which predates devolution in the UK, found that:

- In all four countries, similar economic and demographic trends were increasing the numbers of people cared for at home by relatives.
- No information on children's care giving and its consequences was collected systematically.
- Children were involved to a significant extent in caring.
- In France, Germany and Sweden, policy-makers and professionals were un-aware that, or denied that, children were significantly involved in providing care.
- In none of the countries was support available from the statutory services to any significant extent.
- In Sweden, children's involvement in care-giving was less widespread because support was provided directly to some categories of disabled people. However, Swedish children whose relatives fall into more stigmatised categories are excluded from these arrangements, and frequently act as primary care givers.
- In all four countries, children caring for relatives with mental health or addiction problems, HIV or AIDS, were less likely to be identified and receive support from statutory services.
- At the time, only Great Britain had developed policies aiming specifically to support young carers.

Research evidence on young carers is beginning to accumulate in a number of developed countries: Ireland, Malta, Israel, the United States and, notably, Australia. Of these, only in Australia has there been a systematic attempt to establish the numbers of young carers and to develop policy responses. According to Becker *et al.* (1998), while statistics on young carers in Australia differ from UK figures, overall findings on the experience and impacts of caring are strikingly similar.

Overall, the international evidence on young carers is patchy and weak. However, studies conducted so far indicate that both research and policy in the UK relating to young carers are relatively advanced.

Conclusion

In the decade since young carers were first identified as a source of concern, sufficient research evidence has accumulated to confirm that considerable numbers of children are involved in caring for relatives, that appropriate support is often absent and that caring can have both adverse and positive effects on their well-being and quality of life. Important gaps in knowledge remain. The development of appropriate policies for young carers requires:

- more reliable estimates of their numbers and characteristics, particularly of those in minority ethnic groups
- better knowledge of their lives and circumstances, particularly their financial needs, during transition to adulthood
- better understanding of the impact of care-giving and its longer-term outcomes, both positive and negative, via research based on the general population
- evaluation of local young carers projects
- evidence to support the development of guidelines and quality standards to be used in commissioning services that produce the outcomes young carers want.

Existing studies also identify major gaps in support which should be addressed by social services as a matter of urgency:

- support to ill or disabled parents, to reduce their need to rely heavily on their children
- support specifically to assist them in their role as parents, and sensitive assessment of the needs, both of disabled parents and of children caring for them.

11 Childcare Provision

Christine Skinner

Key statistics:

Approximate number of daycare places in the UK in 2000:

- holiday playschemes   495,438
- playgroups   395,416
- childminders   352,590
- daycare nurseries   280,686
- out-of-school clubs   153,201

Estimated percentage of children attending early education in England, Wales and Scotland:

- 90% in England in 2001
- 88% in Scotland in 2001
- 79% in Wales in 2000

Key trends:

Daycare provision in the UK from 1997 to 2000:

- increase in daycare nursery, out-of-school-clubs and holiday scheme places.
- decrease in childminder and playgroup places.

Early education provision from 1997 to 2000/01:

- increase in numbers of children attending private/voluntary services in England, Wales and Scotland.
- increase in numbers of children attending statutory early education in Scotland and Northern Ireland.
- decrease in numbers of children attending statutory early education in England and Wales.

Key sources:
- Social Services Statistics on daycare
- School Census for early education
- Department for Education and Employment research reports

Introduction

In 1998, the consultation document, *Meeting the Childcare Challenge* marked a sea-change in the status of childcare provision in the UK. A national childcare strategy was introduced based on the key principles of improving the availability, affordability and quality of childcare through locally based partnerships between the public, private and voluntary sectors. Wales, Scotland and Northern Ireland introduced separate papers based on the same key principles (DfEE, 1998a).

Childcare is arguably not an outcome nor a measure of well-being and in this report we have sought to eschew inputs and concentrate on outcomes. However, the aim of the strategy was to increase prosperity through employment, particularly for low-income and lone parent families. It is therefore important to consider childcare services in this report on the grounds that improving provision is central to the government's plans to tackle child poverty. Childcare services are also believed to improve child and family well-being by:
- reducing the risk of child and family poverty by making it easier for parents to take up paid employment
- improving parents' work, educational and social skills through easier access to education and training
- contributing to the development of children's social and educational skills
- enhancing the life chances of children
- reducing the risk of social isolation that can be associated with child-rearing.

However, the effect of different childcare services on children's well-being is not at all clear, partly because of the dual function of childcare. On the one hand, it frees up parents' time to enable them to take up paid work; on the other, it provides developmental opportunities for children. Evidence on the effects of parental labour market participation on child well-being is controversial and contradictory. Some suggest maternal employment when children are under five years old has detrimental effects on their long-term well-being and development (Ermisch and Francesconi, 2001). Others have found that maternal employment can create added family stress (Backett-Milburn *et al.*,

2001). The effects of fathers' participation in paid work is less clear (Ermisch and Francesconi, 2001). By contrast, others have argued there is no evidence of harm to young children resulting from maternal employment (Childcare Commission Report, 2001). Evaluations of integrated childcare programmes have shown positive outcomes for children's educational/social development and well-being (Bertram and Pascal, 2001).

The evidence to date is therefore inconclusive. It is not yet well understood how different forms of childcare affect child well-being, nor how the confounding factors of inadequate family-friendly work practices and the quality and nature of family life interact with childcare. Currently, some longitudinal studies assessing the impacts of early education provision are under way[1] and there is the possibility of more specific studies evaluating individual forms of daycare provision (Munton et al., 2001).

This chapter will therefore focus on formal childcare provision, a potential input to child-rearing. It will set out a baseline of the current level of childcare provision across the four countries of the UK using administrative statistical data. Current and future developments in childcare provision will also be outlined. The chapter will conclude with an assessment of the childcare strategy and a comment on the problems with the data sources.

Development of childcare provision

The Conservative governments of the 1980s and 1990s did little to improve childcare provision. Calls by the Equal Opportunities Commission to develop a national childcare strategy were ignored (Bagilhole and Byrne, 2000) and public nursery daycare provision was allowed to reduce by nearly a half (Harker, 2000). Consequently, the UK lagged behind many of the northern EU countries. In the mid-1990s, only 2 per cent of childcare for children under three years of age was publicly funded in the UK. This compared to:

- 48 per cent in Denmark
- 33 per cent in Sweden
- 30 per cent in Belgium
- around 20 per cent in France and Finland.

Publicly funded provision for children aged between four and six years in the

---

[1] The Department for Education and Skills is conducting a longitudinal survey from 1997 to 2003 – the EPPE project (Effective Provision of Preschool Education).

UK fared better at 60 per cent, but only because the majority of children at this age would be eligible to start primary school education (European Commission Network on Childcare, 1996, cited in Randall, 2000).

Using the latest available data, Moss (2001) describes the trends in publicly funded provision in 15 EU member states in the mid-1990s. These are:

- three years of publicly funded nursery education/kindergarten for children aged 3–6 years
- much lower publicly funded provision for children under three years of age
- the highest levels of publicly funded provision for children under three years of age are in Denmark, Sweden, Finland, Belgium and France
- the lowest levels of publicly funded provision for children under three years of age are in southern Europe, Germany, Ireland and the UK.

Notably, the UK and Ireland are unusual in having a large for-profit sector as opposed to a private non-profit sector (Moss, 2001). Indeed, according to Land (1999, p. 136) there was a threefold increase in childminders and a sevenfold increase in private nurseries in the UK in the mid-1990s. This was in response to rising demand coming from women's increased participation in the labour market. To some extent this offset the fall in public provision, but the Daycare Trust (1999) argued that provision remained woefully inadequate. As described above, the incoming Labour government developed the first national childcare strategy to improve provision.

The main components of the childcare strategy across the four countries of the UK were:

- a New Opportunities Fund from National Lottery monies for the expansion of out-of-school-clubs
- a commitment to guarantee pre-school education for three and four-year-old children where their parents wished it
- financial and other support for the development of childcare partnerships to expand services locally.

The strategy therefore does not provide fully funded childcare services: rather the private/voluntary sectors are expected to fill gaps in provision. Simultaneously, however, childcare subsidies for low-income parents have been increased, making private/voluntary childcare potentially more affordable to these parents. The childcare strategy is therefore primarily a demand-led initiative.

According to the government, the childcare strategy has worked well so far.

It states that new childcare places have been created for half a million children and that by March 2004 the target is to create a million more places (DfES, 2001c). However, assessing the national picture of childcare provision and changes over time is not straightforward:

- Government reports on the 'success' of the strategy tend to relate to England only.
- It is increasingly difficult to measure and identify different forms of provision as multiple services are being provided by single providers and these are not easily recorded.
- Official data sources are not always comparable across countries or across the daycare and pre-school education sectors.

The rest of this chapter will map out a baseline of current provision across all four countries in both the daycare and early education sectors for children aged five or under.

Level of daycare provision across the UK

There are five main types of formal daycare.[2] Full-time care for children under school age[3] is mainly provided by *day nurseries* and *registered childminders,* though both also offer part-time care. *Out-of-school club*s (OOSC) and *holiday schemes* mainly provide care for school-aged children which is wrapped around the school day and school term respectively. This 'wraparound' care fills the gap in school hours/terms and can facilitate parental employment. *Playgroups* offer opportunities for young children (aged from 0–5) to socialise and play. Services are sessional for a few hours per day and are less able to help parents return to work. Generally parents have to pay for all these daycare services. Overall, childminder care offers the greatest flexibility. Childminders can provide out-of-school care, weekend and out-of-hours care, care for all the children in the same family and they can take children to and from other services on behalf of parents.

Table 11.1 describes the number of daycare places across the UK from 1997

---

[2] Informal care is that provided by relatives and friends. Other forms of childcare are excluded from consideration, including care provided in hospital nurseries and care provided in private fee-paying schools.

[3] The age at which children can start school varies slightly across the four countries but is generally between the ages of four and five. Daycare services tend to cover children between the ages of 0 and 14.

until 2001.[4] The data is patchy. England has the most comprehensive and consistent set of data and Scotland the least. The paucity of Scottish data results from changes in data collection methods which audited early education and childcare services together in a new Annual Integrated Census. Data for Northern Ireland is not available for 1997 because of delays resulting from new audit procedures under the Children Order (NI) 1995 which was not implemented until 1996. Northern Ireland data is also distinguished from the rest as it includes services for children up to age 12 (see notes on table), whereas the other countries produce data on children up to age 8 only. Data for 2001 for Scotland, Wales and Northern Ireland was not published at the time of writing. Nevertheless, the identifiable trends for the UK are (see Chart 11.1):

Increases in:

- daycare nursery places (from 227,741 to 285,100)
- out-of-school club places (from 95,279 to 152,800)
- holiday scheme places (from 219,226 to 594,500).

Decreases in:

- childminder places (from 417,527 to 352,590 in 2000)
- playgroup places (from 452,862 to 395,416 in 2000).

The most striking trend for the UK as a whole, is the nearly threefold increase in holiday scheme places.

There are, however, variations across countries in changes over time and in the type of provision that is most common.

Changes over time in daycare across countries

The changes over time across countries are summarised in Chart 11.1. England closely follows the national trend. This is because the greatest number of childcare places across all types of provision is in England (see Chart 11.2). Most notably, the national trend in holiday scheme expansion relates mostly to increases in England.

Wales also closely follows the national trend (see Chart 11.3). There is an expansion in daycare nursery and OOSC places, but a contraction in childminder and playgroup places. There is no distinction made between OOSCs and holiday

---

[4] Data before 1997 predates the national childcare strategy and is therefore not included.

Table 11.1 The numbers of different childcare places across the UK*

	1997	1998	1999	2000	(estimates) 2001
Daycare Nurseries					
England	193,800	223,000	247,700	264,200	285,100
Wales	8,262	8,839	9,894	10,865	**
Scotland	25,679***	**	**	**	#
Northern Ireland##	**	4,229	4,828	5,621	**
Out-of-School Clubs					
England	78,700	92,300	113,800	141,100	152,800
Wales	4,343	5,035	5,620	7,958	**
Scotland	12,236	**	**	**	(18,130)####
Northern Ireland##	**	1,459	#	4,143	**
Holiday Schemes					
England	209,000	256,500	435,000	490,400	594,500
Wales	**	**	**	**	**
Scotland	10,226§	**	**	**	(6,586)
Northern Ireland##	**	3,806	#	5,038	**
Childminders					
England	365,200	370,700	336,600	320,400	304,600
Wales	17,344	17,484	13,923	13,039	**
Scotland	34,983	**	**	**	**
Northern Ireland##	**	18,795	18,807	19,151	**
Playgroups					
England	383,700	383,600	347,200	353,100	330,200
Wales	27,542	26,049	25,067	25,590	**
Scotland	41,620	**	**	**	(29,892)
Northern Ireland##	**	15,892	16,450	16,726	**

* Northern Ireland presents data for children under 12 years of age in relation to childminders, OOSCs, and holiday schemes. All other countries present data for children under 8 years of age.
** Data not available.
*** Statistical returns in 1997 for some daycare nursery providers were sent to both the Social Work Services Group and the Scottish Office Education and Industry Department. Thus there is some double counting between daycare services and early education services. (See Table 11.4 on early education.)
\# No disaggregation of data to identify this provision separately.
\#\# Figures for Northern Ireland not available until 1998 as compiled from Children Order (NI) 1995 returns which was effective from 1996.
\#\#\#\# Numbers in brackets indicate numbers of children attending and not numbers of places available.
§ This is described as the number of *term-time* places and holiday places added together, this does not make sense under this category. It is possible that term-time means half-term holiday care.

schemes in administrative data for Wales. A report by the Wales Out of School Clubs Childcare Co-ordinator, however, states that in June 2000 there were 494 OOSCs also offering holiday play schemes (Fairplay, 2000).

It is extremely difficult to assess changes over time in Scotland because of missing data and the fact that the data is inconsistent. Data for 1997 records the number of places, while 2001 data records the numbers of children attending; these two measures are not fully comparable. Despite this, the data suggests that, as in England and Wales, OOSC provision has expanded while playgroup provision has contracted (see Chart 11.4). Unlike England, however, there is a possible decline in the number of holiday scheme places.

Northern Ireland shows different changes over time. All five types of daycare provision have expanded, with the greatest increase in OOSC places (see Chart 11.5). In that regard it bucks the trend in England and Wales of a decline in both childminder and playgroup places. Part of the explanation for the increase in childminder places may relate to the fact that Northern Ireland data covers children aged up to 12 years. Therefore Northern Ireland may count places for older children that are not counted in England and Wales. It is possible that the increase in playgroup provision is peculiar to Northern Ireland because of the additional funding support for play facilities received through the EU Peace Programme (DHSSPS, 2000b).

Chart 11.1: Number of different childcare places in the UK

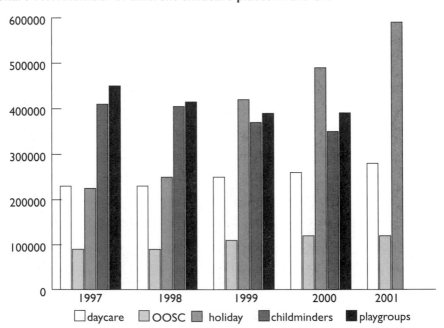

Chart 11.2: Number of different childcare places in England

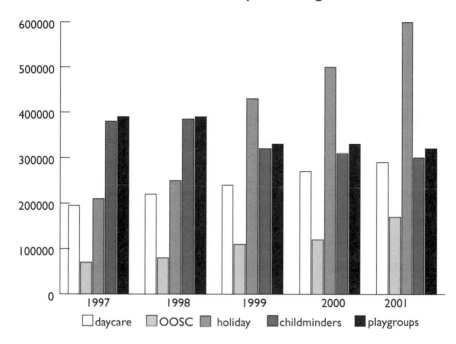

Chart 11.3: Number of different childcare places in Wales

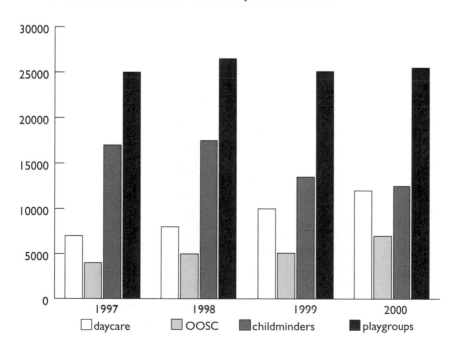

Chart 11.4: Number of different childcare places in Scotland in 1997, number of children attending childcare in Scotland in 2001

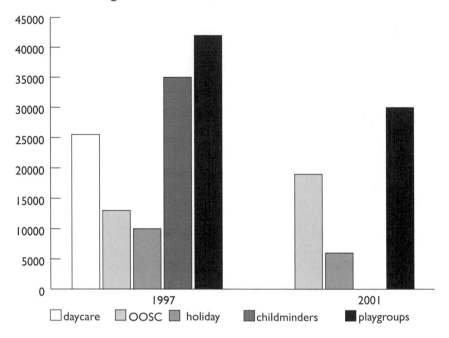

Chart 11.5: Number of different childcare places in Northern Ireland

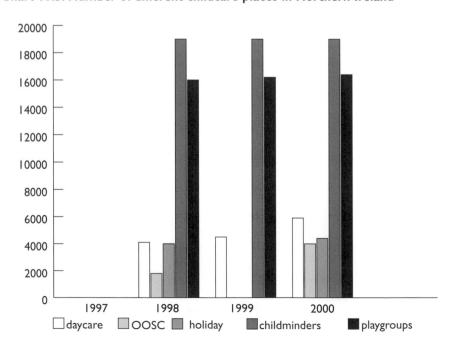

Table 11.2: Changes in childcare places between 1997 and 2001 across the UK

	England	Wales	Scotland	Northern Ireland
Daycare nurseries	Increase, slight but steady	Increase, slight but steady	*	Increase, slight but steady
OOSCs	Increase, nearly double	Increase, nearly double	Increase, possibly slight**	Increase, more than doubled
Holiday playschemes	Increase, nearly threefold	*	Decline, possible loss of a third of places***	Increase, slight but steady**
Childminders	Decline, loss of 60,600 places	Decline, loss of 4,305 places	*	Increase, slight but steady**
Playgroups	Decline, loss of 53,500 places	Decline, loss of 1,952 places	Decline, possible loss of a quarter of places***	Increase, slight but steady

* Data incomplete or not available.
** Increase in places occurs despite a reduction in number of providers (number of providers not shown).
**** Not possible to give an accurate count of loss of places as the data method changed across the years.

Most common types of daycare across countries

Charts 11.2 to 11.5 demonstrate some possible differences across countries in the most common types of provision. These are summarised in Table 11.3. Due to missing data, however, it is difficult to get a true picture. Nevertheless, the data suggests that in England the most common provision is holiday schemes, whereas in Scotland this is ranked third (and is the least common) and in Northern Ireland it is ranked fourth (second from last). In Wales and Scotland, playgroups are the most common types of provision, while in Northern Ireland, childminders are the most common type of provision. Overall, OOSC provision

Table 11.3: Most common types of childcare provision across the UK in 2001

Rank	England	Wales*	Scotland**	Northern Ireland
1	Holiday schemes	Playgroups	Playgroups	Childminders
2	Playgroups	Childminders	OOSCs	Playgroups
3	Childminders	Nursery daycare	Holiday schemes	Nursery daycare
4	Nursery daycare	OOSCs	–	Holiday schemes
5	OOSCs	–	–	OOSCs

seems the least common. It is ranked lowest in three of the four countries (England, Wales and Northern Ireland).

As yet, there is no easy explanation for these apparent differences. They could be due to cultural preferences, to the take-up of funding opportunities and/or differences in the relationship between supply and demand. There will also be regional variations within countries. The government has plans to explore area-based differences in childcare markets and provision in the near future.

Early years education

Early years education is provided mainly through the education system in nursery schools and in nursery/reception classes in primary schools. Provision in the private/voluntary sectors is also available as daycare organisations can now apply for grants to provide early education to 3- and 4-year-old children. The provision is part-time and free, but some parents using private/voluntary services may be charged a fee. Unlike the data on daycare, data for early education measures the *numbers of children* attending and *not the number of places* and therefore describes usage and not actual provision (though these are closely related). Caution must also be exercised in interpreting the data as there is some double counting due to children attending more than one provider, either within the voluntary/private sector itself or also across the statutory sector (see notes to Table 11.4).

As can be seen in Table 11.4, the data is patchy. Despite problems with the Scottish data, the general trends across countries are similar. There has been a considerable increase in the number of children attending voluntary/private early education services in England, Scotland and Northern Ireland (no data for Wales). Chart 11.6 suggests a remarkable, almost fourfold increase in England in just three years. In Scotland and Northern Ireland it appears there has been a doubling in numbers of children attending early education.

The picture is more complex for statutory provision: Scotland and Northern Ireland show modest increases in the numbers of children attending nursery schools/classes, whereas England and Wales show modest decreases (see Charts 11.7 and 11.8). However, when the children attending are considered as a proportion of the whole population of children under five years, there is an apparent overall increase in provision (see Table 11.4). Thus, in 2001, some 90 per cent of children are thought to have attended some form of early education in England and 88 per cent in Scotland. In Wales some 79 per cent of 3- and 4-year-olds were attending statutory early education services in the year 2000

Table 11.4: Number of children under 5 in early education in the UK*, **

	1997	1998	1999	2000	(estimates) 2001
Private/voluntary					
England	***	***	95,100#	364,800	386,200
Wales	***	***	***	***	***
Scotland##	***	14,623	20,458	***	26,040
Northern Ireland	***	1,945	3,407	3,957	***
Nursery schools/classes					
England	713,509	720,478	722,004	713,600	709,600
Wales	55,260	54,720	54,547	54,405	***
Scotland##	***	63,072	66,719	***	72,797
Northern Ireland	11,066	11,371	12,329	13,921	***
% Under 5 in early education####					
England	56	57	58§	88§§	90§§
Wales	74	75	77	79	***
Scotland##	***	***	83§§	***	88§§
Northern Ireland	***	***	***	***	***

* Pre-school education provision in special schools, private/independent schools and hospitals is excluded.
** For England, Scotland and Northern Ireland, there may be double counting as children may attend more than one provider. Thus percentages of total population receiving education likely to be overestimates for these countries.
*** No data available.
# 4-year-old children only.
Scottish data is not comparable across the years; in 1999 results are based on incomplete response and in 2001 a new Annual Integrated Census was introduced. In addition, Scottish data is not easily comparable with other countries because children start primary school at age 5 and entry to school is once per year in August; children not aged 5 in the August have to defer entry for one whole year. Thus Scottish data will include some children aged 5 and over.
Mainly children aged 3 to 4 years, but can include some aged 5. Excludes provision in private voluntary sector unless otherwise stated.
§ In 1999, a further 15 per cent of the 4-year-old population were in education in the private/voluntary sector in England.
§§ Includes private/voluntary provision for 3- and 4-year-old children.

(no data available on private/voluntary attendance). Due to problems of double counting, the overall proportions are likely to be overestimates for England and Scotland.

Assessing the childcare strategy

In relation to expanding daycare, the childcare strategy appears to have been at least partially successful.

Chart 11.6: Numbers of children aged 5 or under in private/voluntary early education in England, Scotland and Northern Ireland

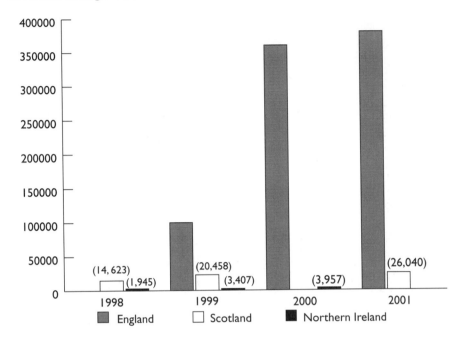

Chart 11.7: Numbers of children aged under 5 in nursery schools/classes in the statutory education sector in England

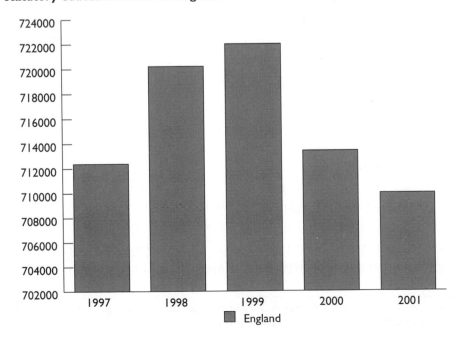

Chart 11.8: Numbers of children aged 5 or under in nursery school/classes in the statutory education sector in Wales, Scotland and Northern Ireland

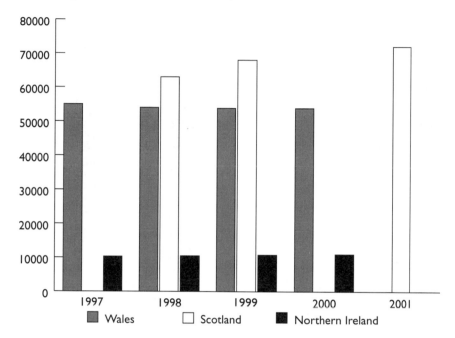

There have been increases in:
- OOSC provision across all countries
- daycare nursery places in England, Wales and Northern Ireland (Scotland no data[5])
- holiday schemes in England and in Northern Ireland (no data for Wales and a possible decline in Scotland)
- childminder places in Northern Ireland only
- playgroup places in Northern Ireland only.

There have been decreases in:
- childminder places in England and Wales (no data for Scotland)
- playgroup places in England, Wales and Scotland.

Potentially, the improvements in OOSCs, daycare nurseries and holiday schemes provide more opportunities for parental employment. The strategy has, however,

---

[5] Analysis of the Integrated Census is not complete and as yet there is no disaggregation of nursery daycare and early education nursery provision.

been unable to halt the decline in childminder and playgroup places, except in Northern Ireland. It is likely that the additional funds available to Northern Ireland through the EU Peace Programme is responsible for this. In 1999, £4.3 million of funds were used to set up 100 PlayCare out-of-school clubs (Ferguson *et al.*, 1999).

In relation to the decline in childminding, arguably the childcare strategy is a victim of its own success. Mooney *et al.* (2001) suggest that anecdotal evidence shows how women are taking up other forms of employment due to the overall expansion in childcare provision. They also suggest other reasons for the decline:

- a reduction in the pool of women who could do childminding
- the low pay and low status of childminding
- the increasing professionalisation of childminding
- the level of bureaucracy surrounding registration and inspection
- a lack of support while doing the job.

However, childminder provision may improve in the future following the introduction of a recruitment campaign and start-up funding for new child-minders launched in 2000.

In relation to the decline in playgroup provision, this results partly from the expansion in public early years education which has forced both sectors to compete to provide for children aged 3–4 years.[6] Simultaneously, however, there has been a rapid expansion in the numbers of children attending private/voluntary sector early education services, much of which is likely to be provided by playgroups. It is difficult to interpret these apparently competing trends.

Clearly, the childcare strategy has been very successful in expanding early education in the private/voluntary sector in all countries (except Wales where

Table 11.5: Attendance of children aged 3 and 4 in early education in England for a specific week

1997		*1998*		*1999*		*2000*	
Age 3	Age 4	Age 3	Age 4	Age 3	Age 4	Age 3	Age 4
88%	96%	91%	98%	90%	99%	91%	98%

Source: Blake *et al.*, 2001

---

[6] Playgroups began to decline under the previous nursery voucher scheme as a result of the introduction of competition with early education providers. This decline has continued under the national childcare strategy for the same reasons.

there is no data). Importantly, this apparent expansion does not necessarily free up parents to enter the labour market, as this service is mainly part-time and is tied to the school day and calendar. It is therefore unlikely that this provision, on its own, will improve opportunities for parental employment. However, there are also problems with the data as there is double counting within early education provision and potentially also across daycare and early education provision. Children can attend more than one provider and this potentially exaggerates the level of expansion in the private/voluntary sector.[7] Survey evidence of parents of 3- and 4-year-old children in England does, however, corroborate the administrative data for England. Attendance for 3-year-olds has increased from 88 per cent in 1997 to 91 per cent in 2000. For 4-year-olds it has increased from 96 per cent to 98 per cent over the same time period (Blake *et al.*, 2001).

Overall, it remains difficult to get a true comparative picture across the four countries in the UK using available administrative data. It is also difficult to understand the level of demand for services and how service use might vary for minority ethnic groups.[8] In order to get a better understanding of demand it is necessary to rely on research evidence.

Research evidence on childcare

Recent research shows that the supply of places does not meet demand. Just under half of all daycare providers (excluding childminders) have waiting lists for places (Callender, 2000). According to the Daycare Trust (2001), there are also insufficient places for children aged under three years, for parents who work shifts or outside normal hours and for minority ethnic groups. In 2000, participation in early education among 3- and 4-year-olds was lower among minority ethnic groups than white groups (91 per cent compared to 95 per cent) (Blake *et al.*, 2001). Also, parents with disabled children are less likely to have access to mainstream childcare services, with demand for places outstripping supply (Childcare Commission Report, 2001, p. 79). Overall, there is little research on the childcare needs of minority ethnic groups and of families with disabled children.

---

[7] Scotland has attempted to tackle some of these problems by introducing a new integrated census which standardises the data collected across daycare and education sectors.
[8] There are also gaps in the data and there is no information on services for children over the age of 8 years, except in Northern Ireland.

It is also important to consider not just the level of provision, but how the type of services might affect demand. It has been found that a lack of flexible care in the form of childminders and out-of-school places actually suppresses demand (Callender, 2000; White and Lissenburgh, 2001). Certainly, in 1999 the most common form of care used by households in England and Wales was informal care (mainly provided by grandparents) as opposed to formal care (La Valle *et al.*, 2000, Table 2.6). In addition, while the numbers of parents in receipt of financial support for childcare costs have risen under the new childcare tax credit scheme from 79,600 in November 1999 to 121,000 in August 2000, these figures are still low, representing only 11 per cent of families in receipt of the Working Families Tax Credit to which the childcare tax credit is attached[9] (Inland Revenue, 2000). This might suggest that the childcare subsidies have a weak potential to generate demand.

This research highlights the importance of convenience, flexibility and quality in childcare provision. The government is attempting to tackle these issues by providing integrated childcare and educational services at the neighbourhood level in England through Early Excellence Centres and Neighbourhood Nursery Centres (DfES, 2001b, 2001c). The Early Excellence Centres pilot initiative was outlined in the 'Excellence in Schools' White Paper in July 1997 and therefore predates the National Childcare Strategy. By December 1999 some 29 centres had been established offering a mix of the following services:

- high quality and integrated early education and childcare
- family support, involvement and learning
- adult education
- health services
- practitioner training
- dissemination of good practice.

Early Excellence Centres are linked to local Early Years Development and Childcare Partnerships and a distinguishing feature is their emphasis on child and adult education. While they are not targeted programmes, the majority cover catchment areas within 20 per cent of the most deprived wards in England within rural, urban and inner city settings (Bertram and Pascal, 2001). The Early Excellence Centres initiative is subject to a detailed local and national evaluation,

---

[9] Receipt of Working Families' Tax Credit (WFTC) is a precondition for receiving the childcare tax credit, but not all families receiving WFTC will be eligible for this support with childcare costs.

with full results becoming available in September 2003. Early results, however, suggest that they are developing a 'one stop shop' concept, with parents and children accessing health, social support, education and care services and that they are well placed to tackle child poverty and social exclusion (Bertram and Pascal, 2001).

The Neighbourhood Nursery Centres initiative was announced by the Department for Education and Skills at the beginning of 2001 and is part of a wider Neighbourhood Childcare Initiative. This initiative is a targeted programme to provide the following new services in 20 per cent of the most disadvantaged areas in England by 2004:

- childminding – 25,000 new places
- out-of-school hours childcare – 50,000 new places
- Neighbourhood Nursery Centres – 45,000 new full-time daycare places.

There is an expectation that the new Neighbourhood Nursery Centres will provide integrated early education, daycare and family support services and will establish links with Early Excellence Centres in their neighbourhoods. Both the Neighbourhood Childcare Initiative and Neighbourhood Nursery Centres Initiative form part of the government's broad strategy to deal with child poverty and social exclusion by providing opportunities for parental employment and by providing early education and support for children to improve their life chances (DfES, 2001e). Wales also plans to develop similar integrated services within 'Children's Centres' in the near future (National Childcare Strategy Task Force, 2001).

These are important developments for disadvantaged families. Alongside these targeted programmes, attempts are also being made to encourage the private/voluntary sectors to provide multiple, fully integrated services in all communities. For example, daycare nurseries are encouraged also to provide out-of-school care and pre-school education. Yet all this falls short of calls made by the Childcare Commission to provide a fully integrated service via a Children's Centre in *every* neighbourhood. Consequently, many parents will continue to face fragmented services in different institutional settings which operate different opening times. Indeed, recent evidence shows that mothers, and particularly lone mothers, still face significant barriers to return to work as a result of a lack of good quality, convenient and affordable childcare (Childcare Commission Report, 2001; La Valle *et al.*, 2000; Finch and Gloyer, 2000).

Conclusion

This chapter has provided baseline data on childcare provision across the four countries of the UK using administrative data. Since the advent of the National Childcare Strategy considerable progress has been made in expanding some forms of daycare provision (mainly OOSCs) and in expanding private/voluntary sector early education provision. However, early education is not the same as daycare, though government spokespersons tend *not* to make the distinction in their drive to demonstrate the success of the strategy. We still have a split system between early education and childcare (Moss, 2001). In part this is evidenced by the different data collection methods across these sectors. Scotland leads the way, however, in introducing an Integrated Census which standardises data collection methods on daycare and early education by counting the numbers of children in each sector. Scottish data is also able to distinguish between the type of provider and the actual kinds of services offered which could include out-of-school care, holiday schemes and early education being provided by playgroups or nurseries. Thus it recognises the increasing diversification of services across providers. However, data on childminding was subsequently not collected. Even so, Scotland may provide a better model for the future.

12 Teenage Pregnancy and Teenage Motherhood

Sharon Tabberer

Key statistics:

- The teenage (under 20) fertility rates for England and Scotland are broadly similar at 29 per 1,000, but higher in Wales at 35 and lower in Northern Ireland at 26.
- The UK has the highest rate of teenage conceptions in Western Europe.

Key trends:

- The teenage conception rate is in decline in England and Wales and Scotland but on the increase in Northern Ireland.

Key sources:

- Population Trends
- *Teenage Pregnancy*, England
- *Myths and Reality*, Northern Ireland
- Welsh Assembly
- Health Education Board for Scotland Research Centre

Introduction

This chapter examines the evidence relating to those young women in the UK who become parents while they are under 20. It examines variations in the conception rate within the UK, compares our rate with that in other countries and examines the associations between the teenage conceptions and teenage parenthood including ethnicity, poverty and deprivation.

Teenage conceptions, abortion, births

Data on teenage pregnancy in England and Wales is readily available through the Office of National Statistics. This data is usually running two years behind, with the most recent data being 1999. This was the same year as the government published its report *Teenage Pregnancy* (SEU, 1999b), which marked the start of the current concern over this issue. While the report provided an action plan only for England, a similar approach seeking a reduction in the teenage pregnancy rate has been adopted in Wales through its Sexual Health Strategy (Welsh Assembly, 2000). In Northern Ireland *Myths and Reality: Teenage pregnancy and parenthood* was published in 2000 (DHSSPS, 2000a). The only country in the UK which has so far not set out its plans to reduce teenage pregnancy in a strategic document is Scotland, although this is currently under consideration.

The ONS publishes data on underage conceptions by age of conception. It can be seen in Table 12.1 that conceptions at all ages in England and Wales fluctuated over the period, but fell between 1998 and 1999. Notably, there was:

- a 7 per cent fall in the underage conception rate (conception per 1,000 girls aged under16).
- a 4 per cent fall in the under-18 conception rate
- a 3 per cent fall in the under-20 conception rate.

Although this data covers a period before new national or local initiatives were up and running, the higher profile of teenage pregnancy at this time might be one reason for the fall in teenage conceptions. The government intends to reduce the teenage pregnancy rate in England by a half by 2010.

In Scotland the Information and Statistical Division collects data on teenage pregnancies. Data here is collected in a different format to that used by the ONS: it is based on year of discharge rather than year of conception and includes miscarriages requiring hospital treatment. Here, the government's headline target,

Table 12.1: Conceptions and births, by age of woman, England and Wales

	1990	1991	1992	1993	1994	1995	1996	1997	1998	1999	2000
Age at conception (1,000s)											
Under 16	8.1	7.5	7.2	7.3	7.8	8.1	8.9	8.3	8.5	7.9	
Under 18	44.8	40.1	37.6	35.8	36.1	37.9	43.5	43.4	44.1	42.0	
Under 20	113.3	101.6	93.4	87.2	85.4	86.6	94.9	96.0	101.6	98.8	

Source: ONS (2001e)

Table 12.2: Teenage pregnancy* by age of mother at conception, year ending 31 March, Scotland

Year	Number in age group			Age group specific rates**		
	13–15	16–19	13–19	13–15	16–19	13–19
1991	796	10,763	11,559	8.8	74.8	49.2
1992	722	10,399	11,121	8.2	77.0	49.8
1993	795	9,468	10,263	9.0	73.4	47.3
1994	728	8,914	9,642	7.9	72.3	44.8
1995	846	8,319	9,165	8.9	68.9	42.4
1996	819	8,240	9,059	8.5	68.5	41.8
1997 (revised)	927	8,564	9,491	9.7	70.8	43.9
1998 (revised)	814	8,,883	9,697	8.7	71.2	44.5
1999 (revised)	841	9,156	9,997	9.0	72.0	45.4
2000*** (provisional)	690	8,622	9,312	7.3	67.4	41.9

* Includes pregnancies resulting in a delivery, miscarriage or therapeutic abortion requiring hospital inpatient or day case treatment.
** Rates per 1,000 females in age group in each age group in each year.
*** Information for year ending 31 March 2000 is incomplete due to a shortfall in data from Glasgow Royal Maternity Hospital and The Queen Mother's Hospital, Glasgow.
Source: ISD (2001)

which was set in 1994 and reaffirmed in the White Paper of 1999 (Scottish Office, 1999) is to reduce the pregnancy rate among 13–15-year-olds by 20 per cent between 1995 and 2010.

The most notable change in Scotland, particularly compared to the data from England and Wales, is with the outcome of pregnancy, with an increasing percentage of pregnancies resulting in abortions or miscarriages. However, because miscarriages and abortions are not disaggregated we do not know whether more women are choosing abortions or experiencing miscarriage.

Recently, the ONS (Griffiths and Kirby, 2000) published an article that brings together data from Scotland with that from England and Wales and allows comparisons to be made between the countries. The data used within the article compares the conception rates over the 1990s for women aged under 18. It does not include miscarriages within the abortion figures and seeks to use the same data sources, although there are some exceptions.

This analysis found:

- Wales had the highest under-18 conception rate in 1992 to 1997 and Scotland the lowest.
- England had the highest percentage of conceptions leading to abortion and Wales the lowest.
- Of the regions in England, those in the north had higher rates of conception

than the Great Britain average, with a lower percentage leading to abortion than the Great Britain average.

- The under-18 conception rate was higher for London than in the other southern regions, with a markedly higher percentage leading to abortion than the Great Britain average.

The one area of the UK missing from this analysis is Northern Ireland. Here, the target for reducing teenage pregnancy was set in 1996 (DHSSPS, 1996) with the aim of a reduction in teenage pregnancies of 10 per cent by 2002. The Department for Health, Social Services and Public Safety's *Myths and Reality: Teenage pregnancy and parenthood* (DHSSPS, 2000a) outlines the strategy for achieving this and points out differences between the rest of the UK and there. In particular, the age of consent for sexual intercourse is 17 years rather than 16, and the 1967 Abortion Act does not cover Northern Ireland. Unlike in the rest of the UK, the teenage pregnancy rate in Northern Ireland continues to be calculated for those under 20. This rate has remained fairly consistent throughout the 1990s. However, unlike the rest of the UK, a steep rise was evident in conceptions for those aged between 15 and 17.

More recent data from Northern Ireland (DHSSPS, 2001) indicates that Northern Ireland is unlikely to meet its targets because, after a fall in the early 1990s, the percentage of teenage births has increased slightly. Again this has been attributed largely to a rise in the number of 16-year-olds giving birth and a fall in 17-, 18- and 19-year-olds. The birth rate is falling in Northern Ireland, as in the rest of the UK, but the percentage of teenage births has shown a slight rise from 15.5 in 1995 to 17.4 in 1999 (DHSSPS, 2000a).

Despite the 1967 Abortion Act not being in force within Northern Ireland, it is accepted within *Myths and Reality* (DHSSPS, 2000a) that both spontaneous and induced abortions do occur. For example, in 1998, 305 women under the age of 20 travelled to England for abortions. Furthermore, this is likely to be an underestimate, as women may not want to give their home address.

The age-specific fertility rates for the under-20s vary within the countries of the UK (see Table 12.3). They are lowest in Northern Ireland at 26.1 per 1,000 women aged 15–44 and highest in Wales at 35.2.

Table 12.3: Fertility rates (per 1,000) of mothers under 20, 2000

	England	Wales	Scotland	Northern Ireland
Fertility rate	28.8	35.2	29.1	26.1

Source: ONS (2001e)

Variations by ethnicity

Generally data comparing teenage pregnancy across ethnic minority groups is sparse. This was noted within the *Teenage Pregnancy* report for England; one consequence of this has been a concentration upon ethnicity as an area for future research.

The most recent analysis of teenage births by ethnicity was that undertaken by Berthoud (2001) who, in the absence of ethnicity data on live births and abortions, used the Labour Force Survey. Working retrospectively on the data, he looked at the age of mothers and children living with them at the time of the survey to calculate any trends. Using this method he found that:

- teenage motherhood is more common among Caribbean, Pakistani and especially Bangladeshi women than among white women
- young Indian women are less likely than white women to have a baby before they are 20
- the rates of teenage births among white and Caribbean women are stable
- there has been a marked decline in early parenthood in South Asian communities in Britain.

Table 12.4: Teenage birth rates per 1,000 by ethnic group, by date of observation

	1976–1982	1983–1989	1990–96
White	27	29	31
Caribbean	46	40	47
Indian	22	17	7
Pakistani	62	41	30
Bangladeshi	83	93	53
(number of observations)	(12)	(92)	(80)
Other	38	26	23

Source: Berthoud (2001)

International variations

Comparative data on teenage pregnancy, teenage births and abortions are difficult to find. Despite promising data collection exercises being under way, gaps in information from some countries and differing bases of analysis make any comparison problematic.

For example, WHO has devised a database of health indicators across Europe, which includes data on teenage conceptions, births and abortions. However, this database does not contain information from all the countries for all years, notable exceptions being France, the UK and Spain on various parameters. Similar problems exist with the information available from the EU using Eurostat. These problems in comparative data were highlighted in the *Teenage Pregnancy* report (SEU, 1999b). Kane and Wellings (1999) found in their comparative research that teenage pregnancy rates in the UK and France were increasing until the early 1970s, when they began to fall sharply. This fall was, however, not sustained in the UK.

The most recent comparative international analysis has been the *League Table of Teenage Births in Rich Nations* compiled by UNICEF (2001a). This shows that the UK has the highest rate of teenage births in Western Europe, and among industrialised countries its rate is less only than that of the USA (see Chart 12.1).

The report also explores the relationship between poverty and teenage pregnancy. It notes that on average, in all countries, teenage mothers are twice as likely to be living in poverty compared to other teenagers. However, there are variations between countries. There is a strong likelihood of teenage mothers living in poverty in later life in some countries (Belgium, France, Germany, the Netherlands and Denmark) and not in others (Austria). This finding, along with the evidence that even those teenagers within the most affluent areas of the UK have a higher birth rate than the average for the Netherlands or France, leads to the suggestion that teenage pregnancy is susceptible to policy interventions. The report goes on to note that any particular model for intervention may not be transferable from country to country, bearing in mind the wider context. However, sex education that enables young people to make informed choices does seem critical in those countries that have succeeded in reducing their rates.

A report looking at the outcomes of teenage motherhood in Europe (Berthoud and Robson, 2001) has found a systematic link between age of childbirth and poverty. This was associated with educational disadvantage – the

Chart 12.1: Under-20 birth rate (1998)

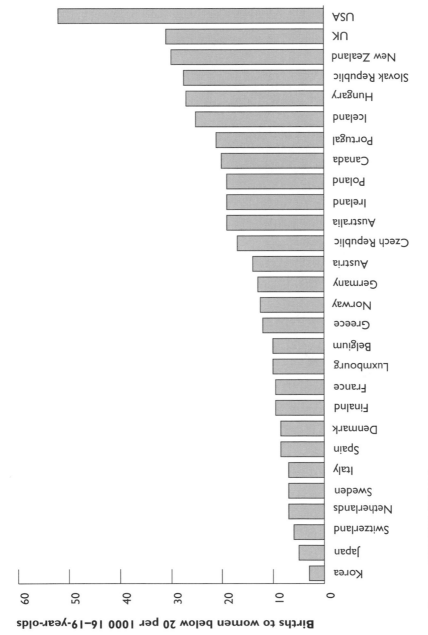

Births to women below 20 per 1000 16–19-year-olds

USA	
UK	
New Zealand	
Slovak Republic	
Hungary	
Iceland	
Portugal	
Canada	
Poland	
Ireland	
Australia	
Czech Republic	
Austria	
Germany	
Norway	
Greece	
Belgium	
Luxembourg	
France	
Finland	
Denmark	
Spain	
Italy	
Sweden	
Netherlands	
Switzerland	
Japan	
Korea	

Source: UNICEF (2001b)

younger the mother at first birth, the fewer qualifications she had. Such a disadvantage could in turn be linked to a higher probability of lone parenthood, which might lead to a lack of family employment and thereby to poverty. There was also a direct correlation between poverty and the age at which she had her first child, regardless of educational achievement. This was particularly notable in those countries (such as the UK) where childbearing at a young age is exceptional and less so in those countries where childbearing at a young age is relatively normal. This suggests that, regardless of other influences, having a child at a young age is likely to result in deprivation.

Teenage pregnancy and associated factors

Research in the UK has associated teenage pregnancy with certain groups being seen as 'vulnerable' (Meyrick and Swann, 1998), and so thought to be 'in danger' of becoming pregnant. These have included young people (Roberts, 2000):

- living in deprived areas
- who do not attend school
- who are looked after by local authority
- who are homeless
- who are the children of young parents.

This work reflects that of Kiernan (1995) who, using data from the National Child Development Study, found that women who become parents at an early age were more likely to have had a mother who was a teenage mother herself. Furthermore, while the experience of poverty as a child was more likely to lead to young motherhood, teenage mothers were also more likely to experience disadvantaged outcomes (Hobcraft and Kiernan, 1999).

The Social Exclusion Unit report (SEU, 1999b) on teenage pregnancy in England found that the poorest areas in England have teenage conception and birth rates up to six times higher than the most affluent areas. They also found, however, that variation existed between areas that suffered from approximately equivalent deprivation. The variation in teenage conceptions could therefore not be solely due to deprivation.

In the other countries of the UK similar area variations have been detected. In the report into teenage pregnancy in Northern Ireland (DHSSPS, 2000a), it was noted that those areas experiencing higher rates of teenage pregnancy were also those recognised as areas of deprivation.

The Health Education Board for Scotland, in a briefing paper designed to inform the future strategy, notes the link between deprivation and teenage pregnancy. It pays particular attention to the association between deprivation and pregnancy outcome, with those from the least deprived areas being more likely to opt for an abortion and those from the most deprived being more likely to continue their pregnancies to delivery.

The Sexual Health Strategy for Wales notes a similar trend to that of the rest of the UK, with a higher rate than for the rest of Europe. It goes on to look at data from the 1991 National Survey of Sexual Attitudes and Lifestyles, which found differences in sexual behaviour between men living in rural and urban areas. Notably, those living in urban areas were five times more likely to report having had sex before the age of 16 than those in rural areas. The strategy for Wales also demonstrates how Wales differs from the rest of the UK, with Wales having an overall conception rate lower than England in 1997, but a consistently higher rate for teenage conceptions.

Teenage motherhood and associated factors

Teenage pregnancy has been associated with increased risk of poor social, economic and health outcomes for both mother and child (NHS Centre for Reviews and Dissemination, 1997). Particular outcomes have been identified, including (SEU, 1999b):
- low birth weight babies
- high infant mortality
- high infant and childhood mortality
- high hospital admissions for children
- high rates of post-natal depression
- low take-up of breastfeeding.

In order to address these outcomes, special emphasis has been placed upon support for young mothers. This has been identified as crucial in the Avon Longitudinal Study of Pregnancy and Childhood (Meadows and Dawson, 1996), which sought to identify factors affecting the health and development of teenage mothers and their children from early pregnancy until the child reached 30 months, and what might help them.

Other research into the support needs of young mothers, this time in relation to education and training, has been funded by the European Union (Dawson,

2000). This study found that a variety of education models existed within the UK, with home tuition and full-time schooling the most favoured in Northern Ireland, home tuition most common in Wales, part-time schooling more common in Scotland and special centres known as pupil referral units being preferred in England.

In order to investigate the situation in Northern Ireland further, Save the Children funded research looking into access to education of school-age mothers (Save the Children, 1996). This research was commissioned in response to concern about the level and type of education received by young mothers in Northern Ireland particularly in relation to the United Nations Convention on the Rights of the Child (Davies *et al.*, 1996). It demonstrated that, while young mothers were keen to continue their education, they could be prevented from doing so by an education system that failed to adequately cater for their needs. This report has been cited in *Myths and Reality* (DHSSPS, 2000) and formed the basis for the recommendations in this document on the education of school-age mothers.

This concentration on the support needs of teenage mothers suggests that young motherhood might not necessarily be a negative experience for both mother and child if other factors are in place. In the Save the Children's report into young mothers and the transition to adulthood (Horgan, 2001), young motherhood was accompanied by the development of a variety of skills such as parenting skills and budgeting skills. These skills can successfully be developed with support on issues to do with money, housing, parenting skills, childcare, education, employment, social life and transport.

Conclusion

With the increased political concern about teenage pregnancy better data on the subject has begun to emerge. In all countries except Northern Ireland the teenage pregnancy rate has begun to fall. However, the link between deprivation and teenage pregnancy remains. Yet this link is not a simple one because many factors can influence the chances of a conception occurring, a conception ending in a termination or birth, and successful teenage motherhood. The success of plans of the different countries within the UK to cut teenage pregnancy will depend as much on more detailed understanding of area, ethnic and family/household variations in teenage pregnancy as they will on better approaches to educational and related services targeted at the young.

The governments of the UK have developed various strategies to reduce the teenage pregnancy rate by up to a half through developing various new initiatives for both young people and young mothers. A reduction in the teenage conception rate is one of the key outcome indicators of the child poverty strategy (DWP, 2001b), it will therefore be interesting to see whether the reduction in 1999 is sustained.

13 The Environment and Children

Deborah Quilgars and Alison Wallace

Key findings:
- Children in lone parent and minority ethnic households and those on low incomes are particularly likely to live in poor housing.
- Neighbourhood dissatisfaction is associated with social housing, social class, region and household type (lone parents most dissatisfied).

Key trends:
- House conditions have improved over time, but lone parents and minority ethnic groups, relative to other households, are now more likely to live in poor housing.
- Children's use of public space has decreased since the 1970s.
- While pollution emissions decreased in the 1990s, traffic volume has tripled over the last 30 years.

Key sources:
- House condition surveys
- Survey of English Housing
- Environment Agency data
- Academic studies

Introduction

This chapter reviews the evidence of the link between environment and the well-being of children and young people in the UK. Four key environmental areas are examined:
- the nature of poor housing and its link with health
- poor neighbourhoods
- children's spatial mobility within their local environments

- the problem and effects of pollution.

While data are patchy, the available literature shows that some children are more likely to be living in poor environments than others. Trends by region and country, and over time, are reviewed wherever possible. Separate chapters examine child health (Chapter 5), unintentional injuries (Chapter 6), child homelessness (Chapter 14) and leisure, recreation and sport (Chapter 16), all of which are relevant to environment.

Poor housing

House conditions

The best data on housing conditions are found in the five-yearly country surveys commissioned by the governments/assemblies in England, Scotland, Wales and Northern Ireland. The surveys, however, use different measures, making comparisons between countries problematic. Since the mid-1990s, the Joseph Rowntree Foundation has funded a review of these data (The State of UK Housing). The most recent report examined data from the 1996 surveys in England, Scotland and Northern Ireland and preliminary data from the 1998 Welsh survey (Revell and Leather, 2000).

In 1996/98, there were 1,455,000 dwellings in the UK that were unfit for human habitation (England, Wales and Northern Ireland) or below a tolerable standard (Scotland) (Revell and Leather, 2000). This represented 6 per cent of the national stock. The levels of unfitness were highest in Wales, at 8.5 per cent of stock. Levels of disrepair were higher, including almost one-third of English stock (repairs needed of over £1,000), nearly three in ten dwellings in Scotland (repairs over £3,000), 14 per cent of dwellings in Northern Ireland (repairs over £3,000) and 23 per cent of dwellings in Wales (over £1,000). In England, unfit dwellings were mostly in urban areas, while in Scotland and Northern Ireland they were most often in rural areas. (There was no clear pattern in Wales.) Within England, unfitness was concentrated in the North, particularly the north-west, as well as in the industrial areas of the Midlands. The private rented sector had the highest proportion of dwellings in poor condition throughout the UK.

Household characteristics

Across the house condition surveys, low-income households were more likely to live in poor conditions (Revell and Leather, 2000). In England, around one in ten households with an income less than £4,000 per annum lived in unfit dwellings, compared to one in 25 of those with an income of over £24,000. In Scotland and Wales at least three-quarters of those living in unfit conditions or in a house with serious disrepair (in England and Northern Ireland about 50 per cent) had incomes below £12,000 per year.

Young and old single people and lone parents were the most likely to experience unfitness or live in dwellings below a tolerable standard (Table 13.1). The picture was less clear for dwellings in disrepair, but in England, for example, lone parent households and families with dependent children were among those most likely to experience poor conditions. A study of housing deprivation in England and Wales (Dale *et al.*, 1996) using the 1991 ONS Longitudinal Study found a high incidence of overcrowding among families with children: compared to 4 per cent of all households, 6 per cent of couples with children were overcrowded, 8 per cent of lone parents, 12 per cent of couples with children with other family members and 35 per cent of households with two or more families.

House condition data in England and Scotland (data was not available in Wales and Northern Ireland) revealed that minority ethnic groups, particularly Asian households, were more likely to live in poor conditions (Revell and Leather, 2000) (Table 13.2). An even higher incidence of overcrowding for Asian households was recorded by the ONS Longitudinal Study (Dale *et al.*, 1996): 57 per cent of Bangladeshi and 46 per cent of Pakistani households were overcrowded. Minority ethnic homeowners, as well as renters, have limited choice of housing (School of Planning and Housing, Edinburgh College of Art/Heriot Watt University, 1997). Locality studies examine minority ethnic groups' housing experiences in detail (eg, Karn *et al.*'s (2001) Manchester study).

In addition, one-off studies have shown that Gypsies/Travellers and asylum seekers are very likely to live in poor-quality housing. On inspection of 154 private sector dwellings of asylum seekers in England, Shelter (Garvie, 2001) found that 17 per cent were unfit for human habitation and 83 per cent of houses in multiple occupation were exposed to unacceptable fire risks. In Northern Ireland, Travellers are eight times as likely to live in overcrowded conditions as the general population, many having limited access to basic services such as water and electricity (NISRA, 2001b). The housing opportunities and

Table 13.1: Households living in poor conditions by type, UK

Household type	% in unfit dwellings	% with urgent repairs over £1,000*
England		
Lone adult under 65/60	7.6	36.2
Two adults	5.8	29.1
Lone parent	11.4	40.7
Family (small and large)	5.1	31.3
Three+ adults	8.7	42.6
Two pensioners	3.8	23.6
One pensioner	8.3	26.6
Northern Ireland		
Lone adult under 65/60	8.6	23.4
Two adults	3.3	17.1
Lone parent	3.9	15.6
Small family	2.6	19.0
Large family	2.3	18.9
Three+ adults	4.3	23.7
Two pensioners	7.5	13.5
One pensioner	10.5	14.6
Wales		
Lone adult under 65/60	14.0	21.0
Two adults	11.3	19.7
Lone parent	14.0	23.2
Small family	12.8	20.4
Large family	14.9	22.8
Three+ adults	13.9	19.3
Two pensioners	11.5	16.8
One pensioner	15.9	21.5
Scotland		
Lone adult under 65/60	1.5	6.2
Two adults	1.1	5.2
Lone parent	0.8	6.2
Small family	0.5	5.2
Large family	0.6	6.4
Three+ adults	1.3	6.1
Two pensioners	1.0	3.9
One pensioner	0.8	4.2

* Repair costs over £1,500 for Wales. Figures for England, Scotland and Northern Ireland are for 1996, figures for Wales are for 1993

Sources: Revell and Leather (2000), Table A5.4, p. 156.

Table 13.2: Households living in poor conditions by ethnic group, 1991, England and Scotland*

Ethnic origin of household head	Per cent in unfit dwellings	Per cent in dwellings with urgent repair costs over £1,000
England		
White	6.1	29.5
Black	7.8	30.6
Asian	12.5	45.6
Other	15.2	44.8
Scotland		
White	1.0	5.3
Black	–	7.8
Asian	2.2	13.4
Other	–	6.6

* Data on ethnic origin not available for Wales and Northern Ireland.
Sources: Revell and Leather (2000), Table A5.9, p. 160.

conditions for Roma and Sinti are generally known to be poor Europe-wide (Organisation for Security and Co-operation in Europe, 2000).

Time trends

House conditions in the UK have improved steadily over time, although the degree of improvement is different for different conditions (Leather and Morrison, 1997). In England, unfitness showed a small reduction from 8.8 per cent of stock in 1986 to 7.2 per cent in 1996. In Wales, unfitness reduced from 19.5 per cent to 13.3 per cent over the period 1986 to 1991 (and to 8.5 per cent in occupied stock in 1998). Northern Ireland saw an improvement from 11 per cent of stock in 1987 to 7.3 per cent in 1996. Finally, in Scotland dwellings below a tolerable standard fell from 4.4 per cent in 1991 to 1.0 per cent in 1996 (Revell and Leather, 2000).

Analysis of the ONS Longitudinal Study (Dale *et al.*, 1996) showed changes in housing deprivation over the period 1971 to 1991 for England and Wales (Table 13.3). Housing deprivation was defined as overcrowding (less than one room per person), lacking amenities (sharing or lacking inside WC or bath/shower) and/or sharing accommodation. Table 13.3 shows that on this measure over nine in ten (94 per cent) of households experienced no deprivation in 1991, compared to three-quarters (75 per cent) in 1971.

Table 13.3: Housing deprivation, residents, England and Wales

	1971	1981	1991
No deprivation	74.9	87.7	94.4
Overcrowding only	9.3	6.6	4.2
Shared accommodation only*	0.7	1.8	0.5
Not sole bath/ WC	9.7	2.2	0.4
> 1 indicator	4.9	1.4	0.4

* In 1981 shared accommodation was defined as shared access from the street. In 1971 and 1991 it was defined as self-contained accommodation (i.e., with the household's accommodation behind its own front door)
Source: Dale et al. (1996), Table 9.4.

While general standards have improved, it is important to note that some type of households have benefited from these improvements more than others. In England, lone parents and minority ethnic households, relative to all households, were more likely to be living in poor housing in 1996 than in 1991, whereas lone persons (younger and older) were less likely (DETR, 1998). The ONS study (Dale et al., 1996) also found that lone parents were twice as likely to be overcrowded than other households in 1991, compared to 1.5 times as likely in 1971.

European comparisons

Data on house conditions is difficult to compare across Europe due to definitional and collection differences. However, the EU collates some statistics on basic housing indicators (Ministry of the Environment, Finland, 2001). The most recent statistics for the UK, however, include England only.[1] England had a higher proportion of older houses (built before 1919) than other European countries (except Denmark and France), and one of the lowest levels of house building since 1980 at 13 per cent of stock (Germany and Sweden being slightly lower). England fared well on the proportion of dwelling stock having a bath/shower (Table 13.4) but performed less well on central heating, with only Belgium and Eire having fewer dwellings with central heating among countries with a similar climate. Space standards in

---

[1] House conditions surveys in the UK show that Wales and Scotland have higher levels of pre-1919 stock than England (with Northern Ireland having slightly lower levels). Figures for central heating are very similar throughout the UK (Revell and Leather, 2000).

Table 13.4: Bath/shower and central heating in dwelling stock, Europe

	Years	Bath/shower, %	Years	Central heating, %
Austria[1]	1999	95	1999	83
Belgium	1994	92	1992	60
Denmark	2000	93	2000	98
Ex-DDR	1993	89	1998	832[2]
Finland	1999	91	1999	92
France	1999	98	1999	842[3]
Germany[4]	1993	98	1998	88[5]
Greece	1991	86	1991	45
Ireland	1998	93	1998	82
Italy	1995	99	1995	79
Luxembourg	1995	98	1995	90
Netherlands	1999	100	1999	89
Portugal	1998	95		n/a
Spain[6]	1996	98	1998	392[7]
Sweden	1995	99	1995	99
UK[8]	1996	99	1996	88

[1] Principal residences only and annual average for 1999. [2] Includes district and storey heating. [3] Includes individual and collective heating. [4] Excludes Ex-DDR. [5] Includes district and storey heating. [6] Based on households. [7] Includes individual and collective heating. [8] Based on England only.
Source: Ministry of the Environment, Finland (2001), Table 2.3, p. 26

English housing also compared unfavourably to most European countries (only Portugal and Finland having smaller floor areas).

The health effects of poor housing

The relationship between health and housing has been the subject of numerous individual studies, but no national data are available. Wilkinson (1999) provides a literature review of the area, and Thomson *et al.* (2001) have systematically reviewed the health effects of housing improvements.

Dampness and hydrothermal growth have been associated with children's health. Platt *et al.* (1989), using a random sample of 597 households (1,169 children) in social housing in Glasgow, Edinburgh and London, found a greater prevalence of respiratory symptoms, fever and headaches among children in houses with damp and/or mould growth, after controlling for other factors such as household income and smoking. Strachan (1988), looking at all tenures in Edinburgh (random sample of 873 children), found that children living in damp housing were three times as likely to have experienced wheeze in the past year, after controlling for other variables. Poor indoor air quality, more generally, gives rise to health risks, including radon, carbon monoxide, house dust mites and tobacco smoke (see later) (Raw and Hamilton, 1995).

Children are more likely to catch infectious diseases in overcrowded circumstances. A strong association exists between housing and childhood accidents (see Chapter 6), and flat dwelling reduces the opportunities for safe play for children (Burridge and Ormandy, 1993). Inaccessible and badly designed housing represents a particular barrier for disabled children, making moving around, playing and learning to look after oneself more difficult (Oldman and Beresford, 1998).

An analysis of the National Child Development Study (following a cohort from 1958 until 1991) concluded that childhood housing played a significant role in adult health outcomes (Marsh et al., 1999). Three housing variables increased the odds of ill health by 1991: living in non-self contained accommodation, past experience of homelessness and dissatisfaction with area. The odds of disability or severe ill health increased by 25 per cent if people suffered multiple housing deprivation.

While research is weak on the effects on health improvements, evidence suggests physical and mental health impacts (Thomson et al., 2001). Somerville et al. (2000) examined the impact of installing central heating on the health of children with asthma, finding that the frequency of all respiratory problems reduced significantly, and days lost from school dropped from a mean of 5.8 days in the previous three months to 1.6. Due to the evidence gaps, Communities Scotland and the Scottish Executive have funded the University of Glasgow to undertake a prospective, controlled study, of the health impacts of new social housing, over 2001 to 2006 (The Scottish Health Housing and Regeneration Research Project SHARP).

Poor neighbourhoods

Defining 'poor neighbourhoods' is not easy (Burrows and Rhodes, 1998). They are often associated with poor council estates, although tenure alone is not a sufficient guide to area deprivation (Lee and Murie, 1997). However, households with children are over-represented in social housing; in 1995/96, 28 per cent of residents in social housing were aged under 16, compared to 21 per cent in owner occupation and 18 per cent of private sector housing (Coles et al., 1998). The odds of lone parents being in social housing has particularly increased over the past few decades (Dale et al., 1996).

Governmental studies such as the Survey of English Housing and House Condition surveys provide some information on neighbourhood concerns. The best study (though only for England) on neighbourhood satisfaction used the 1994/95 Survey of English Housing and specially commissioned data from the 1991 census (Burrows and Rhodes, 1998). Table 13.5 shows that levels of

Table 13.5: Proportion of households with high levels of area dissatisfaction, England

Socio-demographic characteristics	% scoring 4 or more	Total number of households (1,000s)
All	9.7	19,198
Region		
London	14.0	2,699
South East	5.9	2,898
South West	5.8	1,995
Eastern	5.3	2,309
East Midlands	7.9	1,540
West Midlands	10.4	2,017
Yorkshire and Humberside	10.8	2,038
North East	18.1	980
North West	12.9	2,764
Social class of head of household		
I	4.5	1,351
II	7.1	5,048
IIIN	10.1	2,780
IIIM	10.9	5,295
IV	12.5	2,800
V	14.0	1,063
Other	10.3	909
Ethnicity of head of household		
White	9.7	18,319
Black	9.5	329
Indian	9.3	242
Pakistan/Bangladeshi	13.0	136
Other	10.4	216
Household structure		
Couple, no dependent children	8.5	7,002
Couple, with dependent children	9.1	4,694
Lone parent	22.2	1,101
Large adult household	8.8	1,183
Single male	11.1	2,241
Single female	8.3	3,024

Source: Burrows and Rhodes (1998), Table 2.4, p. 9

dissatisfaction were highest in social housing, and that lone parent families were significantly more likely than all other types of household to be dissatisfied. A clear social class gradient and regional variations in area dissatisfaction were also observed (with households in the north-east, north-west, Yorkshire and Humberside and London being less satisfied). There were some differences by ethnicity.

Mumford (2000), focusing on low income areas in east London, also found high levels of neighbourhood dissatisfaction. Between two and three in ten of respondents were dissatisfied with their area, compared to the national Survey of English Housing average of 13 per cent. Concerns for children included safety, drugs, pollution, lack of facilities, lack of play opportunities in flats and paedophiles.

The English House Condition survey (DETR, 1998) used surveyors to identify localities providing 'poor living conditions'. This definition included areas where 10 per cent of dwellings were seriously defective and there were problems such as vacant buildings, litter or vandalism. While 7 per cent of all couples with children were experiencing poor living conditions, twice as many (13 per cent) lone parents were doing so and 10 per cent of households with infants. A high proportion (19 per cent) of minority ethnic households, and unemployed households (18 per cent) were also living in such localities.

Children are being increasingly consulted about their localities, reflecting their genuinely high levels of concern with the local (and global) environment (Adams and Ingham, 1998). The practice of involving young people in community regeneration projects pays particular dividends for the community, providing a sense of ownership of the projects and confidence that is likely to endure beyond the scope of the immediate investment (Matthews, 2001). A project looking at play and leisure facilities for Bangladeshi children in Camden involved young people aged 11–18 years as researchers to canvas views of children aged 8–12 years (Howarth, 1999). Although the study centred on play and leisure opportunities, it provided an often poignant insight into the perceptions and sensibilities of this group of children that may have been missed through other surveys. The study found similar concerns as other young people over their ability to have safe, clean open spaces in which to play, free play activities and the importance of getting information and being consulted. It also found a desire for separate activities and spaces for boys and girls and highlighted their concerns about racism, community safety and their lack of confidence in the police.

A study on Cruddas Park in Newcastle (Speak, 2000) found that children had strong feelings about the physical layout and condition of their neighbour-hood, and had a strong spatial awareness of the area. Best places for them included the shopping centre, school and green areas, while worst places were low-rise flats and terraced housing with gardens (as more fires were started there). Young people have also been recently consulted in East Belfast about their neighbourhoods, identifying changes needed in areas of play and leisure, health, identity, information, training and jobs (Greater East Belfast Youth Strategy Group, 2001).

Robertson and Walford (2000) used children as surveyors (along with a small number of adults) to examine present land use and landscape issues in the UK; 1,037 children participated in surveying a stratified random sampling of 1 km square areas across the UK. The study found a stark contrast between the views of urban and rural 'surveyors': urban 'surveyors' had a great desire for change centring around housing developments, loss of green space, traffic, pollution and litter, recreation and aesthetics, while rural 'surveyors' wanted things to stay the same, preserving green spaces.

The only study to provide some time series data examined the longitudinal elements of the 1991 and 1996 Scottish House Condition Survey (Kearns and Parkes, 2001). Satisfaction with neighbourhood, home and access to facilities were found to have increased overall over between 1991 and 1996. However, in the older and less well-off council areas, there were more people with decreased rather than increased neighbourhood satisfaction, with council areas generally reporting an increase in 'disorder dislike' (which included child-related problems).

Children's use of public space

Children's use of public space has been the subject of detailed one-off studies, but no national data exists in any country. Chapter 16 reviews the evidence on opportunities for active play, which, along with the studies below, suggests that children's use of public space has generally decreased over time as a result of increased anxiety about traffic, as well as stranger-danger outside the home.

O'Brien *et al.* (2000) undertook a survey of 1,378 children (aged 10–14), and their parents, on how children use their local environment in a number of inner and outer London boroughs as well as a New Town (Hatfield). Table 13.6 shows that boys had greater freedom to roam and play outside more independ-ently than girls, with boys more likely to get around by bicycle and use parks. There were also gender differences in perceptions of risk of unsafe places, with

Table 13.6: Selected children's activities and perception of risk by gender and area

	Inner London		Outer London		New Town	
	Female (n=334)	Male (n=334)	Female (n=187)	Male (n=217)	Female (n=199)	Male (n=80)
Activities						
Child plays out without an adult	67%	84%	75%	87%	82%	93%
Visit to park in last week	35%	56%	51%	59%	37%	51%
Child rides bicycle on main road	30%	52%	46%	67%	56%	68%
Child allowed to cross the road	68%	78%	58%	67%	87%	80%
Perceptions of risk						
Feel there are unsafe places	42%	31%	44%	32%	42%	21%
Scared of unknown adults	61%	35%	63%	36%	58%	34%
Scared of young people	51%	46%	58%	49%	54%	47%

Source: O'Brien et al. (2000), Table 3, p. 269

the greatest difference in the New Town area. Some recent research, however, has suggested that the gender gap may be narrowing (Matthews et al., 2001). There were also differences in use of space by age: by the age of 14 the great majority were able to navigate the city freely.

Children from different ethnic backgrounds, and gender within this, were also found to use public space very differently. For example, in London, only 37 per cent of Tower Hamlets older Asian girls were allowed to play outside unaccompanied compared to 92 per cent of older Asian boys. Reasons for this included personal preference as well as fear, racism and parental restraint.

There were also some differences by type of locality, although these were not always consistent. More children were allowed to play on the street outside without an adult (as reported by children) in the New Town area (Table 13.6). Children talked about a harsher and more dangerous physical environment in inner London, with bins being set on fire, shopping trolleys being thrown off balconies and drug-taking in lift shafts. Observational work in New Town suggested that green spaces between home and road supported playing outside in the vicinity of children's homes.

O'Brien et al. (2000) compared their data to Mayer Hillman's of the 1970s and 1990s, finding evidence of a decrease in independent use of public space for 10–11 year olds, but little change for the older group (13–14 year olds). However, some aspects of use of the environment had changed. For example, whereas in

1970 94 per cent children walked to school unaccompanied, in 1998 only 47 per cent did (due to both an increase in being accompanied by a parent and increased car use). An increase in parental anxiety over children's safety in public space was also evident, with fewer parents allowing children out after dark, 6 per cent in 1990 and 2 per cent 1998.

Matthews and Limb (undated) and Matthews (2001) explored how young people (aged 9–16) in Northamptonshire used outdoor space (the 'street'). Less than a third of young people had never used street as a social venue; in summer over a third used it this way daily. Age was important as those over 14 used street space over five times a week to meet friends. However, for many under 10s, the street remained important. There were also differences by social class. For less affluent families the street was the main social forum, as a large proportion could not participate in other leisure and recreational activities. There was little gender difference in the extent to which the street was used (boys did use it slightly more). However, girls used the street for talking with friends while boys used it for informal sport. However, two-thirds of girls and more than a third of boys were afraid to be out alone. Young people living in rural areas highlighted a lack of appropriate services and transport, heightening feelings of boredom and isolation. The authors concluded that local neighbourhoods were still important cultural places for young people, but were always under threat of being reclaimed by adults.

A study of racist victimisation in Belfast, Cardiff, Glasgow and London demonstrated how racial harassment can lead to the loss of children's freedom to play in their local neighbourhood. Children also experienced racist harassment on the journey to and from, and at, school (Chahal and Julienne, 1999). In Northern Ireland, fears of 'the Troubles' are also likely to impact on children's use of public space.

Environment and pollution

The Environment Agency (2000) acknowledges that there are clear links between health and environmental pollution. The Department of Health Committee on the Medical Effects of Air Pollutants (1998) estimated that air pollution in urban areas contributes to 8,100 deaths and 10,500 hospital admissions for respiratory disease a year. Generally, children are more sensitive to pollutants than adults as they are still developing, have less ability to break chemicals down, eat, drink and breathe more for their weight, are more likely to eat things they should not, and also breathe closer to the ground (Friends of the Earth, www.foe.co.uk). Motor vehicle emissions are the main cause of air pollution (Royal Commission on Environmental Pollution, 1997), though pollution also comes from industry, household products and smoking.

Motor vehicle pollution

The volume of traffic on roads and in cities has continued to increase throughout the past three decades. Inner-city areas are most likely to experience high levels of traffic in their neighbourhoods, suggesting that poorer communities experience more air pollution (London Research Centre, 1997).

Many European studies have found a link between the prevalence of asthma and motor vehicle pollution in urban areas, though there is some inconsistency in research results (Burr, 1995). It is, however, generally agreed that pollution is likely to exacerbate existing asthma (Wilson, 1998). One study in Birmingham of children under the age of five found an association between hospital admission rates for asthma and living in an urban area with high traffic flow, particularly when living within 500 metres of a main road (Edwards et al., 1994). Lead poisoning (even at low levels) is known to cause problems with the neurological development of children (Needleman and Gatsonis, 1990).

Government data, however, suggests that vehicle emissions (including nitrogen dioxide, carbon monoxide and lead) have all reduced over the last decade in the UK (Table 13.7), partly as a result of the introduction of catalytic converters and lead-free petrol. Vehicle emission levels, however, vary within the UK. For example, within England and Wales, the north-west and London have the poorest air quality (nitrogen oxides), with the south-west having the best (Environment Agency, 2001).

Industrial pollution

The polluting effects of industrial activity are proven historically. However, evidence on the effects of recent industrial activity is less consistent. For example, a study in East Lancashire of children living within 9 km of a cement works found no significant increased prevalence of respiratory problems in those children compared to those living 20 km or further away (Ginns and Gatrell, 1996). In contrast, a study of 1,872 Merseyside school children found an increased prevalence of respiratory symptoms among those living within 2 km of docks unloading large quantities of coal, as compared to other areas of Liverpool (after controlling for other variables) (Braben *et al.*, 1994). A study looking at mining communities found that children in opencast communities were on average exposed to a small but significant additional amount of particulate matter (PM10) compared to children in control communities. While the overall prevalence and severity of some respiratory illnesses were largely similar in opencast and control communities, GP consultations for respiratory, skin and eye conditions were higher in opencast than in control communities (Pless Mulloli, 1999). A study of women living near landfill sites found that they were a third more likely to have babies with birth defects (cited in Friends of the Earth, www.foe.co.uk).

The annual dose of ultraviolet radiation that reaches the earth has risen by around 11 to 13 per cent over the period 1980 to 1997, in a large part caused by depletion of the ozone layer by chemical emissions. It is considered that the incidence of skin cancer will increase until 2055 despite steps put into place to reverse the trend (Environment Agency, 2001).

Household products

There is some evidence from the USA that chemicals known as PCBs and DDEs, found in inks, paints and electricity transformers act as hormone disrupters and suppress the immune system (though PCBs are no longer produced in Europe). In the USA, exposure of mothers to these chemicals has been shown to produce puberty 11 months earlier in their daughters (cited in Friends of the Earth, www.foe.co.uk). A group of chemicals that make plastic more flexible, phthalates, have also been put forward as having a possible link with asthma. These chemicals leak when chewed and are also present in PVC, in house dust and in food products. Links between childhood leukaemia and paternal exposure to solvents, paints and motor vehicle-related occupations, and between childhood nervous system cancers and paternal exposure to paints are also possible (cited in Friends of the Earth, www.foe.co.uk).

Passive smoking

ONS national survey data for England reveal that non-smoking secondary school children's exposure to passive smoking approximately halved between 1988 and 1998 – from a geometric mean of 0.96 ng/ml to 0.52 ng/ml (Jarvis *et al.*, 2000). This is explained by both the fall in the proportion of parents who are smokers

Table 13.7: Pollutant emissions from transport and other end users in the United Kingdom 1988–1998

	1988	1989	1990	1991	1992	1993	1994	1995	1996	1997	1998	% of total in 1998
Nitrogen oxides	1,000 Tonnes/Percentages											
All transport*	1,385	1,473	1,446	1,442	1,389	1,329	1,267	1,187	1,128	1,013	926	53
Non-transport end users**	1,249	1,310	1,306	1,211	1,183	1,079	1,030	958	932	822	827	47
All emissions	2,634	2,783	2,752	2,653	2,572	2,408	2,297	2,145	2,060	1,835	1,753	100
Carbon monoxide	1,000 Tonnes/Percentages											
All transport	4,859	5,056	4,883	4,781	4,532	4,223	3,955	3,656	3,357	3,838	3,519	74
Non-transport end users	2,032	2,005	1,804	1,821	1,739	1,507	1,408	1,283	1,288	1,252	1,239	26
All emissions	6,891	7,061	6,687	6,602	6,271	5,730	5,363	4,939	4,645	5,090	4,758	100
Lead	1,000 Tonnes/Percentages											
Road transport	3.1	2.6	2.2	2.0	1.7	1.5	1.3	1.1	0.9	0.8	0.6	57
Non-transport end users	0.6	0.5	0.5	0.5	0.6	0.5	0.5	0.4	–	0.5	0.4	43
All emissions	3.7	3.1	2.7	2.5	2.3	2.0	1.8	1.5	0.9	1.3	1.0	100

* "All transport" includes road transport, railways, civil aircraft and shipping.
** 'Non-transport end users' includes domestic, industry, commercial/public service, exports, and other emissions.

Source: DETR/ Scottish Executive and Welsh Assembly (2000), Table 2.8, p. 63

and the reduction of smoking in public places (see Chapter 19 for rates of smoking among children). As well as higher risks for perinatal and sudden infant death among the children of smokers, and of lower birth weight, there is also evidence of poorer respiratory health, increased risk of asthma and ear and throat problems from passive smoking (Smith and Phillips, 1996).

Conclusions

Data on house conditions are generally reliable, although they are not standardised by country. These national surveys, along with other data such as the ONS Longitudinal Study, demonstrate that certain 'types' of households are more likely to live in poor-quality housing, including lone parents, minority ethnic households and those on low incomes. While all households, including those with children, are more likely to be living in better-quality housing in the 1990s compared to the 1970s, lone parents and minority ethnic groups now live in worse housing *relative* to other groups. There are no national datasets available on the health effects of housing, and while individual academic studies are numerous, they do not allow causal links to be established. Nonetheless, the weight of evidence indicates that poor housing contributes to poor health, particularly higher rates of respiratory diseases.

Some data exists on neighbourhood satisfaction, for example within the Survey of English Housing. However, data is not available for all countries. Families with children are spatially concentrated in social housing, which is often, though not exclusively, associated with poor neighbourhoods. Area dissatisfaction is associated with household type, social class and region. Limited trend data suggests that overall satisfaction levels may have increased, but not for certain areas such as poor council estates.

A number of one-off studies suggest that children are now more restricted in movement within their environments than their predecessors, particularly in inner-city areas, and that age, gender and ethnicity are all related to freedom of movement. No national data, however, is available in this area.

Evidence also exists that suggests that children may suffer detrimental effects from pollution caused by traffic, industrial activities, household chemicals and smoking. Environment Agency and allied statistics show that some key emissions have fallen over the 1990s in the UK (despite regional differences), but ultraviolet radiation levels are increasing, and traffic volume continues to grow. ONS national survey data show a reduction in exposure to passive smoking among children.

14 Homeless Children

Anwen Jones

Key statistics:

- In 2000, 119,950 households were accepted as homeless in Great Britain.
- In the same year 12,694 households were presented as homeless in Northern Ireland.

Key trends:

- The number of homeless households in Great Britain peaked at 179,410 in the early 1990s and then gradually declined.
- More recently the number of homeless households has risen in all four countries of the UK.
- The number of households in temporary accommodation in England is at its highest since the early 1990s.

Key sources:

- Department of Transport, Local Government and the Regions
- Welsh Assembly Housing Directorate
- Scottish Housing Executive
- Northern Ireland Housing Executive
- Academic research

Introduction

This chapter is concerned with child homelessness in the UK. The chapter begins with a brief summary of the homelessness legislation and the protection this offers to children and young people. It then goes on to consider the extent of child homelessness and trends in homelessness figures in recent years in the UK as a whole and in the countries of the UK. The final part of the chapter presents an overview of the research evidence on the causes and consequences of child homelessness.

Homelessness legislation in the UK

Article 27 of the UN Convention on the Rights of the Child (United Nations, 1989) states that children have the right to the conditions of living necessary for their development. It also states that "States Parties, in accordance with national conditions and within their means, shall take appropriate measures to assist parents and others responsible for the child to implement this right and shall in case of need provide material assistance and support programmes, particularly with regard to nutrition, clothing and housing". In the UK, local authorities have a legal responsibility to accommodate families with children who are found to be statutorily homeless. The statutory definition of homelessness (used by local housing authorities when making decisions on applications for assistance) broadly states that a person or household is homeless if they:

- have no accommodation in the UK (for England and Wales the household is only homeless if they have no accommodation anywhere in the world) or
- have no accommodation which they can reasonably occupy (for example without threat of violence or abuse) or
- have nowhere to lawfully place a mobile home.

In order to be accepted for the main housing duty under the terms of the legislation, households must show that they are in priority need and have not made themselves homeless intentionally. They must usually prove that they have a local connection to the housing authority to which they are applying. Households with dependent children represent one of the main priority need categories, along with households containing a pregnant woman. In Scotland, all households which are believed to be homeless, whether in priority need or not, are eligible for temporary accommodation.

The position of young people

Until recently most single homeless young people aged 16 and 17 were not automatically accepted as being in priority need under the legislation, although there were exceptions. Young care leavers in Scotland have been accepted as in priority need and under the Housing (Northern Ireland) Order 1988 young people at risk of sexual or financial exploitation are deemed to be in priority need. More recently the position of young people in terms of their statutory rights to housing has improved in England and Wales. The Welsh Assembly has recently extended the priority need categories so that they now include 16- and 17-year-olds and young people aged between 18 and 21 who have spent any time in the care of a local authority or who are at particular risk of sexual or financial exploitation (Welsh Assembly, 2001d). In England the most recent version of the Homelessness Code of Guidance states that 16- and 17-year-olds and care leavers are likely to be at risk as a result of their age and circumstances and it is expected that local authorities would normally find them vulnerable. This position will be strengthened by a forthcoming Statutory Instrument.

The extent of child homelessness

While it is widely accepted that the number of households experiencing homelessness has increased in many European countries, there is no precise or generally accepted measure of the size and nature of the problem. At national level, targeted primary research on homelessness is uneven and lacks comparability (FEANTSA, 1998). Nevertheless, the European Observatory on Homelessness estimates that across the EU, 3 million people have no fixed home of their own and 15 million people live in sub-standard or overcrowded accommodation. Marsh and Kennett (1999) suggest two main reasons for the paucity of data. First, homelessness, and child homelessness in particular, is a politically sensitive issue. Housing is seen as a basic right and the presence of homeless families is an indication that the social system and/or government are failing in one of their key tasks. Statistical measures of homelessness, like those of other politically sensitive issues such as crime and unemployment, are socially negotiated and societies with different socio-political traditions are likely to come to very different understandings of the term. Second, research in England has demonstrated the existence of a considerable degree of local discretion in the interpretation of the legal framework. Whether a household is accepted as homeless by a local authority depends on the locality it finds itself in (Hoffman, 1996; Marsh and Kennett, 1999; Pawson, 2000).

The extent of child homelessness in the UK and the regions

The main statistical sources on the incidence of statutory homelessness in the UK are the returns submitted quarterly by local authorities to the Department of Transport, Local Government and the Regions, the Welsh Assembly Housing

Directorate, the Northern Ireland Housing Executive and the Scottish Executive. These returns provide information on applications and acceptances under the homelessness legislation, the main reason for homelessness and the use of temporary accommodation including bed and breakfast accommodation (B&B), registered social landlord accommodation, hostels, private sector leases and 'other' temporary accommodation. These returns represent the best available dataset on the incidence of family homelessness, but there are limitations. In England these statistics only measure the incidence of official homelessness, that is, households found to be homeless by the local authority. In Scotland, Wales and Northern Ireland, the homelessness returns record all homeless applications. As Quilgars (2001a) has noted, nothing is known of those households that do not present themselves to the local authority as homeless. The main limitation of the datasets when considering child homelessness is the fact that the returns only record the number of households with dependent children accepted as homeless, but not the number of children or other detailed information about the characteristics of the family. There are no official statistics for youth homelessness, although the government has recently commissioned research to produce them.

Trends over time

Homelessness acceptances in England, Scotland and Wales increased from the 1980s to the early 1990s, when total homelessness acceptances in the three countries peaked at 179,410 in 1992 (see Table 14.1). There were a number of reasons for the rise in homelessness in the UK and the rest of Europe during this period: the economic recession and the subsequent rise in home repossessions as well as the increased demand for housing from the rising number of newly formed households. In addition, since the early 1980s public investment in housing has decreased substantially in most of the 15 member states. In the UK, the situation was exacerbated by the diminishing stock of affordable housing to rent, both in the private sector and, as a consequence of the Right to Buy policy, in the social sector. Homelessness acceptances then gradually declined through most of the 1990s to a total of 117,001 in 1999; this figure increased slightly to 119,950 in 2000 (Wilcox, 2001). The pattern in Northern Ireland is rather different (see Table 14.2) – here homeless presentations remained relatively constant through the 1990s.

Area differences

Northern Ireland: In Northern Ireland, all homelessness presentations have been around 10,000–11,000 per annum (see Table 14.2) and the number of homeless families presenting has also remained constant at around 4,500 or 40 per cent of all presentations. In 2000/01, however, there was a significant increase in the numbers of presenters to 12,694. On average 41 per cent of those presenting as homeless are families. With a total population in Northern Ireland of 626,000, households accepted as homeless represent 1.1 per cent of all households. This is a significantly higher proportion than in the rest of the UK, but the higher figure is partly due to the introduction of a new Housing Selection Scheme (in effect householders can be assessed as homeless without presenting as such) and feuds. Comparative homeless rates are higher than the remainder of the UK primarily because of the different legislative base and method of identifying homeless people (NIHE, 2001). In Northern Ireland 6 to 7 per cent of homelessness presentations cite domestic violence as a cause of homelessness. Intimidation, ranging from neighbour intimidation to that arising from civil disturbances, accounts for around 15 per cent of presentations – this increased to 22 per cent in 2000/01. The highest incidences of homelessness are to be found in the urban Housing Executive Districts in Belfast and surrounding Greater Belfast. There are also pressures in the provincial cities and towns, particularly in (London) Derry, Newry and Ballymena. In Northern Ireland around 20 per cent of families accepted as homeless are placed in temporary accommodation. Overall the average length of stay is 135 days. The Northern Ireland Executive has set a specific target to secure permanent tenancies within three months for 7 per cent of applicants accepted as homeless (NIHE, 2001).

Wales: In Wales, homelessness acceptances have fluctuated between a high of 11,125 in 1993 and a low of 4,171 in 1999 (see Table 14.1). In 2000 local authorities decided that a total of 4,143 households were unintentionally homeless and in priority need; 63 per cent of these households were households with dependent children. The rate of homelessness varies between unitary authorities. The numbers found to be unintentionally homeless and in priority need per 1,000 of the population ranged from 0.2 in Newport to 4.1 in Torfaen. Twenty-nine per cent of homelessness occurred as a result of relationship

Table 14.1: Local authority homeless acceptances, number of households

	1980	1985	1986	1987	1988	1989	1990*	1991	1992	1993	1994	1995	1996	1997**	1998**	1999	2000
Not held to be intentionally homeless																	
England	60,400	91,010	100,490	109,170	113,770	122,180	140,350	144,780	142,890	132,380	122,460	121,280	116,870	102,410	104,490	105,490	106,160
Scotland***	7,038	10,992	11,056	10,417	10,463	12,396	14,233	15,500	17,700	17,000	16,000	15,200	15,500	15,600	16,200	–	–
Wales	4,772	4,825	5,262	5,198	6,286	7,111	9,226	9,293	9,818	10,792	9,897	8,638	8,334	4,297	4,380	3,695	4,143
Great Britain	72,210	106,827	116,808	124,785	130,519	141,687	163,809	169,573	170,408	160,172	148,357	145,118	140,704	122,307	125,070	109,185	110,303
Held to be intentionally homeless																	
England	2,520	2,970	3,070	3,270	3,730	4,500	5,450	6,940	6,350	5,660	4,570	4,690	5,120	4,970	6,140	7,340	9,140
Scotland	938	980	1,144	1,030	1,128	1,271	1,580	1,800	2,200	2,000	1,800	1,700	1,700	1,800	2,000	–	–
Wales	674	546	703	485	532	694	737	550	452	333	396	362	815	343	380	476	507
Great Britain	4,132	4,496	4,917	4,785	5,390	6,465	7,767	9,290	9,002	7,993	6,766	6,752	7,635	7,113	8,520	7,816	9,647
All homeless acceptances																	
England	62,920	93,980	103,560	112,440	117,500	126,680	145,800	151,720	149,240	138,040	127,030	125,500	121,990	107,380	110,630	112,830	115,300
Scotland	7,976	11,972	12,200	11,447	11,591	13,667	15,813	17,300	19,900	19,000	17,800	16,900	17,200	17,400	18,200	–	–
Wales	5,446	5,371	5,965	5,683	6,818	7,805	9,963	9,843	10,270	11,125	10,293	9,001	9,149	4,640	4,760	4,171	4,650
Great Britain	76,342	111,323	121,725	129,570	135,909	148,152	171,576	178,863	179,410	168,165	155,123	151,401	148,339	129,420	133,590	117,001	119,950

* The 1990 figures for Wales include 2,000 households made homeless in Colwyn Bay by flooding in the February of that year.

** The England and Wales figures for 1997 and 1998 reflect the changes in homeless legislation, and as a result no longer include 'non priority acceptances'. In 1996 these accounted for 3,310 acceptances in England and 3,501 acceptances in Wales.

*** Scottish figures are for priority need homeless and potentially homeless cases only; 1999 and 2000 figures were not available at the time of compilation.

Sources: Department of the Environment, Transport and the Regions, Scottish Executive, Welsh Executive.

Table 14.2: Northern Ireland Housing Executive lettings and homelessness in Northern Ireland

	1980/81	1981/82	1982/83	1983/84	1984/85	1985/86	1986/87	1987/88	1988/89	1989/90	1990/91
Allocations to Applicants/priority groups*	9,966	10,621	12,824	13,152	12,491	12,417	11,877	10,940	11,357	11,357	11,637
Homelessness:											
presenting										6,675	9,187
accepted AI**										3,110	4,404
Placed in temporary accommodation										741	1,849

Table 14.2: continued

	1991/92	1992/93	1993/94	1994/95	1995/96	1996/97	1997/98	1998/99	1999/00	2000/01
Allocations to Applicants/priority groups*	11,170	10,489	10,280	10,455	8,826	10,164	10,946	10,643	8,496	8,588
Homelessness:										
presenting	10,081	10,099	9,731	10,068	10,468	11,092	11,672	11,552	10,997	12,694
accepted AI**	4,158	4,061	3,971	4,014	4,319	4,708	4,956	4,997	5,192	6,457
Placed in temporary accommodation	1,771	1,790	1,865	1,747	2,151	2,141	2,123	2,249	1,937	2,455

* Allocations to Applicants ("allocation to priority groups" before 2000/01) comprise lettings to new tenants, and exclude transfers.
** Accepted AI= priority need corresponds to acceptances as priority need case elsewhere in the UK.
Homeless legislation was only extended to Northern Ireland in April 1989. A new selection scheme was introduced in November 2000 resulting in a change in allocation headings to: Allocations to Applicants, Housing Executive transfers and Housing Association combined transfers.
Source: Department of the Environment for Northern Ireland

Table 14.3: Homeless households in temporary accommodation in England under the provisions of the 1985 and the 1996 Housing Acts (numbers of households)

	1980	1985	1986	1987	1988	1989	1990	1991	1992	1993	1994	1995	1996	1997	1998	1999	2000
Bed and breakfast	1,330	5,360	8,990	10,370	10,970	11,480	11,130	12,150	7,630	4,900	4,130	4,500	4,160	4,520	6,930	8,120	9,860
+ Hostels*	3,380	4,730	4,610	5,150	6,240	8,020	9,010	9,990	10,840	10,210	9,730	9,660	9,640	8,860	9,060	8,920	10,320
+ Private sector leasing								23,740	27,910	23,270	15,800	11,530	10,980	14,320	16,220	22,390	25,390
+ Other**		5,830	7,190	9,240	12,890	18,400	25,130	14,050	16,690	15,200	15,970	18,450	17,410	17,330	19,310	22,750	26,870
+ Homeless at home***								8,700	10,420	8,640	8,370	8,890	9,500	9,900	9,150	9,330	11,050
= Total	4,710	15,920	20,790	24,760	30,100	37,900	45,270	68,630	73,490	62,220	54,000	53,030	51,690	54,930	60,670	71,510	83,490

* Includes women's refuges.

** Includes dwellings leased by local authorities from private landlords for years prior to 1991.

*** Figures for households accepted as homeless, but that remain in their existing accommodation pending rehousing, were not collected before 1991.

Sources: Homelessness Statistics, Department of the Environment, Transport and the Regions, Hansard 18/4/91, Column 186

breakdown, 39 per cent occurred as a result of the loss of accommodation through mortgage or rent arrears or through other reasons for losing rented accommodation. Only 2 per cent resulted directly as a result of leaving institutional care. At the end of 2000 some 910 homeless households were in temporary accommodation. Around 150 were placed either in hostels or in B&B accommodation. In the first quarter of 2001, 1,262 households were accepted as in priority need compared with 1,028 in the first quarter of 2000 and this trend continued through the first half of 2001, which saw a growth of 24 per cent in the number of households officially considered as homeless. However, it should be noted that some of this increase is due to the expansion of the priority need categories (Welsh Assembly, 2001e; *Housing Today*, 31 January 2002).

Scotland: Homelessness acceptances in Scotland through the latter part of the 1990s were around 7,000–8,000 (see Table 14.1). During the second quarter of 2001 local authorities reported 11,558 applications under the homelessness legislation. This represented an increase of 3 per cent compared with the same quarter of 2000. At the end of June 2001 there were 4,006 households in temporary accommodation, having been placed there by a local authority under the homelessness legislation. This figure represents a small decrease (2 per cent) compared with the number at the end of June 2000. In Scotland information is available for the first time on the type of temporary accommodation occupied by children. Of the 1,406 households (containing 2,625 children) with children in temporary accommodation at the end of June 2001, the majority (83 per cent) were in local authority accommodation, 6 per cent (88) were in B&B accommodation and 7 per cent (101) in hostels. The local authorities with the highest number of families in temporary accommodation are Glasgow (300), Edinburgh (135) and Fife (107) (Scottish Housing Executive, 2001). The main reported causes of homelessness in Scotland are new household formation (32.2 per cent), loss of independent accommodation (20.2 per cent), household dissolution (34.4 per cent) and discharge from an institution (7.9 per cent). The relative importance of various recorded causes of homelessness vary widely between different authorities. For example, the percentage accounted for by new household formation ranges from nearly half in East Renfrewshire to only a sixth in Orkney. Relationship breakdown is the most common cause of homelessness for families with children, while the loss of independent accommodation is the immediate cause of homelessness for more than half of priority homeless households consisting of two adults and children (Pawson *et al.*, 2001).

England: Homelessness acceptances in England have fluctuated between 113,000 and 122,000 since the mid-1990s (see Table 14.1) but increased from 112,830 in 1999 to 115,300 in 2000. In England, around 70 per cent of households accepted for rehousing are families with children or families including a pregnant woman. At the end of March 2001 there were 75,120 households living in temporary accommodation in England, the highest number since the first figures were compiled in 1977 (Wilcox, 2001). Of these, nearly 1,100 were placed in B&B accommodation – an increase of 32 per cent for the same period in 2000 and the highest number since the home repossession crisis in the early 1990s (Shelter, 2001; Wilcox, 2001). Table 14.4 details the use of B&B and other forms of temporary accommodation for all homeless households in the nine regions of England.

As Table 14.4 shows, the increase in B&B use has been greatest in London, which accounts for almost a quarter (24 per cent) of all homeless applications in England. But numbers are also rising in areas of high housing demand in the south-east and south-west. In response, the government has set up a Bed and Breakfast Unit that has a national remit to deal with the increasing use of B&B in England (Weaver, 2001). In 2000 there were 10,000 asylum seeker and refugee households living in temporary accommodation in London boroughs as well as 4,000 unaccompanied asylum-seeking children, about three-quarters of whom were aged 16 or 17 years old.

Table 14.4: Homeless households in temporary accommodation in English regions March 2001, numbers of households

Region	In registered social landlord	In B&B	In other* temporary accommodation	Total
North East	1,180	50	230	1,460
Yorkshire and Humberside	1,860	250	720	2,830
North West and Merseyside	610	120	1,230	1,960
East	2,950	490	1,820	5,260
West Midlands	1,230	110	460	1,800
East Midlands	1,370	50	390	1,810
South West	2,100	960	2,550	5,610
South East	5,150	1,250	5,430	11,830
London	8,970	7,570	26,110	42,650

These figures do not include people placed in temporary accommodation by social services or those who placed themselves in temporary accommodation.
* Including private rental sector and hostels.
Source: Shelter Regional Statistics http://www.shelter.org.uk/housing/statistics compiled from DETR Homelessness Statistics 2000/01.

The causes of child homelessness

It is widely acknowledged that the causes of homelessness among all households are multi-faceted and complex, but the key precipitating factors are violence, relationship breakdown and harassment or intimidation. A longitudinal study of 168 homeless families with 249 children (Vostanis *et al.*, 1998) found that 89 per cent of families became homeless to escape violence, either in the form of direct assaults (53 per cent), threats of violence (14 per cent) or from sustained harassment (11 per cent). Smaller numbers left to avoid the sexual or other physical abuse of children in the family (5 per cent) or following the destruction of household property (5 per cent). Three families became homeless because their house was burned down by others. Ongoing research for Shelter (Jones *et al.*, 2002) found the main reason for homelessness among families using resettlement services in Bristol, Sheffield and Birmingham was domestic violence. In 41 per cent of cases families had become homeless as a result of male violence, in 9 per cent because of harassment from neighbours, in 14 per cent as a result of relationship breakdown and in 10 per cent because of a loss of private rented tenancy. Families do become homeless for other reasons: for example, because of mortgage repossession. An increasing problem in some areas such as London and Birmingham is that asylum-seeking families become homeless once they have been granted refugee status and National Asylum Support Service support is withdrawn. Gypsy and Traveller families are often homeless under the law because there are insufficient campsites where they may legally park.

Other risk factors associated with homelessness

While violence, harassment and relationship breakdown are precipitating factors, research suggests a number of other associated risk factors including poverty and deprivation, young parenthood and single parenthood, and poor educational achievement (Anderson and Tulloch, 2000; Motion, 2000). The early experiences of parents are also thought to be significant and research has found that many homeless families are headed by parents who had disrupted family backgrounds and/or who have experienced violence and/or sexual abuse as children. (Vostanis and Cumella, 1999; Jones *et al.*, 2002; Bassuk and Perloff, 2001). Little is known about the dynamics of homelessness among families who have been homeless more than once, but the incidence of repeat homelessness among families is becoming evident (see for example, Pawson *et al.*, 2001). The UK research, although limited, suggests that domestic violence, relationship breakdown and antisocial behaviour are important contributory factors in repeat homelessness. Recent research conducted by Walters and East (2001) suggests that homelessness and/or unsettled lives can undermine parenting skills and that a possible reason for a loss of tenancy after rehousing is the disruptive behaviour of children, leading to tensions with neighbours and difficulties in entering community support networks. Research also suggests that people who have experienced homelessness as children or as young people are likely to become homeless again in later life (Jones, 1999; Motion, 2000).

Older children and young people

The best current estimate (based on a number of existing studies) of youth homelessness in Britain is 32,000 16–21-year-olds (NCH, 2001). Care leavers are hugely over-represented among homeless youth: they are 60 times more likely to be homeless than other young people. Nearly half of young homeless people in London are from Black, Black Caribbean and other minority ethnic groups (NCH, 2001). A third of a homeless young people group in a Safe in the City study (Bruegel and Smith, 1999) left home before the age of 16. Research conducted by the Safe on the Streets Research Team (1999) suggests that 10,000 young people aged 16 had been 'on the run' for a continuous period of six months or more before they were 16 years old. The Children's Society has estimated that 100,000 children aged under 16 run away each year in the UK. A recent report found that 80 children under the age of 16 become homeless every day in Scotland and, in any one year, approximately 11,500 young people aged 16–24 years old apply to their local authority for housing support as homeless – a quarter of all homeless applications (HMSO, 2001). It has also been estimated that over 2,000 children under the age of 16 run away in Northern Ireland each year (see Chapter 9).

Cause of homelessness among older children and young people

For older children, the evidence of family and relationship breakdown as a contributory cause of homelessness is overwhelming and the number of young people leaving home because of family problems is increasing (NCH, 2001). In the UK as a whole, it is estimated that one in nine young people run away or are forced to leave and stay away overnight before the age of 16 (Raws, 2001). In Scotland, in 80 per cent of cases involving young people aged under 18, homelessness results from being asked to leave the home of parents, friends or relatives and a survey of young homeless people in Nottingham found that just under three-quarters left home because of family conflict (Lemos and Crane, 2001). Most young homeless people report deprived family backgrounds, and in British studies up to half of single young homeless people had experience of being looked after. It is thought that the care system fosters reliance on others and that children are ill-prepared for independent living. Furthermore, support for young people leaving care is often inadequate (Wrate and Blair, 1999; Jones *et al.*, 2001). Bruegel and Smith (1999) estimated the risks to young people of becoming homeless. Their study involved interviews with 195 homeless young people from London and 155 young people living in deprived areas. They found, in common with other research (see for example, Smith *et al.*, 1998) that the young homeless people were far more likely to be poor than the comparison group and to have experienced violence more than once (45 per cent compared with 29 per cent of the comparison group). The homeless young people were also more likely to have experienced family disruption and far fewer said they had enjoyed a good relationship with their mother (40 per cent compared to 80 per cent of the comparison group).

The consequences of homelessness for children

Living in temporary accommodation

As Quilgars (2001a) has noted, most early reports on the effects of homelessness on the well-being of children were based on information gathered by health visitors and other professionals and centred on the use of B&Bs (Hague and Mallos, 1999; HVA and GMSC, 1988; Taylor and Jones, 1990; Thomas and Niner, 1989). B&B accommodation is often below standard, dangerous and lacking facilities for cooking and washing (GLA, 2001b). Added to this, overcrowded conditions and limited space for play can hamper children's development and exacerbate an already stressful situation, all of which take a toll on physical and mental well-being. In addition, the location of temporary accommodation is often a problem; in London one in every seven households in temporary accommodation is located outside the home borough (GLA, 2001a). It is often necessary to place homeless families in areas away from their previous home (for example, when the cause of homelessness is domestic violence or harassment). Although necessary, this has implications in terms of access to education, health and social services as well as the loss of informal support networks of friends and family (Jones *et al.*, 2002; McCrum, 2001; Victor *et al.*, 1989).

No robust national studies exist of the effects of homelessness on the well-being of children. In the absence of such data it is impossible to determine whether homelessness is the cause of physical and/or mental ill health or whether it exacerbates existing conditions. A study of homeless children living in B&Bs in London (Parsons, 1991), for example, found that a high proportion of children born in B&Bs had low birth weights and 30 per cent of homeless children were considered not to be in normal health. However, the relative poverty of the area meant that 20 per cent of children living in permanent accommodation were also in this category. Where comparative research has been conducted, there is evidence that homeless children suffer higher levels of mental ill health, psychosocial stress, behavioural problems and delayed development than children who are not homeless (Davey, 1998; Vostanis and Cumella, 1999).

More recent research suggests that the effects of homelessness on children depend on the reasons for homelessness, the age of the child and the type of accommodation and area where they are housed (McCrum, 2001; Hall *et al.*, 2000; Vostanis and Cumella, 1999). Where families are housed in self-contained accommodation in an area they know and where parents are coping well, children are largely unaffected. However, where parents are not coping well or suffering stress or where families are living in shared accommodation in a strange area then children are likely to be affected in a number of ways. These effects could manifest themselves fairly quickly or take some time to develop and include behavioural changes, bed wetting, physical health problems, reluctance to eat, a general failure to thrive and the worsening of existing conditions such as asthma and insomnia (McCrum, 2001; Hall *et al.*, 2000). The effects of homelessness on older children are also dependent on their circumstances. Research studies have consistently shown that the health of people sleeping rough is extremely poor (Anderson *et al.*, 1993; Mental Health Foundation, 1996). Young people sleeping rough expose themselves to danger, to hunger and ill health, to alcohol and drug abuse and to physical and sexual abuse (Palmer, 2001; Pleace *et al.*, 2000; Jones, 1999). The Children's Society (Stein *et al.*, 1994) found that a large majority of young people who ran away from home or from care did so before the age of 16 and one in seven of these young people had become involved in prostitution as a survival strategy. There is also emerging evidence of a link between running away under the age of 16 and repeated episodes of homelessness in later years (see Chapter 9 and Jones, 1999).

The experience of becoming homeless and events leading up to homelessness

Most research has focused on children's experiences of *being* homeless rather that their experiences of *becoming* homeless. One study (Nettleton *et al.*, 2000; Nettleton and Burrows, 2000) looked at the consequences of losing the family home through repossession. It found that children often worried about their parents' well-being and articulated concerns about the loss of their 'home' and school, about not being able to control the situation and about arguments and tension within the household. Vostanis and Cumella (1999) questioned the extent to which homeless children's mental health problems were related to previous experiences prior to homelessness or to the experience of homelessness itself. The authors conclude: 'Children and parents who become homeless constitute a high risk group for the development of mental health problems and disorders. These problems are often caused by life events and adversities that precipitate homelessness, but also by subsequent losses and the removal of protective factors' (Vostanis and Cumella, 1999, p. 34). Other studies suggest that the events leading up to homelessness, for example witnessing or experiencing abuse and violence, may continue to affect children for some time after rehousing (McGee, 2000; Jones *et al.*, 2002).

Conclusion

This chapter has considered the extent of homelessness among children in the four countries of the UK. It has been seen that there is limited evidence on the extent of homelessness in the EU. However, the European Federation of National Organisations Working with the Homeless has recommended that research should be carried out in a systematic and comprehensive fashion in all 15 member states, based on common criteria defined at European level, and allowing for the regular publication of comparable data concerning access to housing and the quality and costs of housing.

Data from the UK shows that homelessness is still a significant problem and that the number of homelessness acceptances has increased. It has also been seen that homelessness can have detrimental long-term effects on children's well-being, although there is only limited data which allows comparisons to be made between the well-being of homeless children and housed children. It is likely that there are numerous factors in addition to homelessness which impact on children's well-being. There has only recently been a renewed interest in the problem of child and family homelessness and evidence is limited. However, emerging evidence suggests that many homeless families have complex needs and that, without support, they may experience homelessness again in the future. All the research suggests that homeless children and young people are, for the most part, from deprived and/or disrupted backgrounds and homelessness is only one manifestation of, if the most extreme form of, their social exclusion.

15 Educational Achievement

Bob Coles and Helen Kenwright

Key facts:

- There are differences in the type of schools children attend in the different countries of the UK.
- Girls obtain higher qualifications than boys.
- Children in Scotland and Northern Ireland do better than children in England and Wales.
- About 8 per cent of 16- and 17-year-olds are not in education, employment or training.
- Attainment varies by gender, ethnicity and social class.

Key trends:

- More young people are achieving better qualifications at school leaving age and fewer are leaving with no qualifications.
- The numbers of students in post-16 education have increased, but the drop-out rate is stable.
- Improvements in Key Stage 2 scores have not been sustained over the last two years.
- The gap in attainment by social class increased in the late 1980s and 1990s, but shows some signs of closing.

Key sources:

- Youth Cohort Studies and Scottish and Northern Ireland School Leaver Surveys
- OFSTED reports
- Education statistics

Introduction

Educational achievement is fundamentally important to the life chances of most children and young people. The right to education is enshrined in the UN

Convention on the Rights of the Child, and attaining success in education is a graduated staircase to success in adulthood in terms of occupation, income and lifestyle. All children in the UK are entitled to 'free' full-time education between the ages of 5 and 16. Public examinations taken at the age of 16 plus are seen as a crucial indicator of educational 'success', and therefore much of this chapter will focus on what research evidence can tell us about these results.

Research also indicates that examination success is strongly influenced by educational experiences throughout childhood, which are in turn shaped by the social and economic circumstances in which a child is brought up. Success is also related to social class, ethnicity and gender in a pronounced way. This chapter reviews some of this evidence. Yet it must also be recognised that the attainment of qualifications is not the only achievement children and young people reach through their experience of education.

Education in the four countries of the UK

Since the beginning of the century most of the education of teenage children has been funded by the state. Over the last century, the UK has developed four separate but related education systems (Croxford, 2000; Raffe, 2000). Based upon a major study of 'The Home Internationals', Croxford points to differences between the four countries according to the degree to which pupils are educated in schools which are comprehensive or selective, independent, denominational, single sex and socially segregated. This study was based on surveys in all four countries carried out in 1990/91, but many of its broad findings still hold.

The greatest differences in types of schools across the UK is of different patterns of comprehensive versus selective schools. Comprehensive schooling is the experience of the vast majority of young people over the age of 11 in both Scotland and Wales. In England a small minority of around 7 per cent of pupils attend either grammar schools or secondary modern schools. Although there are proposals to abolish the 11 plus system, at the time of writing Northern Ireland largely retains the selective system, although in the face of considerable controversy (Leonard and Davey, 2001). Northern Ireland also still has a huge majority of pupils (97 per cent) who are educated in schools associated with religious denominations.

Single-sex schools are most common in Northern Ireland (33 per cent), then England (18 per cent) and Wales (15 per cent) while only 3 per cent of Scotland's schools are single-sex. Independent schools are most common in England, where they comprise more than one in ten of all schools, compared with just 3 per cent of Welsh schools and 6 per cent of Scottish provision. The 'Home International' studies report that these differences between types of school have an impact on forms of social segregation within schooling, with more social segregation in England and Northern Ireland, ie, children are most likely to be educated with children of a similar social background (Croxford, 2000).

There are also marked differences between the curriculum followed in the four countries. Following the 1988 Education Reform Act, England, Wales and Northern Ireland adopted a National Curriculum. Scotland has its own distinctive education system and a recommended 5–14 curriculum which is followed by most schools. It also has its own qualification system which is different from that in the other three countries. Post-compulsory education and training has also gone through a series of changes over the past century, especially the last 20 years. All four counties have further education colleges of various types, although they are funded differently (Raffe, 2000).

It is perhaps important at the beginning of this chapter to remind the reader that formal qualifications are not the be-all and end-all of the value of schooling. While qualifications are important currency in terms of economic success, all forms of learning can contribute to social cohesion, personal growth and quality of life (Kennedy, 1997). Sex education, education on drugs, health and other forms of social education are delivered through Personal and Social Education. Physical education is often a primary means through which children and young people of school age keep fit, learn teamwork skills and thrive. Citizenship education is also to be introduced in England at Key Stages 3 and 4 from August 2002. Yet these important aspects of the curricula are not very amenable to formal testing and the beneficial results do not appear in published statistics. The Wider Benefits of Learning Research Centre is currently investigating these relationships (the Centre's information can be accessed through the website at www.learningbenefits.net). While this chapter will focus on formal measures of educational outcome, these wider implications of education should not be forgotten.

The rest of this chapter, however, examines patterns of learner achievement for children and young people within the structures described above and highlights some of the problems that remain in systems which continue to fail many learners.

Sources of evidence

Unlike some topic areas covered by other chapters, we can be reasonably confident that the evidence on school achievements is relatively robust. Schools, local authorities and government routinely collect information about public examination results and publish these in league tables. The government also sponsors major sample surveys of young people. The Youth Cohort Studies and the Scottish School Leavers' Surveys, for instance, allow for the systematic examination of the relationship between school qualifications and socio-economic background.

Attainment

One short chapter cannot do justice to all the different measures of education attainment between the four countries of the UK, nor show how all these are socially patterned. The tables below illustrate the qualifications young people attained at the end of Year 11 (the age of 15).

Qualifications at the age of 15

Table 15.1 indicates quite marked differences between the qualifications attained in the different countries of the UK and between girls and boys. In all countries girls out-perform boys, with a higher proportion obtaining five or more of the top grades and a smaller proportion of girls than boys obtaining no qualifications. Both boys and girls in Scotland and Northern Ireland are obtaining better qualifications at the age of 16 than their contemporaries in England and Wales, with Wales having the highest proportion of 16-year-olds with no qualifications. Within England, there are relatively small differences between the qualifications obtained in the different regions, but pupils in the south and east do slightly better than pupils in the north.

Participation in post-compulsory education and training

Although qualifications at the age of 15 are the most commonly quoted measure of educational attainment, increasingly participation and achievement beyond the end of compulsory schooling is seen as being important. Overall, 'staying on' rates are highest in Scotland and Northern Ireland, lower in England and Wales,

Table 15.1: Attainment level at Year 11, 1999–2000

Country-region	5 or more A*–C	1–4 A*–C	D–G only	No graded qualifications	2 or more A levels 3 SCE/NQ highers
England	49.2	24.4	20.8	5.6	30.0
Male	44.0	24.6	24.9	6.5	26.7
Female	55.8	24.1	16.6	4.6	33.5
Wales	49.1	19.5	19.5	7.7	27.2
Male	43.4	24.3	23.3	8.9	23.3
Female	54.9	23.0	15.7	6.4	31.2
Scotland	58.3	25.8	10.3	5.6	31.4
Male	53.1	28.3	12.4	6.2	27.4
Female	63.5	23.2	8.2	5.0	35.4
Northern Ireland	56.9	22.9	16.5	3.6	37.7
Male	48.7	24.8	21.4	5.3	30.5
Female	65.4	21.0	11.7	1.9	45.2
Regions of England					
North East	43.2	24.4	25.7	6.7	22.0
North West	47.5	25.0	21.7	5.8	27.6
Yorks and Humb	43.6	24.0	25.6	6.8	25.3
East Midlands	47.8	24.0	22.6	5.7	28.8
West Midlands	46.5	25.1	22.7	5.7	27.8
East	53.0	23.9	18.5	4.6	33.9
London	48.1	27.0	19.2	5.7	30.1
South East	54.8	22.7	17.3	5.2	35.6
South West	54.0	23.3	18.2	4.5	32.8

England figures include GNVQ equivalents. Scottish figures include National Qualifications (NQs) from 99–00 onwards
Sources: Regional Trends, DfES, Welsh Assembly, Scottish Executive, Northern Ireland Department of Education.

although the pattern is quite complicated. Table 15.2 indicates participation rates in the different forms of post-compulsory education and government-supported training in the four countries of the UK and across the different regions of England at the ages of 16 and 17.

Table 15.2 shows marked differences between the countries and between regions in England. Participation in school-based education is particularly strong in Scotland, slightly less so in Northern Ireland and significantly less in England and Wales. In Scotland, whereas involvement in education at the age of 16 is strong, there is little competition from the further education sector and by the age of 17 a large proportion have completed their schooling. Further education accounts for a much higher proportion of students in England, Wales and Northern Ireland than in Scotland, by a factor of around three. Aggregating all full-time, post-compulsory education together (school and full-time further

Table 15.2: 16- and 17-year-olds participating in post-compulsory education and government-supported training, 1998/99

	16-year-olds School	FT	FE PT	GST	All ed & GST	17-year-olds School	FT	FE PT	GST	All† ed & GST
Country-region										
England	34.5	35.0	6.5	8.9	82.6	27.4	29.6	8.4	11.1	73.7
Wales	37.7	31.0	7.6	16.1	92.5	28.4	26.3	9.4	15.7	79.8
Scotland	67.4	11.2	11.0	9.4	88.0	37.6	10.9	13.4	14.9	63.4
N. Ireland	45.5	27.9	13.3	37.0		25.9	13.7			
English regions										
North East	25.9	35.3	7.8	13.9	81.2	19.8	29.0	9.4	15.8	72.5
North West	24.5	40.5	8.4	12.3	82.0	19.8	33.5	9.9	14.7	73.7
Yorkshire and Humberside	29.6	33.9	9.7	13.1	83.3	23.8	27.6	11.6	14.7	73.9
E Midlands	37.2	29.4	7.4	10.6	82.2	29.8	24.9	9.2	13.3	74.1
W Midlands	31.1	36.4	7.9	9.8	82.5	24.7	30.3	10.0	11.6	73.7
East	40.9	33.2	5.0	6.4	83.0	32.6	27.9	7.1	8.2	72.7
London	39.4	34.6	4.2	4.5	81.9	29.8	31.7	5.8	5.9	72.3
South East	39.3	34.9	4.5	5.9	82.9	31.7	29.8	6.1	8.2	73.8
South West	39.2	33.9	5.8	8.2	84.4	31.1	28.7	7.9	12.0	76.4

† All is not always the aggregation of all the figures because some categories may not be mutually exclusive.

Figures given are of the percentages of 16- and 17-year-olds respectively.

FE=further education; FT=full-time; PT=part-time; GST=government-supported training

Figures for England and Wales exclude overlap between full-time education and government-supported training.

Data for training in Northern Ireland is not equivalent as data is only provided on school leavers as a whole rather than each separate age cohort.

Sources: Regional Trends, DfES, Welsh Assembly, Scottish Executive, Northern Ireland Department of Education.

education) still leaves Scotland top of the league with 78.6 per cent involved, followed by Northern Ireland (74.4 per cent), England (69.5 per cent) and Wales (68.7 per cent).

All four countries share a UK pattern of relatively low participation at age 17 relative to participation rates at the age of 16. In Scotland this relates to the curriculum pattern for 16–17-year-olds, although this changed in 2000. But by the age of 17, less than half (49.5 per cent) of 17-year-olds were still at school or in full-time further education in Scotland, compared to 57 per cent in England and 54.7 per cent in Wales. Participation rates in Northern Ireland were by the far the highest at 62.9 per cent.

The proportion of both 16- and 17-year-olds involved in government-supported training is much higher in Wales and northern regions of England than it is the in the south-east of England. Involvement in government-supported training in Scotland shows marked increases between the ages of 16 and 17, suggesting that significant proportions progress from post-16 education to government-supported training at age 17.

Participation, however, does not directly indicate that the young person involved will achieve their chosen qualification. Indeed, we comment below on a very significant problem of drop-out and failure to obtain the qualification for which the young person initially registered. In England and Wales DfES figures put national retention rates at 78 per cent, and success (ie, the percentage of those who enrolling for a qualification who achieved it) at only 56 per cent.

The disengagement of 16- and 17-year-olds

In the late 1980s researchers, particularly in south Wales, identified a significant proportion of 16-year-olds who left school but did not either find work or become involved in training. At the time, this group were referred to as 'status zero', a technical term drawn from careers records indicating that they were not in education, employment or training. The researchers, however, used the term as a powerful metaphor for the fact that this group appeared to "count for nothing and were going nowhere" (Williamson, 1997). In England, the group became more officially recognised in the influential Social Exclusion Unit report *Bridging the Gap* (SEU, 1999a). This estimated that around 160,000 16- and 17-year-olds were 'NEET' – not in education, employment or training – around 8 per cent of the age cohort. Some doubts have been expressed about the robustness of this estimate, however, as official records and school-based and household-based surveys are least likely to include disaffected young people and those who may have already 'dropped-out' of school and/or home (Britton *et al.*, 2002; Coles, 2000). There is also some indication that minority ethnic groups are over-represented within 16- and 17-year-olds who disappear from the systems of education, training and work (Britton *et al.*, 2002).

While first 'discovered in Wales' and subsequently rediscovered as a national problem in England, 'status zero' has also been the subject of serious attention in Northern Ireland and Scotland. Existing data sources initially suggested that only 4 to 6 per cent of the age cohort might be disengaged. But a survey of those eligible to leave school in 1993 found that a quarter of the cohort had experience of at least one spell of 'status zero' between 1993 and 1995, with two-fifths of these being a period of inactivity of over six months. In Northern Ireland, while the same background factors found to be correlated with disengagement as in the rest of the UK were significant, 'status zero' was also found predominantly in Catholic areas (Istance and Rees, 1997). A more recent follow-up survey has helped to examine the more dynamic picture of movements into and out of inactivity between the ages of 16 and 22 (McVicar, 2000). This concludes that young people are most likely to experience a long spell of inactivity at the age of 18+ if:

- they are Catholic
- they are poorly qualified at 16
- they come from families with experience of unemployment
- they come from disadvantaged areas
- they come from single parent families (males)
- they have children (females).

The Social Exclusion Unit report (SEU, 1999a) makes it clear that routes into NEET include drop-out from employment, education and training, and that disengagement is strongly correlated with pre-16 educational disadvantage and disaffection. Those NEET are highly likely to be unqualified, to have truanted from, or been excluded from, school, and that groups which figure strongly include care leavers, teenage mothers, young carers and those living in 'deprived circumstances' including lone parent families and those in social housing. Being disengaged at the age of 16 was also found to be highly predictive of long-term unemployment later in life. But the evidence also suggests that routes into disengagement can be traced back to much earlier patterns of dissaffection and disadvantage both at school and in the home (Britton et al., 2002)

Attainment at earlier ages

The introduction of class-based testing at Key Stages at the ages of 7 (8 in Northern Ireland) 11, and 13 allows for some comparison between performances earlier in school careers. Key Stage tests are increasingly being used as educational 'targets' to improve performance. Table 15.3 shows the proportion of pupils reaching or exceeding expected standards at each Key Stage for three of the four countries of the UK. Scotland does not produce such data, as it does not follow the same National Curriculum. Data for Wales is available for the first time in 2001 and Northern Ireland does not publish test results for science. But this data should prove a valuable base line for comparison in subsequent years.

Table 15.3: Percentage of pupils reaching or exceeding expected standards at Key Stage teacher assessments, summer 2000

Country	Key Stage 1			Key Stage 2			Key Stage 3		
	English	Maths	Science	English	Maths	Science	English	Maths	Science
England	84	88	88	70	72	79	64	66	62
Wales	82	88	87	70	71	78	63	64	62
Northern Ireland *	95	95	–	71	75	–	73	72	–

* Pupils are not assessed in Science in Northern Ireland.
Source: Regional Trends, 36 (2001)

Trends

Increases in levels of attainment

There is clear evidence in the results obtained in the four countries of the UK that more and more young people (both boys and girls) are obtaining better qualifications by the minimum school leaving age and fewer are leaving with no qualifications.

Charts 15.1 and 15.2 indicate that the percentage of young people obtaining five or more A*-C grades increased in all countries, with more girls doing better than boys in every country. More boys and girls in Scotland and Northern

Chart 15.1: Percentage of boys obtaining 5 or more A*-C grades in the final year of compulsory schooling, 1994–2000

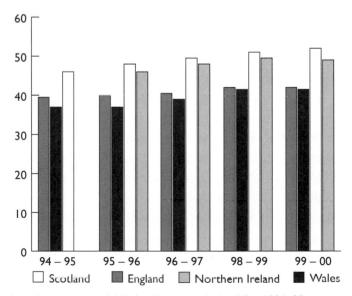

□ Scotland   ■ England   ▨ Northern Ireland   ■ Wales

Note: Equivalent data is not available for Northern Ireland for 1994–95.

Chart 15.2: Percentage of girls obtaining 5 or more A*-C grades in the final year of compulsory schooling, 1994–2000

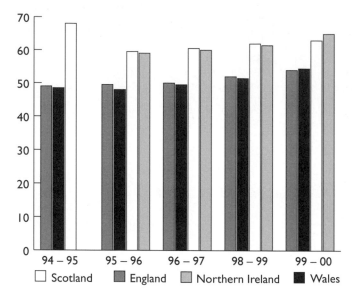

Note: Equivalent data is not available for Northern Ireland for 1994–95.

Ireland have obtained these qualifications that their peers in England and Wales throughout the period.

The proportion of boys gaining these qualifications increased between 1994 and 2000:

- in England from 39 per cent to 44 per cent
- in Wales from 35.9 per cent to 43.4per cent
- in Scotland from 46.4 per cent to 53.1 per cent
- in Northern Ireland from 44.5 per cent (1995–96) to 48.9 per cent. (Equivalent data is not available for Northern Ireland for 1994. The Northern Ireland Office reports on data on all school leavers rather than year groups.)

The proportion of girls obtaining the same qualifications increased between 1994 and 2000:

- in England from 48.1 per cent to 54.6 per cent
- in Wales from 46.3 per cent to 53.1 per cent
- in Scotland from 56.4 per cent to 63.6 per cent
- in Northern Ireland from 58.8 per cent (1995–96) to 63.4 per cent.

In England it might be suspected that the introduction of league tables for schools in which A*-C grades are published in newspapers might induce schools to concentrate considerable effort in trying to get those just failing to obtain five of these grades to obtain them. Were this the case, one would expect this to result in a lower proportion obtaining 1–4 A-C grades. But the published data does not indicate that this is the case either in England or in the other three countries. Rather, standards appear to be rising across the board.

Charts 15.3 and 15.4 illustrate trends in the proportions of young people reaching minimum school leaving age without any graded passes. In both England and Wales there has been a steady decline in the numbers of boys and girls reaching the end of Year 11 without any qualifications – a decline between 1994 and 2000 from:

- 9.3 per cent to 6.5 per cent of boys in England
- 6.8 per cent to 4.6 per cent of girls in England
- 13 per cent to 6.4 per cent of boys in Wales
- 5.8 per cent to 5 per cent of girls in Wales

The proportion of boys obtaining no graded passes in Northern Ireland is much smaller but the decline has been less steep, from 6.7 per cent in 1996 to 5.3 per

Chart 15.3: Percentage of boys obtaining no graded pass school qualifications by the end of compulsory schooling, 1994–2000

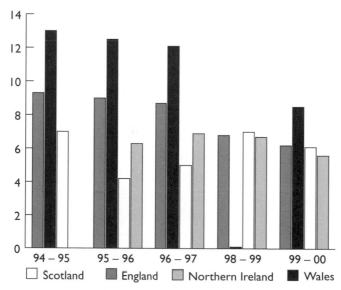

Note: Equivalent data is not available for Northern Ireland for 1994–95.

Chart 15.4: Percentage of girls obtaining no graded pass school qualifications by the end of compulsory schooling, 1994–2000

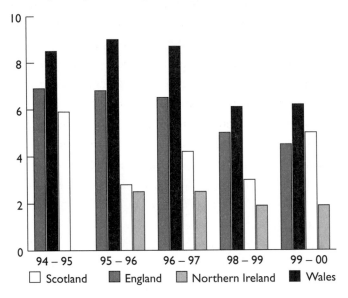

Note: Equivalent data is not available for Northern Ireland for 1994–95.

cent in 2000. Less than 2 per cent of girls in Northern Ireland (1.9 per cent) obtain no graded qualifications at 16 and the percentage has been below 3 per cent throughout the period.

Drop-out post 16: the dynamic picture

Student drop-out from full-time post-compulsory education is seen as an indicator of college performance on the one hand, and a factor increasing the risk of young people becoming socially excluded on the other. The SEU's report *Bridging the Gap* quotes Youth Cohort Study data which shows that nearly 10 per cent of those who were out of work and education at the age of 18 had embarked on a course of full-time education at 16, but failed to complete it. Drop-out is seen as dangerous to young people, especially those who have already had negative experiences of education, because it is another in a series of failures, and will further sap the individual's confidence. Drop-out is regarded as hugely wasteful, not only of a young person's potential but of public expenditure: "much, if not all, of the cost of the course is wasted" (SEU, 1999a, p. 36). This echoes the observations made in the Audit Commission's report *Unfinished Business* six years earlier, which described drop-out as 'a source of significant waste in 16–19 education' (Audit Commission, 1993, p. 36).

Although the numbers of students in post-16 education have increased, retention has remained more or less constant overall, at around 85 per cent. The National Audit Office reports that there is significant variation between different institutions – figures of between 98 per cent and 70 per cent retention, with sixth form colleges (which typically attract those with better GCSE results) generally being better performers. Variation in drop-out is related to previous achievements, just as participation and qualifications are related. The Audit Commission found that 42 per cent of students from vocational courses holding 10 or less GCSE points drop out, compared with just 15 per cent of those holding 21–40 points. Similar trends were observed for students on vocational courses. Payne (1998) reports similar findings for A-level students.

There is little gender difference, or variation between ethnic groups, but young people living in areas with 'high deprivation factors' are more likely to drop out. Retention generally improves the higher the qualification being studied. Schools and colleges continue to strive to improve retention and some have seen dramatic results. But overall the rates remain static. Unfortunately, little data is available on the reasons for drop-out, although surveys commonly cite 'finding employment', 'personal issues' and 'financial problems' as key causes (for example, Martinez and Munday, 1998; Kenwright, 1997). Nor can we be sure how drop-out relates to young peoples' future success.

Improvements in attainment during early schooling

The government notes encouraging trends from its own educational indicators in England. In *Opportunity for All: Making Progress* (DWP, 2001b), improvements are noted for 11-, 16- and 19-year-olds. The proportion of 11-year-olds achieving Level 4 or higher in Key Stage 2 tests have improved from 63 per cent to 75 per cent for literacy and from 62 per cent to 71 per cent in numeracy, although it should be noted that the trend has shown a plateau for the literacy measure in the past year, and a 1 per cent decline in the numeracy measure (see Chart 15.5).

The DfES National Learning Targets are 80 per cent for literacy and 75 per cent for numeracy by 2002, which appear by no means certain to be attained if the 2000–2001 trend continues. The measure for 16-year-olds is the proportion with one or more GCSEs. This indicator has shown steady improvements of half a per cent or so from 1998 to 2000, with an overall rise of 2.1 per cent from 92.3

Chart 15.5   Trends in the proportion of 11-year-olds achieving Level 4 or above in Key Stage 2 tests for literacy and numeracy, England

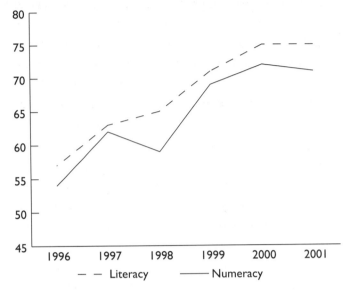

Source: DWP (2001b)

per cent in 1997 to 94.4 per cent in 2000. The number of 19-year-olds with at least one Level 2 qualification has also risen, from 69.7 per cent in 1996 to 75.3 per cent in 2000. The National Learning Target of 85 per cent by 2002, however, still appears optimistic.

Differences of attainment: gender, ethnicity and class

The official statistics of educational attainment can reveal some different patterns of attainment over time. But to examine background factors in more detail we have to turn to survey-based data on attainment, such as that collected by cohort studies and school leaver surveys. In England there was significant increase in educational performance following the introduction of GCSEs in 1988. This change is also associated with an increase in the so-called gender divide, whereby girls have increasingly out-performed boys in 16-plus examinations. Prior to GCSEs girls were on average 1.3 percentage points better than boys, and this had increased to 6 percentage points by the mid-1990s (Dolton *et al.*, 1999).

Compared to gender differences, differences between socio-economic and ethnic groups are much more marked. Recent studies of the attainment of different ethnic groups in England illustrate the complexity of these relationships. The highest achieving ethnic groups are Indian and Chinese. The lowest include Pakistani, Bangladeshi and African-Caribbean young people. Yet as Gillborn and Mirza (2000) point out, this variation is not consistent between local authorities. In some schools any one of the nationally under-performing ethnic groups may be 'top of the class'. The government has made much of both between-school and within-school differences of performance in order to emphasise the mutability of educational disadvantage. Yet it is too easy to write off educational performance differences as the result of good or bad teaching or willingness to learn. Most of the research evidence points to the systematic under-performance of African-Caribbean boys in particular, and recent OFSTED inspection reports point to many LEAs having "uncertainty which verges on helplessness" about strategies to raise the standards achieved by these groups (OFSTED, 1999).

It is also important to recognise that the least well achieving group are children from Gypsy and Traveller families. The problems faced by children from Roma and Sinti communities was the subject of an extensive report by the Organisation for Security and Co-operation in Europe (2000). Save the Children also published a report about education provision for Roma/Gypsy and Traveller children in Europe (2001). Both reports highlighted that poor and inadequate educational provision for such children is in contravention of numerous conventions including the UN Convention on the Rights of the Child. Yet throughout eastern and western Europe such children were subjected to discriminatory treatment, despite the fact that there was evidence that their parents wished for them to be properly educated. Both reports make reference to the UK. Moreover, the 1999 OFSTED report which concluded that 'the level of hostility faced by gypsy traveller [sic] children [in England] is probably greater than for any other minority ethnic group. Although there was evidence of some school attendance by children in the early years of schooling many were reported as simply absent from education altogether by the age of 14 and they were invariably never entered for any formal qualifications' (OFSTED, 1999).

Most progress has been made by Indian pupils, who now exceed the attainments of white pupils, while African-Caribbean and Pakistani pupils have widened the gap in the opposite direction. Bangladeshi pupils, meanwhile, have improved, but the attainment gap between them and white pupils remains (Gillborn and Mirza, 2000). Demie (2001) describes variations in attainment related to levels of fluency in English. As might be expected, children with little

English tend not to do as well as those from the same ethnic group but with better fluency. Furthermore, bilingual children who are fluent in English tend to do better than English-only speakers.

One of the difficulties in reaching simple conclusions about the relationship between ethnicity and educational performance is that there are sometimes marked gender differences and some ethnic groups have a very different socio-economic profile to others. The better performance of Indian young people is sometimes attributed to the occupational background of their parents as much as to family support and cultures of expectation. Both Dolton *et al.* (1999) and Gillborn and Mirza (2000) have made recent attempts to examine how 'in general improvement' has been distributed to different genders, ethnicity and socio-economic groups.

Dolton *et al.* (1999), for instance, have looked at changes in the proportion of young men and women obtaining qualifications from 'poor and good backgrounds' between 1986 and 1992. This indicates that all groups improved following the introduction of the GCSE examinations. But by far and away the biggest improvements were to be found in boys and girls from more privileged home backgrounds, who showed more than a 20 per cent improvement during this time compared to the 3 or 4 per cent increases from those from poor home backgrounds.

Table 15.4 shows a summary of changes since 1992. This shows that increasing proportions of all groups are gaining the top grades at GCSE, with 2000 results from those from skilled and semi-skilled manual and unskilled manual backgrounds showing very marked improvements.

A review of survey evidence across all four countries of the UK was carried out as part of the 'Home International' studies by the Centre for Educational

Table 15.4: Changes in educational attainment in England and Wales by parents' occupation, 1992–2000

	% achieving 5 or more GCSE Grades A*-C in Year 11				
	1992	1994	1996	1998	2000
All	37	42	44	46	49
Managerial/professional	60	66	68	69	69
Other non-manual	51	58	58	60	61
Skilled manual	29	36	36	40	45
Semi-skilled manual	23	26	29	32	37
Unskilled manual	16	16	24	20	30

Source: Youth Cohort Study, Cohorts 5–10

Sociology at the University of Edinburgh (Croxford, 2000). This concluded that the impact of social class was weaker in Scotland (and to a lesser extent in Wales) than it was in England. It suggested that part of the reason for this was the greater extent of social segregation within the schooling system in England. The lack of comparable data for Northern Ireland precluded firm conclusions about the impact of social class on educational attainment there. However, the study found greater variation between schools in England and Northern Ireland than in Scotland and Wales. In part this 'school effect' was seen to be connected to the social composition of the school, with schools in Wales and Scotland 'more comprehensive' in every sense – with less variance in the socio-economic status of the intakes (Croxford, 2000).

Attainment and indicators of poverty

Early studies such as that by the Plowden Committee (1967) established a clear relationship between educational attainment and social class, and their evidence fuelled the drive towards comprehensive education in the 1970s. However, recent work shows that the trends persist despite the considerable changes in the education system over the past quarter of a century.

In more recent research a range of indicators has been developed to identify and compare different levels of deprivation, such as the percentage of pupils receiving free school meals and the proportion of households in the local education authority (LEA) area with low or unskilled workers. Educational performance is also now typically measured by Standard Assessment Test (SAT) scores at the ages of 7 and 11, and GCSE results, although as Smith and Noble (1995) observe, this raises some problems as the SATs were disrupted by industrial action in the early 1990s. Nonetheless, clear relationships have been found. McCallum (1993) describes a variance of between 25 and 50 per cent in SAT scores at the age of 7, being associated with the predominating social class of households with children in the LEA area. Sammons (1995) found that children receiving free school meals were likely to perform more poorly in SATs at the age of 7 than their peers. In a large and complex study in 55 schools in Wandsworth, Strand (1999) found that pupils eligible for free school meals made less progress between base line assessment in the reception class to Key Stage 1 (KS1) assessment. However, African, Caribbean and Indian children within the free school meals group did better than children from other ethnic backgrounds. Sammons et al. (1997) also found that, within inner city London schools, children eligible for free school meals had poorer results at Key Stage 1, but Thomas (1995) did not find such an association in shire counties in England.

Shuttleworth (1995) found similar relationships in Northern Ireland between free school meal entitlement and GCSE results, and Patterson (1992) found similar trends in Fife. This analysis also revealed that parental education and occupation were independently associated with educational attainment, both factors being indicators of deprivation.

Gray *et al.* (1993) found that the Youth Cohort Study data revealed an association between socio-economic background and post-16 participation rates, with the most likely stayers-on being from non-manual and well-educated backgrounds. The Youth Cohort Study also shows that attainment at 16-plus is still related to deprivation factors. The effect of deprivation seems to have a long-term effect, as Smith and Noble (1995) argue. They show that while individuals and their families may move in and out of social disadvantage, the association between deprivation and educational attainment in primary school is likely to persist throughout an individual's school career.

It would also appear that the attainment gap between the poor and the better-off has persisted, despite improvements in school performance overall. Studies such as that by Mortimore and Blackstone (1982) show that social background has an association with educational attainment independently of the impact of the school attended. Smith and Noble (1995) present an example of school performance, as measured by the percentage of a cohort getting five or more GCSEs. Between 1988 and 1994 all LEAs improved significantly, but the gap between the LEAs with 'disadvantaged' status and those with 'medium' and 'advantaged' status was found to have widened.

The links between educational attainment and social background are complex. As Smith and Noble (1995) suggest, it seems likely that an accumulation of factors, such as family problems, health issues and discrimination serve to limit most severely the chances of poorer children to achieve their potential.

Conclusions

On the basis of the evidence reviewed in this chapter, it is fair to conclude that more young people appear to be achieving more in terms of formal qualifications than ever before. However, inequalities of achievement persist and some argue that they have intensified. There are still some groups who statistically under-perform.

There are also some young people who appear to have been left beached by socio-economic change, which increasingly rewards educational achievement and consigns the unqualified and early school leavers to insecure, badly paid work or no work at all. Educational achievements are strongly related to social class and disadvantage on the one hand, and later labour market positions on the other, which in turn link to other aspects of welfare and well-being. This raises significant concerns that cycles of deprivation and disadvantage are still being reinforced through our system of education.

16 Physical Activity: Structured Sport vs Active Play

Naomi Finch

Key statistics:
- In 1994, girls and older children were most likely to be overweight, and girls of all ages were more likely to be obese than boys.
- Girls and older children are less likely to undertake both sport and active play.
- Children are more likely to participate in active play than sport.
- International and regional analysis shows that participation in sport in England is comparatively low.

Key trends:
- The proportions of overweight and obese children have increased for all age groups and for both sexes across Scotland and England between the years 1974 and 1994, with the exception of English boys aged 4–6.
- Between 1995 and 1998, sporting participation increased in all UK countries, except Wales.
- 'The Play Surveys' suggest that participation in play has decreased over time and that free play has become restricted as a result of increasing anxiety about the consequences of playing outside.

Key sources:
- National Study of Health and Growth in England and Scotland
- Health Behaviour in School-Aged Children: A WHO Cross-National Study
- National Diets and Nutrition Survey
- Health Survey for England
- Scottish Health Survey
- Disability and Sport 2000: Young people with a disability and sport
- The Play Space Survey

Introduction

In 1991, the UN Convention on the Rights of the Child made it the child's right to rest and leisure, and to engage in play and recreational activities appropriate to the age of the child. It also stipulated that States' Parties should encourage the provision of appropriate and equal opportunities for cultural, artistic, recreational and leisure activity.

The benefits of physical activity include (National Playing Fields Association, 2000):

- psychological benefits: release of stress, confidence-building and self-esteem etc.
- social benefits: a domain in which to build relationships, meet friends etc.
- community benefits: facilitates social inclusion, promotes social cohesion, offer opportunities for exploring differences
- educational benefits: a cognitive tool through which children learn life skills such as risk-taking.

Article 24 in the UN Convention on the Rights of the Child also made it the child's right to enjoy the highest level of health possible. Chapter 5 examines child health and Chapter 4, diet and nutrition intake (energy intake) of young people. But in order to understand the extent to which children lead a healthy life style, it is important to examine their participation in physical activity (energy expenditure). Before we do this, we shall review childhood obesity.

Childhood obesity

Evidence of direct relationships between physical activity and health among children is generally weak. However, small but beneficial associations have been demonstrated between physical activity, reduced obesity, the extent to which a child becomes an active adult (Prescott-Clarke and Primatesta, 1998) and the associated risk factors of heart disease and other chronic diseases (Cole *et al.*, 2000). Until recently there has been no generally accepted definition of overweight and obese children. Different studies have used a variety of Body Mass Index percentile cut-offs to define 'overweight' and 'obese'[1] (Prescott-Clarke and Primatesta, 1998). However, these percentile cut-off points are

---

[1] Usually children are defined as overweight if their Body Mass Index is above the 85th centile of the 1990 BMI reference curves for the UK and obese if above the 95th centile.

somewhat arbitrary. In 2000, the Childhood Obesity Working Group established an internationally accepted definition of 'overweight' and 'obese' for children that identifies age- and sex-specific cut-off points[2] (Cole *et al.*, 2000). These have opened the opportunity to provide baseline information and trends in overweight and obese children. A longitudinal study using the National Study of Health and Growth in England and Scotland has provided trends over a 20 year period

Table 16.1: Trends in percentage overweight by age and sex, England and Scotland, 1974–1994

	1974	*1984*	*1994*	*Change 1974–1994*
English boys				
No.	4,139	3,259	3,016	
Age (years)				
4 to 6	6.8	4.6	5.4	−1.4
7 to 8	6.2	5.7	9.0	2.8
9 to 11	6.2	5.8	12.7	6.5
Total	6.4	5.4	9.0	2.6
English girls				
No.	3,871	3,008	2,858	
Age (years)				
4 to 6	9.5	7.5	10.9	1.4
7 to 8	7.6	10.6	12.5	4.9
9 to 11	9.9	9.9	16.7	6.8
Total	9.1	9.3	13.5	4.4
Scottish boys				
No.	1,172	2,141	2,072	
Age (years)				
4 to 6	7.0	5.7	7.6	0.6
7 to 8	4.2	6.4	8.0	3.8
9 to 11	5.0	6.9	13.4	8.4
Total	5.4	6.4	10.0	4.6
Scottish girls				
No.	1,078	2,105	2,036	
Age (years)				
4 to 6	10.1	9.3	11.9	1.8
7 to 8	7.0	11.3	15.1	8.1
9 to 11	9.1	10.6	19.6	10.5
Total	8.8	10.4	15.8	7.0

Source: Chinn and Rona (2001)

---

[2] Adult cut-off points were linked to body mass index centiles for children in order to produce the child cut-off points. For adult populations, the body mass index (weight/height2) is widely used, and a cut-off point of 30 kg/m2 is recognised internationally as a definition of adult obesity and 25 kg/m2 for overweight. (Cole *et al.*, 2000).

Table 16.2: Trends in percentage obese by sex, England and Scotland, 1974–1994

	1974	1984	1994	Change 1984–1994
English boys	1.4	0.6	1.7	0.3
English girls	1.5	1.3	2.6	1.1
Scottish boys	1.7	0.9	2.1	0.4
Scottish girls	1.9	1.8	3.2	1.3

Source: Chinn and Rona (2001)

using the new cut-off points (Chinn and Rona, 2001). Table 16.1 and 16.2 demonstrate that the proportions of overweight and obese children[3] have increased for all age groups and for both sexes across Scotland and England between the years 1974 and 1994, with the exception of English boys aged 4–6 years. The 1994 data demonstrates that girls and older children are most likely to be overweight and that girls are more likely to be obese.

The definition of physical activity: Sport vs Active play

There are two different forms of physical activity: sport and active play. They are distinct since "play, leisure, and recreation, but not sports, have in common the voluntary commitment of the participant" (Sutton-Smith in Dyck, 2000, p. 19). Play is subjective, "freely chosen, personally directed, intrinsically motivated behaviour that actively engages the child" (National Playing Fields Association, 2000). Sport, on the other hand, "is defined by the presence of an external reward" and is "carried out by actors who represent or who are part of formally organised association" (Edwards, 1973). Play therefore gives children the oppor-tunities to enjoy freedom and exercise control over their actions (National Playing Fields Association, 2000). Sport, controlled by adults, potentially reduces the freedom of the child.

Children's physical activity is far more diverse than that of adults. It is characterised by short bouts of activity and is less likely to involve clearly defined periods of specific activities (Armstrong *et al.*, 1990). Research has focused upon the more quantifiable structured sporting participation, and data on children's participation in active play is relatively sparse.

---

[3] This includes only white children aged 4–11. Minority ethnic groups were included in a separate inner-city sample not reported here.

Physical activity: sources
'The Sport Surveys'

The Sports Council in each UK country funds Sport Surveys with young people (England: Sport England, 2000; Finch *et al.*, 2001; Wales: Sports Council for Wales, 2001a and 2001b; Scotland: Allison *et al.*, 1999 and Martin and Coalter, 2000; Northern Ireland: Kremer *et al.*, 1997), which provide data on participation, attitudes and motivations towards sport.

Advantages
- Data exist for all UK countries.
- With the exception of Northern Ireland, trend analysis is available.
- The disability sports survey 2000 (Finch *et al.*, 2001) provides the only data available on sport, disability and young people.

Disadvantages
- There is no differentiation between active play and sport.
- There is no collaboration between the surveys.
- The Northern Irish survey did not specifically measure current sporting participation.

'The Health Surveys'
The National Diet and Nutrition Survey for Great Britain

The survey was undertaken in 1997 with 2,127 children and young people aged 4–18 years. For those aged 7 or over, a 7-day diary method was used to assess the duration, intensity and frequency of physical activity.

Advantages
- The sample was found to be generally representative of the population in terms of social and demographic characteristics as assessed by reference to the 1996/97 General Household Survey.

Disadvantages
- It is a one-off survey; no trend data.
- There is only limited analysis on the separate countries in Great Britain.
- Northern Ireland is not included in the sample.

Health Survey for England and the Scottish Health Survey

Since 1995 in England and 1998 in Scotland, the health surveys have asked children about participation in *out-of-school* physical activity in five areas in the seven days prior to interview: sport and exercise; active play; walking; housework and gardening; and sitting.

Advantages
- Sport and active play are differentiated.
- They are directly comparable.
- They are undertaken each year in England and every three years in Scotland so there is potential for trend analysis.

Disadvantages
- The data are available for England and Scotland only.[4]
- They are less comprehensive than the Sports Surveys.
- Data collected was limited to activities lasting at least 15 minutes duration which, given the sporadic nature of children's activity patterns, may be too long a period.

'The Play Surveys'

'The Play Surveys' provide data on a variety of issues associated with (active) play, including the factors that prevent children from undertaking play. The most important survey is The Play Space Survey (The Children's Society and the Children's Play Council, 2001) – a survey undertaken with 800 4–16-year-olds in England and Scotland.

Advantages
- They provide data in an area with limited research.

Disadvantages
- There is no data on participation in active play.
- They are small one-off studies.

---

[4] A health survey exists for Wales but the sample does not include children.

Cross-national data

The COMPASS project

The COMPASS project seeks to promote harmonisation of sports participation statistics in Europe. Taking differences in methodologies, etc, into account, COMPASS has used a basic approach to make comparisons between England, Finland, Italy, Netherlands and Sweden and has created seven groups to reflect level of participation. (For an explanation of these groups, see COMPASS (1999).)

The Health and Behaviour of School Children Survey

The World Health Organization's 'Health and Behaviour of School Children Survey' (HBSC), established in 1985/96, is the only data source currently available which contains *international* comparative data on exercise (which could be interpreted by children to include active play) in 27 countries (Currie *et al.*, 2000).

Advantages
- Identical questions are asked in each country.
- It is conducted at 4-yearly intervals, so trend analysis is available.
- Data is available for all UK countries.

Disadvantages
- Only 11-, 13- and 15-year-olds are included in the sample.
- Questions on physical activity are limited.

In this chapter, we have used the HBSC survey for comparative analysis. The HBSC survey has also been used for trend and regional analysis.

Participation in physical activity

The Health Education Authority (HEA, 1998) recommends that people aged 5–18 should participate in physical activity of at least moderate intensity for one hour per day. Moderate intensity activity is defined as activity equivalent to walking which might be expected to leave the participant feeling warm and slightly out of breath. It is further recommended that at least twice a week, some of this activity should be vigorous. Vigorous activity is usually equivalent to at least slow jogging which might be expected to leave the participant feeling out of breath and sweaty. It is therefore important not only to examine basic

Table 16.3: Proportions who had undertaken moderate or vigorous activity in the 7-day recording period, by sex and age, Great Britain,[1] 1997

	Moderate activity[2]	Vigorous activity[3]	Base
Boys			
7–10	99	77	263
11–14	96	83	254
15–18	84	68	194
All boys	93	76	711
Girls			
7–10	95	74	236
11–14	96	78	255
15–18	91	53	222
All girls	94	69	713

[1] This survey did not include Northern Ireland.
[2] This includes people who participated in any moderate intensity activity during the recording period. Young people who did not take part in any moderate intensity activity may have taken part in a vigorous/very vigorous intensity activity.
[3] This category includes people who participated in any vigorous or very vigorous intensity activity during the recording period. Young people who had not taken part in vigorous/very vigorous activity may have taken part in moderate intensity activity
Source: Gregory and Lowe (2000)

participation rates but also to identify the intensity and duration of the activity.

The National Diet and Nutrition Survey for Great Britain measured duration of activity using the above definitions. Table 16.3 shows that:

- boys were more likely than girls to have undertaken vigorous activity, but no variation is apparent between the sexes for moderate activity
- a decline in participation for both categories is evident with age.

Table 16.4: Mean hours spent in activity of at least moderate intensity per day by sex and age, Great Britain, 1997

Hours	Boys				Girls			
	7–10	11–14	15–18	All	7–10	11–14	15–18	All
No time	0	2	9	4	4	1	5	3
< ½ hour	10	12	29	17	16	24	41	27
<1 hr	30	32	56	39	51	56	69	58
< 1.5 hrs	52	55	78	62	75	81	84	80
<2 hrs	73	78	89	80	91	92	92	92
Mean	1.6	1.5	1.0	1.4	1.1	1.0	0.8	1.0
Base	263	254	194	711	236	255	222	713

Source: Gregory and Lowe (2000)

Analysis by duration (Table 16.4) shows that:

- girls were more likely than boys to spend less than one hour per day in activity of at least moderate intensity
- older children were more likely than younger children to spend less than one hour in activity of moderate intensity.

Regional variation

The HBSC survey provides regional data for the number of hours spent in vigorous exercise in the reference week. Table 16.5 shows that:

- young people in England were the least likely to have taken part in vigorous exercise
- young people in Northern Ireland were the most likely to have undertaken seven hours or more vigorous activity
- regional variation is more marked between boys than between girls.

Health Surveys have been carried out in England and Scotland, but not in Northern Ireland or Wales. The Health Survey for England and the Scottish Health Survey do not differentiate between moderate and vigorous activity, but do compare sport and active play. Table 16.6 (basic participation) and 16.7 (duration) show the following:

- Participation rates are higher for active play than for sport regardless of age, sex or region.
- The greatest variations between regions were found for sport – variations which reflect the findings from the HBSC survey, i.e. that children in England were the least likely to have undertaken sport.
- Reflecting both the HBSC survey and the Diet and Nutrition Survey, girls and older children were less likely to have undertaken either sport or active play. However, the drop in sporting participation occurs at a later age than the drop in active play participation.
- English children, especially girls, were least likely to have undertaken sport for seven hours or more in the reference week.
- English girls were significantly less likely than Scottish girls to undertaken active play for seven hours or more, but little variation is apparent between English and Scottish boys.

Table 16.5: Number of hours per week of vigorous exercise[1] in free time by region, age and sex, 1997/98

	Sex			Age		
	Boys	Girls	11	13	15	All
England						
No time	5	8	6	6	7	7
About ½ an hour	17	25	26	19	18	21
I hour or less	23	26	25	25	24	25
2–3 hours	26	24	22	26	27	25
4–6 hours	15	10	10	14	14	13
> 7 hours	12	5	7	9	9	9
Base	5,063[2]	5,241[2]	2,193[3]	2,102[3]	1,891[3]	10,407[4]
Wales						
No time	3	8	4	5	7	5
About ½ an hour	7	15	14	11	9	11
I hour or less	18	29	27	22	22	23
2–3 hours	36	32	36	36	30	34
4–6 hours	20	12	13	16	19	16
> 7 hours	16	5	8	11	13	10
Base	2,054	2,024	1,376	1,424	1,278	4,078
Scotland						
No time	2	6	2	5	6	4
About ½ an hour	10	17	15	14	12	14
I hour or less	17	24	22	19	20	20
2–3 hours	28	30	26	30	23	29
4–6 hours	22	15	19	19	17	19
> 7 hours	21	8	16	14	13	14
Base	2,723	2,827	2,062	1,778	1,710	5,550
Northern Ireland						
No time	3	5	3	3	7	4
About ½ an hour	10	19	17	13	13	14
I hour or less	19	25	23	22	20	22
2–3 hours	30	28	27	29	30	29
4–6 hours	18	14	16	17	15	16
> 7 hours	21	9	16	16	15	16
Base	1,796	1,550	1,068	1,197	1,081	3,346

[1] Exercise may be interpreted by the children to include active play

[2] The base for boys and girls do not add up to the overall base due to some respondents not stating their sex. However, these respondents have been included in the overall base.

[3] In the English 1997/8 HSBC survey, from which this figures have been obtained, age groups between 11 and 16 were interviewed. However, only the results for selected aged groups are shown here. Therefore, the base for age group does not add up to the overall base. The overall base also includes some respondents whose age group is unknown.

[4] The overall base includes those respondents who did not state their sex and/or whose age is unknown.

Sources: HEA (1997); Data provided by the Health Promotion Agency for Wales; own analysis of the 1998 HBSC survey for Northern Ireland; Research Unit in Health and Behavioural Changes, University of Edinburgh.

Table 16.6: Percentages participating in sport and active play by sex, age and region, 1998

Age	England		North England		Scotland	
	Boys	Girls	Boys	Girls	Boys	Girls
Sport[1]						
2–3 years	35	39	37	46	44	47
4–5 years	48	44	48	47	53	56
6–7 years	58	55	62	57	68	59
8–9 years	70	64	70	73	72	72
10–11 years	73	70	79	70	82	70
12–13 years	74	53	79	50	79	66
14–15 years	68	45	68	39	78	51
All	60	53	63	55	69	60
Active play[2]						
2–3 years	90	90	90	86	88	87
4–5 years	93	89	92	92	92	91
6–7 years	91	89	93	86	94	91
8–9 years	88	86	81	83	95	89
10–11 years	90	81	91	86	93	86
12–13 years	80	63	80	67	84	74
14–15 years	79	53	78	46	81	50
All	88	80	87	77	90	81
Base (weighted)	2,146	2,077	591	613	1,096	1,045

[1] Sport and exercise activities included more "organised" or "structured sporting activities".
[2] Active play included "active things like" (younger children) "play active games, run about, kick a ball about, ride a bike"; (older children) "cycle about, run about, kick a ball about".
Source: Shaw et al. (2000)

The characteristics of participants in physical activity

The Health Survey for England, the Scottish Health Survey and the Diet and Nutrition Survey undertook analysis by various characteristics, in addition to age and sex. None of these surveys include Northern Ireland, for which no data could be found that undertook analysis by various characteristics (other than sex and age).

Social class

For basic participation, analysis has been undertaken according to social class using the Health Survey for England and the Scottish Health Survey (Tables 16.8 and 16.9):

- In England, there is evidence of socio-economic gradients in the participation rates in sport for both sexes and age groups.

Table 16.7: Number of hours participated in sport and active play in the last week by sex

| | England (1995–97) | | Scotland (1998) | |
	Boys	Girls	Boys	Girls
Sport				
No time	42	49	31	40
Less than an hour	10	14	8	9
1, less than 3 hours	20	21	20	23
3, less than 5 hours	11	8	13	12
5, less than 7 hours	6	4	7	5
More than 7 hours	11	5	21	11
Mean	2.6	1.5	3.8	2.4
Active play				
No time	15	28	10	19
Less than an hour	8	10	4	5
1, less than 3 hours	17	17	12	15
3, less than 5 hours	11	10	13	12
5, less than 7 hours	11	7	9	8
More than 7 hours	54	28	53	41
Mean	10.41	5.45	8.8	7.1
Base (weighted)	2,146	2,077	1,096	1,045

Sources: Prescott-Clarke and Primatesta (1999); Shaw *et al.* (2000)

- In Scotland, there is some evidence of socio-economic gradients in sporting participation rates for girls, but no pattern is evident for boys.
- For active play, there is no clear relationship between social class and participation.

Table 16.8: Participation rates in sport by social class

| **England (1995–7)** | Boys | | Girls | |
	2–10	11–15	2–10	11–15
I and II	60	73	63	63
III non-manual	57	78	53	59
III manual	44	75	46	53
IV and V	45	71	35	47
Scotland (1998)	Boys		Girls	
I and II	70		66	
III non-manual	69		58	
III manual	71		58	
IV and V	63		55	

Sources: Prescott-Clarke and Primatesta (1999); Shaw *et al.* (2000)

Table 16.9: Participation rates in active play by social class

England (1997)	Boys		Girls	
	2–10	11–15	2–10	11–15
I and II	89	80	78	56
III non-manual	87	78	81	48
III manual	86	83	80	54
IV and V	85	81	80	55
Scotland (1998)	Boys		Girls	
I and II	88		81	
III non-manual	91		84	
III manual	91		82	
IV and V	90		80	

Sources: Prescott-Clarke and Primatesta (1999); Shaw *et al.* (2000)

Income

For basic participation, analysis has been undertaken according to equivalised household income using the Health Survey for England and the Scottish Health Survey (Table 16.10):

● With the exception of boys aged 11–15, the higher the income the higher the likelihood of sporting participation;

Table 16.10: Participation rates in sport and active play by income, England, 1995–1997

	Boys		Girls	
	2–10	11–15	2–10	11–15
Sport				
Up to £6,500	40	75	34	43
Over £6,500 to £10, 655	43	69	37	52
Over £10, 655 to £15,899	52	71	56	61
Over £15,899 to £24,381	65	78	63	62
Over £24,381	66	75	64	69
Active play				
Up to £6,500	84	84	78	56
Over £6,500 to £10, 655	84	81	80	51
Over £10, 655 to £15,899	86	78	80	60
Over £15,899 to £24,381	93	84	82	57
Over £24,381	89	75	79	48

Source: Prescott-Clarke and Primatesta (1999)

- On the other hand, for active play, a decrease in participation is evident for those in the higher income bands.
- The data suggests that families with higher incomes may neglect free play in favour of more structured sporting activity.

Family type

The National Diet and Nutrition Survey for Great Britain is the only survey for which analysis is available by family type. Table 16.11 demonstrates that having a sibling positively affects duration spent on physical activity.

Table 16.11: Hours spent in activity of at least moderate intensity per day young people aged 7–18 by sex and family type, Great Britain, 1997

	Males		Females	
	Mean	Median	Mean	Median
Young person living with:				
Both parents and other children	1.4 hours	1.3 hours	1.0 hours	0.9 hours
Both parents, no other children	1.2 hours	1.0 hours	0.9 hours	0.7 hours
Single parent	1.4 hours	1.2 hours	1.0 hours	1.0 hours
Base		711		713

Source: Gregory and Lowe (2000)

Ethnicity

Matthews (1992) hypothesised that children from minority groups are perhaps more restricted because their families tend to concentrate in inner-city localities, live in poor housing and be at the lower end of the income range, thus restricting participation in both sport and active play. The 1999 Health Survey for England focused upon ethnicity. The findings for basic participation (Table 16.12) show that:

- Girls were less likely to have participated in either sport or play, regardless of ethnicity.
- Generally, South Asian children (with the exception of Indian boys) were the least likely to have taken part in sport.
- For active play, there is little variation by ethnicity.

Table 16.12: Participation rates in sport and active play by ethnicity, England, 1999

	Black Caribbean	Indian	Pakistani	Bangla-deshi	Chinese	Irish	General population (1998)
			Ethnic group				
Sport							
Boys							
% participating	68	59	46	48	51	64	63
Ratios for participation	1.08	0.94	0.74	0.76	0.82	1.03	1
Girls							
% participating	55	34	31	27	53	59	56
Ratios for participation	0.98	0.62	0.55	0.48	0.95	1.05	1
Active play							
Boys							
% participating	92	87	87	87	89	91	92
Ratios for participation	0.99	0.94	0.94	0.95	0.96	0.98	1
Girls							
% participating	83	81	81	81	81	89	86
Ratios for participation	0.96	0.94	0.94	0.94	0.94	1.03	1
Bases (unweighted)							
Boys	300	268	397	385	138	270	1,905
Girls	312	203	393	358	126	265	1,841

Source: Erens *et al.* (2001)

Table 16.13: Mean hours participating in sport and active play in the week prior to interview by ethnicity, England, 1999

	Black Caribbean	Indian	Pakistani	Bangla-deshi	Chinese	Irish	General population (1998)
			Ethnic group				
Sport and exercise							
Boys	4.94	3.51	2.36	2.61	1.45	4.41	3.36
Girls	2.13	0.86	1.44	0.89	1.60	2.36	2.33
Active play							
Boys	11.01	8.11	7.70	4.93	7.29	11.25	11.04
Girls	7.20	4.96	6.10	3.29	4.73	9.32	8.90
Bases (unweighted)							
Boys	300	268	397	385	138	270	1,905
Girls	312	203	393	358	126	265	1,841

Source: Erens *et al.* (2001)

Analysis by duration of activity (Table 16.13) shows that:

- Regardless of ethnicity, children had spent more hours participating in active play than in sport.
- Chinese boys and Indian and Bangladeshi girls had spent the least amount of time, on average, participating in sport in the reference week.
- Bangladeshi boys and girls had spent the least number of hours, on average, participating in active play.

Disability

Sport and play are just as beneficial for disabled children as for all children and can serve to empower and counteract stigma (Finch *et al.*, 2001). No data is available on active play and disability. Finch *et al.* (2001) undertook a quantitative survey on disabled children (aged 6–16) and sport in England and Scotland. The results of the survey were compared with the 1999 survey undertaken with the general population of children (Table 16.14):

- Disabled children were less likely to participate in sport than all children, and the gap between the two increased with more frequent participation.
- Those with a self-care related or mobility disability were less likely to participate in sport than those with other disabilities.
- Those in special schools were generally more likely to participate than those in mainstream schools.

Table 16.14: A comparison between disabled children and all children of the participation rates and mean number of sports undertaken in the 12 months prior to interview

	In or out of school		In school		Out of school	
	Disabled	All (1999)	Disabled	All (1999)	Disabled	All (1999)
Sports undertaken at least once						
Participation rate	95	99	90	99	85	98
Mean no. of sports undertaken	7.9	14.4	5.7	8.4	4.7	10.3
Sport undertaken 10 times or more						
Participation rate	74	94	64	83	56	87
Mean no. of sports undertaken	3.0	6.8	2.1	3.6	1.7	4.4
Base	2,293	3,319	2,293	3,319	2,293	3,319

Source: Finch et al. (2001)

Finch *et al.* concluded that low participation of disabled children is only partly attributed to lack of motivation; only 10 per cent of children cited this as a reason for not participating in sport. Rather, a link can be made with external barriers. Those who were least likely to undertake sport (i.e. those with a self-care related or mobility disability) were the most likely to cite barriers such as lack of facilities for disabled children and lack of trained staff at sport centres as reasons for not undertaking sport. By contrast, those who were most likely to undertake sport (those with a hearing disability) were least likely to cite reasons associated with their disability.

The dynamics of sport and active play

Sport

Table 16.15 shows changes in sport participation over time using the HBSC survey. Data for 1990 has not been included for Northern Ireland because limited data analysis was undertaken for this year. England did not take part in the 1990 survey. Between 1994/96 and 1997/98:

- The proportion of young people exercising for at least four hours a week

Table 16.15: Percentage exercising for at least 4 hours per week outside school, by sex, 11–16-year-olds, 1990–1998

	England (base)	Wales (base)	Scotland (base)	Northern Ireland (base)
Males				
1990	*	37 (3,121)	37 (1,924)	**
1994/95	28 (3,396)	33 (1,791)	36 (2,373)	34 (1,944)
1997/98	27 (5,241)	37 (2,054)	42 (2,723)	39 (1,796)
Females				
1990	*	15 (3,367)	19 (2,126)	**
1994/95	10 (2,976)	14 (2,109)	18 (2,504)	16 (1,940)
1997/98	15 (5,241)	15 (2,024)	24 (2,827)	23 (1,550)
Both sexes				
1990	*	26 (6,488)	28 (4,050)	**
1994/95	19 (6,406)	24 (3,900)	27 (4,877)	25 (3,932)
1997/98	22 (10,407)	26 (4,078)	33 (5,550)	31 (3,346)

* England did not take part in the 1990 survey.
** Data for 1990 has not been included for Northern Ireland because limited data analysis was undertaken for this year.
Sources: HEA (1997 and 1999); Data provided by the Health Promotion Agency for Wales; Health Promotion Agency for Northern Ireland (1994 and 1995); own analysis of the 1998 HBSC survey for Northern Ireland; Todd *et al.* (2000).

increased in England, Scotland and Northern Ireland, but stayed generally stable in Wales.

- In all countries except England the proportion of boys exercising for at least four hours a week increased.
- In all countries except Wales the proportion of girls exercising for at least four hours a week increased.

Active Play

The results from the English and Scottish Health Surveys indicate that children are more likely to participate in active play than sport. However, lack of spontaneous play opportunities has been suggested as one of the causes of the increase in child obesity in England (Dietz, 2001). Indeed, evidence from 'The Play Surveys' suggest that participation in play has decreased over time and that free play has become restricted as a result of increasing anxiety about the consequences of playing outside.

In a recent survey with 38 play professionals (Cole-Hamilton, 2001), 22 said they think that children have less access to dedicated play spaces than five years ago. In a separate survey asking parents' views on play, 80 per cent said that they think children now spend less time playing outside than they did when they themselves were young and 78 per cent said the main reason for this was fear from harm from strangers (The Children's Society, 2001). Furthermore, in the last 20 years, car traffic has almost doubled and cars now dominate outdoor public places where children could once play relatively safely (Hillman, 1999). While the UK has one of the lowest rates of road traffic deaths internationally (UNICEF, 2001a), it has the highest number of child pedestrian fatalities in Europe, relative to the number of children in the population (DETR, 2000).

There is also evidence that children are restricted from playing where they want. In 1996, a study (Wheway and Millward, 1997) made over 3,500 observations of children under 18 at 12 housing estates in England. It observed that children mostly play where adults can see them. Also, in the same study, interviews were undertaken with 236 children between the ages of 5 and 18. While these revealed that children's favourite locations to play were open spaces (56 per cent), the observations demonstrated that low proportions were actually undertaking play in these areas. Likewise, The Play Space Survey (The Children's Society and the Children's Play Council, 2001) undertaken with 800 children aged 4–16 in England and Scotland showed that, while children's favourite play areas were the park (31 per cent), they were most likely to play in the street (27 per cent) or the garden (27 per cent).

The Play Space Survey also revealed that children themselves are aware of problems restricting play. Although 65 per cent said that there are enough places to play *in the way* they want to, 61 per cent said that certain things stop them from playing *where* they would like to. Their biggest concerns were bullying from older children (25 per cent), fear of traffic (17 per cent), parents' fear of strangers (15 per cent), dirty play areas (10 per cent), drug dealers (8 per cent) and their own fear of strangers (7 per cent). A small study with 171 Pakistani children in Sheffield (Woolley and Amin, 1995) revealed that children's activities in public open spaces had been restricted because of a lack of facilities or public spaces in the vicinity (66 per cent), because they felt unsafe or scared (17 per cent) and because of racism (12 per cent) and bullying (3 per cent).

Cross-country comparison

No data has been found that compares active play participation across countries. This section undertakes international comparison of participation in exercise (which may be interpreted by children to include active play) using the HBSC. Analysis undertaken in Chapter 4 (Diet and Nutrition) using the same survey shows that young people in the UK countries have the worst diets of all countries in the study. Analysis of the physical activity data (Table 16.16) shows that:

- In all countries, girls age 11–15 are less likely than boys to undertake sport for two or more hours a week.
- England has one of the worse records of all countries.
- Scotland is the only UK country ranking within the top ten.

Conclusion

Until recently, in an effort to lower obesity levels and increase fitness among children, official documents have placed greater emphasis on increased participation in structured sports rather than informal play (Department for Culture, Media and Sport, 2000; DoH, 1999). To an extent this focus is supported by the data; the results of 'The Health Surveys' show that active play participation is higher than participation in sport and, while low sporting participation is

Table 16.16: A cross-country comparison of participation of 11–15-year-olds in vigorous exercise two or more hours a week, 1997/98

Country	Girls %	Boys %	Rank
Austria	69	84	1
Germany	69	83	2
Denmark	65	77	3
Switzerland	57	80	4
France	53	79	5
Finland	58	73	6
Norway	63	65	7
Canada	53	71	8
Scotland	53	71	9
USA	54	67	10
Wales	48	72	11
N Ireland	51	68	12
Poland	48	67	13
Sweden	50	64	14
Ireland	49	63	15
Belgium	45	66	16
Czech Republic	48	57	17
Greece	39	66	18
Estonia	42	62	19
Hungary	43	58	20
Israel	34	64	21
Greenland	40	56	22
Lithuania	32	56	23
England	27	54	24
Russia	28	47	25
Portugal	23	44	26
Latvia	21	41	27

Source: Currie *et al.* (2000) and author's own calculations

associated with socio-economic characteristics and geographical area, little variation is apparent for active play. However, the data link obesity with low sport and active play participation, and girls and older children are more likely to be overweight and less likely to participate in either sport or active play. Furthermore, while participation in sport has generally increased, 'The Play Surveys' suggest that participation in play has declined and that anxieties over safety issues and limited (suitable) play provision and open spaces restrict children from playing where they would like and as much as they would like. If play, as opposed to sport, is considered a right, children are only partially enjoying that right.

Nevertheless, it is difficult to monitor adequately articipation in active play because few sources presently exist that enable us to do so. The Health Survey for England and the Scottish Health Survey offer a valuable data source, but no trend analysis has been undertaken. Moreover, no data can be found for Wales and Northern Ireland that treat active play separately from sport, although The Health Survey for Wales (which currently only includes adults) offers a potential source. More extensive data exist for sport, but comparable data between the UK countries is limited in scope. Comprehensive data exist in the form of 'The Sport Surveys', but greater collaboration is needed between the surveys for more useful data. Active play is clearly an important source of physical activity for children but, in order to develop our understanding of this, more data is needed on children's participation in and attitudes towards active play *vis à vis* sport.

17 Truancy and School Exclusions

Eirian Edwards and Bob Coles

Key facts:

- The percentage of half-days missed as a result of unauthorised absences from secondary school was 1 per cent in England and Scotland and 1.5 per cent in Wales.
- The number of permanent exclusions/expulsions from schools was 8,323 in England, 337 in Wales, 360 in Scotland and 85 in Northern Ireland in 1999/2000.

Key trends:

- In England unauthorised absence from all maintained schools has remained at around 0.7 per cent since 1994 and progress has yet to be made to meet the target of reducing the overall truancy rate by a third by 2002, and a further 10 per cent by 2004.
- Permanent exclusions hugely increased in England in the 1990s to reach a peak in 1995/96, since when official rates of permanent exclusions have declined.

Key sources:

- DfES
- Welsh Assembly
- Scottish Executive
- The five Education and Library Boards in Northern Ireland

Introduction

Truancy and school exclusion were the subject of the first report of the Social Exclusion Unit (SEU) set up by the Prime Minister shortly after the General Election in 1997. The introductory remarks in the report illustrate why the topics received such high profile attention at the turn of the century:

"Truancy and exclusions have reached a crisis point. The thousands of children who are not in school on most schooldays have become a significant cause of crime. Many of today's non-attenders are in danger of becoming tomorrow's criminals and unemployed. No one knows precisely how many children are out of school at any time because of truancy or exclusion. But each year at least 1 million children truant, and over 100,000 children are excluded temporarily. Some 13,000 are excluded permanently."
(SEU, 1998b, p. 1)

The sources of evidence

Despite truancy and school exclusions being of such high profile importance, comparing the four countries of the UK is not straightforward as they operate under different systems. England and Wales operate under the same school exclusion legislation, but Northern Ireland and Scotland each has its own legislation and regulations (Parsons, 1999). The terminology used is also different. In England and Wales, exclusions are divided into 'permanent' and 'fixed-term' exclusions, in Scotland they are divided into 'permanent' and 'temporary' exclusions, while Northern Ireland uses the terms 'expulsion' and 'suspension'.

Technically, truancy means self-exclusion – a pupil not attending school when legally required to do so. School exclusion usually refers to decisions made by the school to require a pupil not to attend, either for a fixed period of time or permanently. In England and Wales, in the case of permanent exclusion, the child's parents can appeal to a special panel of the local education authority (LEA), and the LEA has a responsibility for providing alternative education (although until very recently, this was unlikely to be more than a few hours a week in a Pupil Referral Unit). Scotland has its own distinctive education system. Here the responsibility for school exclusion lies with the education authority and not the head teacher of the school, as in England and Wales, although this responsibility can be devolved to schools. In Northern Ireland, as in England and Wales, the head teacher may suspend a pupil, but under the Northern Ireland regulations, expulsion is more difficult. Consultations must take place between the head teacher, the parent of the pupil, the chief executive of the Education Board and the chair of the Board of Governors before a pupil can be expelled. These expulsion meetings must "include consultations about the future provision of suitable education for the pupil concerned" (Parsons, 1999, p. 33).

Issues about truancy and school exclusions will be covered later in the chapter.

First we turn to what the data can, and cannot, tell us about the scale and nature of the problems.

Truancy rates

In England, Wales and Scotland, official truancy rates are based upon schools reporting unauthorised absence, usually based on those who fail to register without authorisation, usually at the beginning of each half-day. But, especially since these rates now appear in school league tables, LEA tables in England and Wales and education authority tables in Scotland, they are highly sensitive and subject to various means of manipulation (NCH, 2000; Mittler, 2000). In Northern Ireland, no distinction is made between authorised and unauthorised absence from school. Data on absence is collected by each of the five Education and Library Boards (ELBs), but it is not published. Northern Ireland does not have league tables (Edwards, 2001). Truancy rates in England are one of the key *Opportunity for All* indicators used to measure progress made to tackle poverty and social exclusion, with a target of reducing the overall truancy rate by a third by 2002 and by a further 10 per cent by 2004 (DWP, 2001b). In Wales, the National Assembly has set targets to reduce the level of unauthorised absences from secondary schools from 1.5 per cent in 1997 to 1 per cent by the year 2002 (Welsh Assembly, 2001a). In Scotland, the Executive aims to reduce the number of days lost through truancy from secondary schools by a third (Lloyd *et al.*, 2001, p. 1). In Northern Ireland, the Department of Education has introduced a measurement of social need, of attendance of 85 per cent or less, as a result of the New Targeting Social Need (New TSN) policy, which requires all departments to focus their attention on those most deprived. This data will be collected by all five ELBs from 2000/01 and first comparisons will be available after data for 2001/02 are collated (Edwards, 2001). The New TSN Action Plan has set a target to reduce by 30 per cent the number of pupils identified as persistent non-attenders by 2003, compared to 1998/99 (New TSN Unit, 2000).

In England, secondary schools reported double the truancy rates (at 1.0%) compared to primary schools (at 0.5%) in 1999/2000. Both the Department for Work and Pensions (DWP) and the Department for Education and Skills (DfES) report that in England, unauthorised absence from maintained schools for half a day or more has remained constant (DWP, 2001b) at around 0.7 per cent since 1994 (DfEE, 2000a, p. 4). Progress has yet to be made on meeting the *Opportunity for All* truancy target by 2002 (DWP, 2001b). Unauthorised absences from secondary schools in England have remained constant at 1 per cent since 1994/95, rising to 1.1 per cent in 1997/98 and 1998/99 (DfEE, 2000a, p. 8). There are, however, marked differences between LEAs (DfEE, 2000a) as Table 17.1 illustrates. Scotland also reports unauthorised absence from secondary schools at 1 per cent, which has remained stable between 1997 and 2000. In contrast to England, almost all absence from primary schools in Scotland was authorised (Scottish Executive, 2001a). In Wales, the official unauthorised absence rate for secondary pupils was 1.5 per cent for 1998/99 and 1999/2000 (Welsh Assembly, 2001a). Both Scotland and Wales also report wide variations in unauthorised absence as illustrated in Table 17.1.

Yet these official rates are not the only indicator of the size or nature of the problem. Official truancy rates are known to underestimate hugely unauthorised absence. OFSTED reports huge variation between schools in what is meant by 'unauthorised' absence. Some absences are recorded by schools as 'authorised' – these might involve parents' taking a child on holiday during term time for instance. OFSTED reports that two schools with the same overall official rates of absence are markedly different in allocating these to 'truancy' or 'authorised absence' (OFSTED, 2001). The official rates can thus be distorted and misinterpreted in several ways. Firstly, if a few individuals persistently truant for weeks at a time, this will affect the official rates. It will have a marked effect on the educational performance of these individuals, but potentially little effect on the attainments of the school as a whole. On the other hand, where a large number of pupils truant occasionally and irregularly, this may have an effect on their classes and school (Scottish Executive, 2001a). Furthermore, it is known that some pupils truant after registration; they are marked present on the register but then leave school (Cullingford, 1999). Some truants forge notes from the

Table 17.1: Percentage of half-days missed as a result of unauthorised absence from secondary schools in England, Wales and Scotland, including the highest and lowest rate within each country, 1999–2000

	England	Wales	Scotland
Average	1.0	1.5	1.0
Highest	Westminster 3.1	Cardiff 3.6	Clackmannanshire 5.6
Lowest	Isle of Scilly 0.1	Merthyr Tydfil 0.4	East Renfrewshire 0.1
			Orkney Islands 0.1
			Shetland Islands 0.1

Note: No data are available for Northern Ireland
Sources: DfEE (2000a), Welsh Assembly (2001a), Scottish Executive (2001a)

parents for their non-attendance, while other parents actively collude with their children in condoning absence (Cullingford, 1999; Britton *et al.*, 2002). Some pupils in England and Wales were excluded from school for persistent non-attendance – and such chronic non-attenders, once excluded, would not appear in the truancy figures (Milner and Blyth, 1999). However, under guidelines issued by the DfEE in 1999, pupils in England can no longer be excluded for truanting (DfEE, 1999a), but there is evidence that a number of schools remove absent pupils from the school roll in order to manipulate the attendance figures (Milner and Blyth, 1999).

A further source of data on absences is from truancy sweeps conducted by the police and educational welfare officers. This indicates that the vast majority (around 80 per cent) of young people stopped did not have valid reason for not being in school, but were often in the company of an adult, such as a parent. OFSTED have estimated that there are approximately one million 'lost days' of 'unauthorised absence' annually (Audit Commission, 1999, p. 5; OFSTED, 2001, p. 2). Yet another source of evidence on unauthorised absence from school are self-report studies. In England and Wales, the Youth Cohort Study collects information on young people's self-reported absence. These surveys ask respondents whether they have been absent from school in Years 10 and 11. Reviewing this evidence, Newburn reports that around 5 per cent of young people in England and Wales truant for days or weeks at a time and a 'hardcore' of around 11,000 pupils truant in their final year of schooling (Newburn, 1999). In his annual report, the Chief Inspector of Schools for England draws attention to the fact that "we are becoming increasingly aware from data that there is a significant group of 'missing pupils' who should be in school, but are not, and about whom, almost by definition, we know very little. In total, these groups represent a significant number of pupils who are still being failed by the system" (OFSTED, 2002, p. 19).

School exclusion

Perhaps surprisingly, systematic data on school exclusions were not published at all until the mid-1990s (Parsons, 1999). There were small-scale studies, but there was little national data until Parsons drew attention to the escalating rates of permanent exclusions (DfE, 1995). Based on this work, and official rates on permanent exclusion published since then, it can be seen that permanent exclusions in England did indeed hugely increase in the 1990s to reach a peak in

1995/96 since when official rates of permanent exclusions have declined. Table 17.2 is compiled from two main sources. Since 1995/96 the DfEE (renamed the Department for Education and Skills (DfES) in 2001) has published national statistics on permanent exclusion for England. Before 1993, LEAs were not required to keep accurate data on permanent exclusions and the government's National Exclusions Recording System was known to have had incomplete data. However, one independent scholar, Carl Parsons, conducted his own survey of local authorities in England for the DfEE and the table below gives his estimates for England for 1990-1996 (Parsons, 1999), followed by figures released from the DfEE from 1995/96 and more recently the DfES. Since devolution, data for Wales is published by the Welsh Assembly.

There is some suggestion that this rise in permanent exclusions is a particularly English phenomenon, at least in part the result of reforms in education introduced by the 1988 Education Reform Act, including local management of schools and the publication of league tables for examination successes in 16-plus examinations. The same legislation applied in Wales, but not in Scotland or Northern Ireland (Parsons, 1999). The figures are affected by directives and policy changes. Following the SEU report, which set a target of reducing permanent exclusions in England by a third by 2002, the DfEE issued two circulars to schools and LEAs (in October and November 1999) in England, designed to reduce exclusions, especially permanent exclusions (DfEE, 1999a

Table 17.2: Permanent exclusions from schools in England, including type of school, and Wales

	England Primary	England Secondary	England Special	England Total	Wales Total
Parsons' estimates					
1990/91	378	2,532	*	2,910	
1991/92	537	3,296	*	3,833	
1992/93	1,215	7,421	*	8,636	
1993/94	1,291	9,433	457	11,181	
1994/95	1,438	10,519	501	13,581	543
DfEE/DfES figures				**Welsh Assembly**	
1995/96	1,608	10,344	524	12,476	543
1996/97	1,573	10,463	632	12,668	473
1997/98	1,539	10,187	572	12,298	503
1998/99	1,366	8,636	436	10,438	390
1999/2000	1,266	6,713	384	8,323	337

Sources: Data for England: Parsons (1999) p. 23; DfEE (2000b); DfES (2001a).
Data for Wales: Parsons (1999) p. 32; Welsh Assembly (2001b).

and 1999b). In England, the number of permanent exclusions is also an *Opportunity for All* indicator. As the figures in Table 17.2 illustrate, the number of permanent exclusions has fallen from 12,668 in 1996/97 (the baseline year) to 8,323 in 1999/2000, thus meeting the government target of reducing the number of permanent exclusions by a third (DWP, 2001b). No new target has been set by the government for England. In January 2002, the DfES issued a Revised Draft Guidance on School Exclusions for England, for consultation, and the accompanying press release states that the government is now "focusing on prevention, early intervention and the provision of education for long-term excluded children" (DfES, 2002b, p. 2). Wales has also set a target to reduce permanent exclusions by one-third, from 473 in 1996/97 to 313 by March 2003, and as Table 17.2 illustrates, they are on track to meet this target by 2003 (Welsh Assembly, 2001b).

However, anecdotal evidence suggests that self-withdrawal and long-term truancy have increased as exclusion figures fall in England, and also that fixed-term exclusions are used repeatedly in place of permanent exclusion (Osler *et al.*, 2001). In England, fixed-term exclusions are not recorded systematically as there is no legal requirement for schools in England to report fixed-term exclusions "of less than five days to the local education authority" (Smith, 1998, p. 6). A study carried out by The Children's Society of 64 education authorities estimated that 30,000 individual pupils were given fixed-term exclusions (Smith, 1998). Data on fixed-term exclusions of between five days and a maximum of 45 days has to be reported by the school to the LEA but this data is not collated by the DfES. The SEU cites OFSTED's estimate that there are around 100,000 fixed-term exclusions a year in England (SEU, 1998b, p. 8). Throughout the 1990s, numerous studies found evidence that schools across the country were using informal exclusions, which were not recorded officially (Munn *et al.*, 2000). More recently, research conducted by Osler *et al* into reasons behind school exclusions found similar evidence of schools using unofficial exclusions, but in some instances recording it as authorised absence, for example, disguising informal exclusions as 'medical problems' (Osler *et al.*, 2001, p. 21). They also found that unofficial and unrecorded exclusions were used by some schools in order to cover up the level of exclusion or to meet their targets for a reduction in exclusion. In some cases, schools justified using unofficial exclusions as being in the best interests of the pupil as it was not recorded on the pupil's school record. Schools, in general, only used unofficial exclusion as a short-term measure, but Osler *et al.* found evidence to suggest that schools used unofficial permanent exclusions for some pupils in their final year of compulsory education, which amounted to long-term truancy "encouraged and condoned by the school" (Osler *et al.*, 2001, p. 3).

In Scotland a circular to local authorities (February 1998) required them to report, record and monitor all information on exclusions from school, starting in 1998/99. In the light of this additional guidance, some local authorities' education departments re-assessed their procedures on exclusions and some authorities began to report permanent exclusions for the first time. This helps explain an apparent increase, as shown in Table 17.3, in the numbers of permanent exclusions in Scotland at a time when rates were falling in England (Scottish Executive, 2001d, pp. 3–4). In Scotland, as in Northern Ireland, the number of permanent exclusions is dwarfed by the number of temporary exclusions. In England and Wales, a pupil can only be given fixed-term exclusions "for up to 45 days in a school year" (DfEE, 1999a, p. 32). Similarly, in Northern Ireland, a pupil may only be "suspended for a maximum of 45 days in any one school year" (Geraghty, 1999, p. 24) but in Scotland there is "no national fixed term period for exclusion" (Munn *et al.*, 2000, p. 18). Over 99 per cent of exclusions in Scotland were 'temporary' in 1999/2000 (Scottish Executive, 2001d, p. 1). The number of pupils temporarily excluded is available from 1999/2000. The Scottish Executive has set a target of reducing the number of days lost by exclusions by one-third (Lloyd *et al.*, 2001, p. 1).

The education system and procedures for exclusion and suspension in Northern Ireland are different again. Northern Ireland has, of course, a very small pupil population compared to other countries in the UK, with fewer than 349,000 pupils overall. A regulation introduced in 1995 was intended to make

Table 17.3: Temporary exclusions, including the number of pupils temporarily excluded in 1999/2000, and permanent exclusions, Scotland

	Temporary exclusions	No. of pupils temporarily excluded	Permanent exclusions
Parsons' estimates			
1994/95			343
1995/96			185
1996/97			117
Scottish Executive			
1998/99	36,856		344
1999/2000	38,409	20,869	360

Sources: Parsons (1999) p. 32; Scottish Executive, (2001d), p. 6

Table 17.4: Suspensions, including number of pupils suspended, and expulsions in Northern Ireland

	No. of suspensions	No. of pupils	No. of expulsions
1996/97	3,748	2,631	76
1999/00	6,299	4,289	85

Sources: Data for 1996/97 – Kilpatrick *et al.* (1999); Data for 1999/00 – Edwards (2001)

exclusions more difficult. Northern Ireland has five Education and Library Boards (ELBs) and each keeps its own data on exclusions and suspensions: the data is not collated nationally. Research carried out on the academic year 1996/97 found that there were 76 permanent exclusions in 1996/97, a tiny proportion compared to the English figures. However, while exclusions are low, there are a considerable number of 'suspensions' as Table 17.4 illustrates, with some pupils experiencing multiple suspensions (Kilpatrick *et al.*, 1999). Recent research conducted by contacting the five ELBs found that the number of expulsions in 1999/2000 remains low (as shown in Table 17.4), but the number of pupils receiving suspensions has increased since 1996/97 (Edwards, 2001). The New TSN to promote social inclusion has set a target to "reduce by 20 per cent the number of pupils with multiple suspensions by 2003 compared to 1998/99", and to "reduce by 30 per cent the number of pupils expelled from school by 2003 compared to 1998/99" (New TSN Unit, 2000, p. 4).

In all countries in the UK there is anecdotal evidence at the very least of some schools 'encouraging' parents to withdraw their children before formal permanent exclusion procedures are instigated and being excluded is recorded on a young person's file (Britton *et al.*, 2002; Vulliamy and Webb, 2000; Hayden, 2000; Geraghty, 1999; Edwards, 2001).

Comparison with Europe

In contrast to the UK, permanent exclusion from school is almost unheard of in most countries in Western Europe (Parsons, 1999; Parsons, 2000; Munn *et al.*, 2000). A study conducted by Parsons found that if a school is planning to exclude a pupil, it is the responsibility of the head teacher to first find a place for the child in another school. This is the case in Austria, Belgium, Denmark, France, Germany, Luxembourg, the Netherlands, the Republic of Ireland and Spain (Parsons, 1999, p. 34). This means that there are no comparative statistics on permanent exclusions. Indeed, as Parsons emphasises, this is not because they have found an easy answer to the problem but that it is a *"fundamental principle"* (author's italics) in these countries that children "should be receiving a full-time education" (Parsons, 1999, p. 33). One of the main issues concerning school exclusion in the UK is that when a pupil is excluded, it can be many months before he/she is reintegrated into full-time education. A recent study of LEAs in England found that only 62 per cent of pupils permanently excluded from primary school, and 54 per cent of pupils permanently excluded from secondary school, were reintegrated into mainstream education (Parsons and Howlett, 2000). Similarly, in Scotland the rate of reintegration of excluded pupils into mainstream education is low (Lloyd *et al.*, 2001), while in Northern Ireland only five expelled pupils out of 76 pupils returned to full-time education (Kilpatrick *et al.*, 1999). This violates the UN Convention on the Rights of the Child (Article 28) which states that no one should be denied the right to education, although having a disruptive pupil in the class may also violate the rights of others to an adequate education (Harris *et al.*, 2000). This is perhaps the reason for the government policy that, from 2002, it is accepted as the statutory responsibility of all LEAs in England to ensure that all excluded pupils receive *full-time* education (DfEE, 1999b; SEU, 1998b).

Characteristics of those who are excluded and reasons for exclusion

Although truancy and school exclusions are widespread, they are by no means evenly spread throughout the population. Most, but by no means all, truancy and school exclusions occur in pupils of secondary school age. Hayden has recently pointed to significant increases in exclusion of children of primary school age, including some as young as four and five years old. Among primary school exclusions, boys outnumber girls by ten to one in England (Hayden, 1997, 2000), and in Scotland 92 per cent of pupils excluded from primary school in 1999/2000 were boys (Scottish Executive, 2001d, p. 1). Over all age ranges in England, 84 per cent of permanent exclusions were boys (DfES, 2001a, p. 2), while in Wales four-fifths of permanent exclusions are of boys (Welsh Assembly, 2001b). In Scotland the figure is very similar, with boys accounting for 81 per cent of exclusions (Scottish Executive, 2001d, p. 1). Northern Ireland reports that the majority of pupils expelled were secondary school boys, of whom most were in Year 11, but just under 40 per cent were in Years 8, 9 and 10

(Kilpatrick *et al.*, 1999). In England about two-thirds of pupils undergoing permanent exclusions are aged 13 and over (DfES, 2001a). In Scotland and Wales, 85 per cent of pupils excluded were from secondary school (Scottish Executive, 2001d, p. 1; Welsh Assembly, 2001b).

In England there has been concern for some time about the over-representation of minority ethnic groups among those permanently excluded from school. The SEU report accepted that, although accounting for no more than 1 per cent of the school population in England, African-Caribbean children accounted for around 8 per cent of all those permanently excluded (SEU, 1998b). Estimates of the over- and under-representation of different groups have varied significantly. It is widely accepted that Chinese and Indian pupils are rarely excluded, whereas African-Caribbean boys are over-represented, with some estimates suggesting that this may be by a factor of eight (Hayden, 2000). The DfES, in its more recent report, estimates that black pupils are three times more likely to be permanently excluded than their white counterparts (DfES, 2001a). Wales and Northern Ireland do not publish the breakdown of exclusion figures by ethnic groups (Welsh Assembly, 2001b; Kilpatrick *et al.*, 1999; Edwards, 2001, 2002), while in Scotland only 2.11 per cent of pupils excluded in 1999/2000 were from a minority ethnic group (Scottish Executive, 2001d, p. 8). However, as Lloyd *et al.* puts forward, this could be a result of Scotland's different demographic structure, rather than a sign of a "more inclusive educational system" (Lloyd *et al.*, 2001, p. 10).

There is increasing evidence of the relationship between poverty and living in poor neighbourhoods, and school exclusions (OFSTED, 1996) and truancy (SEU, 1998b). In Scotland, just under half of all school exclusions involve children who are entitled to free school meals – often used as a proxy measure of poverty (Scottish Executive, 2001d). In Northern Ireland, just over half of all those expelled are entitled to free school meals (Kilpatrick *et al.*, 1999). In Wales, data on whether excluded pupils are in receipt of free school meals is not published (Edwards, 2002), but in both Wales and England there is a correlation between the proportion of pupils entitled to free school meals and the rate of unauthorised absenteeism (DfEE, 2000a, p. 5; Welsh Assembly, 2001a, p. 1). In England, it is accepted that there is spatial clustering of school exclusions, with schools serving poor neighbourhoods as also proving to be schools with high exclusion rates (OFSTED, 1996). Godfrey and Parsons (1999) estimated that low levels of home ownership and other indicators of social deprivation were also correlated with school exclusions. Hayden's research on children excluded from primary school found a correlation between exclusion and particular family patterns, namely single parent households and households which included a step-parent (Hayden, 1997). These patterns are also factors relating to the likelihood of young people being 'looked after' in care, although there is other evidence that being looked after exacerbates educational disaffection. Those looked after (by local authorities) in England are ten times more likely to be permanently excluded from school than those who are not (SEU, 1998b; Smith, 1998). In Scotland, 8 per cent of all pupils excluded in 1999/2000 were children looked after by the local authority (Scottish Executive, 2001d, p. 2).

Other over-represented groups among those excluded from school include pregnant schoolgirls. The SEU report on teenage pregnancy in England pointed to the complex relationship between pregnancy and various forms of educational disaffection. On the one hand, young women who truanted regularly or were excluded were more likely to become pregnant than their peers. On the other hand, becoming pregnant often resulted in the termination of schooling and the consequent lack of qualification at 16 (SEU, 1999b) despite the fact that following Circular 10/99 it is illegal for a school in England to use "pregnancy on its own" as a "reason for exclusion from school" (DfEE, 1999a, p. 14). One study found that more girls in secondary schools in England and Wales were out of school because of pregnancy than because of permanent exclusion (Audit Commission, 1999, p. 61). A study in Northern Ireland highlighted how school-age mothers were fighting prejudice and discrimination in education (Save the Children, 1996).

As Table 17.2 indicates, in England a considerable amount of exclusion occurs from special education, including attendance at special schools. In Wales, just under 4 per cent of pupils excluded in 1999/2000 were from special schools (Welsh Assembly, 2001b). The DfES report that in 1999/2000 a pupil with a statement of special educational need in England was seven times more likely to be permanently excluded than a pupil without a statement (DfES, 2001a). However, under government guidelines, pupils in England who have statements should only be excluded in the "most exceptional circumstances" (DfEE, 1999a, p. 33). It should be remembered, however, that some young people who are 'statemented' (or have a 'Record of Need' in Scotland), will have emotional or behavioural difficulties (Hayden, 1997). In Scotland, 4 per cent of all exclusions in 1999/2000 involved pupils with a Record of Needs (Scottish Executive, 2001d, p. 2). In Northern Ireland, 10.5 per cent of all pupils expelled in 1996/97 had a statement of special educational needs (Kilpatrick et al., 1999, p. 3).

The SEU report in England and Kilpatrick *et al.*'s study of suspension and expulsion in Northern Ireland make it clear that reasons for exclusions (in England) and suspensions (in Northern Ireland) vary from relatively trivial offences to more serious acts of violence, often against other children (SEU, 1998b; Kilpatrick *et al.*, 1999). Officially recorded reasons are precisely that and may disguise a hidden history of disruptive behaviour or difficult relationships and incidents within the school. A student may be excluded for theft or violence (terms with a criminal connotation), but these could refer to stealing a chocolate bar from a lunch box or a fight in the playground following provocation from others (Hayden, 2000). Where local authorities record reasons, bullying, fighting and assault on peers top the list, covering a third of all exclusions. One study found that abuse and assault on staff accounted for just over 1 per cent of exclusions, although an OFSTED report found a slightly higher rate of just under 4 per cent (Imich, 1994; OFSTED, 1996). In Northern Ireland, 2 per cent of suspensions in 1996/97 were for acts of violence against a teacher (Kilpatrick *et al.*, 1999, p. 2), while in Scotland, 2.7 per cent of exclusions in 1999/2000 were for physical abuse of members of staff (Scottish Executive, 2001d, p. 8). In Wales, data on the reasons for exclusions is not published (Edwards, 2002).

Much research makes it clear that the underlying causes for school exclusion throughout the UK are connected to issues which are taking place in the home as well as things happening at school, and there is often a complex interaction between the two (Brodie and Berridge, 1996; Hayden, 1997). Children and young people often experience a range of traumas at home, including bereavements, the divorce or separation of parents, abuse, family stress and disrupted home circumstances (Britton *et al.*, 2002). Other factors involve aspects of family lifestyle such as watching television late, leaving children over-tired the next day. Within school, factors include changes in school management (a new head) sometimes determined to change the ethos of the school, often resulting in new forms of classroom management and a low tolerance of difficult pupils (Bates, 1999; Coles, 2000). The combination of all these factors also lies behind the rise in the formal diagnosis of 'learning disabilities' including child psychiatric disorders, Attention Deficit Disorder (ADD) or Attention Deficit Hyperactivity Disorder (ADHD) (Blyth and Milner, 1997). Since the 1988 reforms in England and Wales, teachers and schools are under pressure to increase standards and in this environment there is a disincentive to give sufficient time to understanding the root causes of the problematic behaviour of disturbed or disturbing children

(Mittler, 2000). In addition, possible causes for differences in exclusion rates in England and Wales include: different LEA policies, which can make all the difference in minimising school exclusions (Osler *et al.*, 2001); variation in resources of individual LEA educational welfare services (Audit Commission, 1999) and a lack of alternative education provision in some LEAs (Audit Commission, 1999; OFSTED, 2002).

Characteristics of those who truant and their reasons

Although school exclusion and truancy are regarded as different aspects of educational disaffection, the characteristics of those who truant do not mirror the characteristics of those who are excluded from school. For instance, although boys outnumber girls among those who are excluded, self-reported truancy rates indicate that there are few differences between boys and girls (O'Keefe, 1994; SEU, 1998b). Part of the problem of examining the characteristics of truants is that much of the 'more reliable' estimates are themselves based on surveys of school-aged children – 17 per cent were absent from school at the time of O'Keefe's survey (O'Keefe, 1994). Persistent truants will of course be the least likely to take part. However, some groups are known to be over-represented among those absent from school, but not likely to be excluded from school.

Attendance rates for Gypsies and Travellers are relatively low in all four countries of the UK, especially in secondary school. A third of Traveller children of secondary school age in England are reported as having an attendance record of less than 50 per cent (SEU, 1998b), with many others unlikely to be registered with school authorities. In Scotland, Save the Children estimates that only about 20 per cent of Gypsy and Traveller children of secondary school age attend school "with any degree of regularity" (Save the Children, 2001, p. 206). In Northern Ireland, a working group has been set up to consider difficulties which Travellers face (New TSN Unit, 2001, p. 1). Similarly, in Scotland the report of an inquiry into Travelling people and public sector policies has recently been published and has been debated by the Scottish Parliament (Save the Children, 2001). In Wales, prosecution for non-registration and non-attendance has led to an improvement in attendance rates of Traveller children (Save the Children, 2001, p. 246). The Welsh Assembly is undertaking a review of services for Gypsies/Travellers, including a review of education and strategies for increasing the number of Gypsy/Traveller children receiving secondary education.

Young people performing significant caring tasks at home for other family members are known to be among those absent from school but not excluded, often at the cost of their own education. One study found that a fifth of young carers of compulsory school age surveyed were missing school (Dearden and Becker, 1998).

Young people looked after are over-represented among truants. A joint report by OFSTED and the Social Service Inspectorate reported that in England almost 12 per cent of looked after children of statutory school age were not in school, rising to 26 per cent of 14–16-year-olds who should have been studying for their GCSEs (Coles, 2000; Social Services Inspectorate and OFSTED, 1995).

The reasons for and explanations of truancy are often a mixture of negative feelings about schooling (including a dislike of some teachers and some lessons) and positive reasons for wanting to do something else (hanging about or doing things with friends, shopping and sometimes criminal activity). There is some evidence that some young people truant to avoid bullying, while others stay away from school to avoid the sometimes painful experience of humiliation because of being a weak reader, for instance (DfEE, 1999f; Reid, 1999; Save the Children, 2001).

Costs and consequences of school exclusion and truancy

As the quotation at the beginning of this chapter makes clear, the Labour government's concern with truancy and school exclusions is largely because of the financial and human costs involved – and especially because of the link between various forms of educational disaffection and later economic disengagement (unemployment) and criminal behaviour (Vulliamy and Webb, 2000). According to the Audit Commission, nearly a half of all school-age offenders had been excluded from school and a quarter had truanted significantly (Audit Commission, 1996). There is some evidence that the criminal justice system is harsher on those who are either excluded or truant, by imposing custodial sentences (SEU, 1998b, p. 17). Although it is difficult to find direct links between educational disaffection and criminal behaviour, many have argued that being left in an unsupervised and unstructured environment adds to the temptations to offend. The SEU report concluded that "Exclusion and truancy have costly effects, whether those costs are borne by the police, courts and prisons, by the social security budget or by the victims of crime" (SEU, 1998b, p. 18).

A number of authors have tried to be more precise about the costs of exclusion and truancy. Parsons estimated that the cost of excluding children from school in 1996/97 was £81 million. The cost of excluding a single child is estimated to be £4,300, whereas the cost of extra support for those at risk of exclusion was £2,800 (Donovan and Kenway, 1998, p. 6; Parsons, 1998).

One factor to have emerged in a number of studies of social exclusion is the relationship between truancy and school exclusion pre-16, disengagement between the ages of 16 and 18 and long-term unemployment thereafter (SEU, 1999a). Truancy and school exclusion are highly likely to result in poor educational qualifications at the age of 16. The National Children's Homes (NCH) report that 38 per cent of truants left school with no qualifications at all compared to only 3 per cent of non-truants (NCH, 2000; Mittler, 2000). The fifth Social Exclusion Unit report (SEU, 1999a) concerned those 16- and 17-year-olds who were not in any form of education, employment or training (NEET). Among the 160,000 who are NEET, those who truant or who have been excluded are highly over-represented. A quarter of those truanting persistently in Year 11 in 1996/97 were NEET subsequently, compared to only 3 per cent of those who had not truanted at all. Those who had been permanently excluded in Years 10 or 11 were two-and-a-half times more likely to be NEET, and those who had fixed-term exclusions were twice as likely to be inactive at age 16 and 17. And 40 per cent of those who were inactive at the age of 16 and 17 were still inactive at the age of 21 (SEU, 1999a, p. 39; Coles, 2000). Calculating the long-term cost of exclusion at the age of 16 and 17, researchers at the University of York have estimated that the unit cost is of the order of £52,000 and the total financial lifetime cost is a staggering £7.2 billion (Godfrey *et al.*, 2001).

Conclusions

This chapter has reviewed a range of evidence on truancy and school exclusion. It has emphasised that, while evidence is at times suspect and unreliable, there is a strong indication that both increased during the 1990s. Even though permanent exclusions have begun to decrease in England and Wales since 1998, truancy and school exclusions continue to present a serious challenge to policy-makers and practitioners in all four countries of the UK.

As this chapter has identified, there are gaps in the data on truancy and school exclusion. Further research is needed to close these gaps. Research needs to be undertaken in all four countries on the use of unofficial exclusions. In England and Wales, research is needed on the use and number of fixed-term exclusions. As stated earlier in the chapter, data on fixed-term exclusions is not collated by the DfES. In Northern Ireland, data on suspension and exclusion is not collated by the Department of Education and is not published by any of the five ELBs. The last project undertaken for the Department of Education was the Kilpatrick *et al.* (1999) study of suspensions and expulsions for the academic year 1996/97. A similar study undertaken now would close a major gap in the data on suspensions and expulsions from schools in Northern Ireland. In Scotland, England and Wales, further research is needed on the use of authorised and unauthorised absences, and whether using unauthorised absence gives a true picture of the amount of truancy from school. In Northern Ireland, no distinction is made between unauthorised and authorised absence.

Although the government has appeared to take a strong stand to reduce truancy and school exclusions, it has also been caught in what a number of critics have described as a series of policy dilemmas (Parsons, 2000; Vulliamy and Webb, 2000). One key concern of the government has been to try to raise standards in schools. In order to do this, head teachers are encouraged to show strong leadership, yet be tough on discipline *and* create a demanding *and* inclusive school ethos. Yet when in doing this they exclude troublesome pupils, they undermine another government objective of reducing school exclusions and truancy because of the impact of this on crime, underachievement and long-term social exclusion.

18 Children, Young People and Crime

Bob Coles and Suzanne Maile

Key statistics:

- Those young people cautioned or found guilty of an offence constitute only a tiny fraction of those who commit crime.
- Relatively few young people are responsible for a large number of offences. For instance, in Scotland in 2000, 890 children under the age of 16 had more than 10 offences reported against them.
- Some criminal behaviour is self-reported by 57 per cent of young men aged 12–30 in England and Wales and by 37 per cent of young women in that age group. Around one in five admit to an offence in the last year.
- Self-reported crime in Scotland is much more widespread than in England and Wales, with 85 per cent of young men and 67 per cent of young women saying they committed an offence in the last year.
- While official crime levels in Northern Ireland are half that in England and Wales, 75 per cent of young people self-report criminal behaviour.
- The vast majority of known offenders are male, although gender differences narrow where evidence is based on self-reported crime. This is especially true in Northern Ireland where the official crime ratio is 9:1 compared to 3:1 for self-reported crime.
- The peak ages of offending are in the late teenage years between 18 and 19, although self-report studies suggest a much younger age (14) for young women.
- Many children and young people are the victims of crime, including assault, theft and harassment, with different reports suggesting that, across the UK, between a third and a half of them experience such crimes every year.

Key trends:

- There are some signs that recorded crime has reached a plateau and is beginning to decline in all countries.

- However, there are also signs of some increases in persistent offending, particularly among the young. In Scotland, those under the age of 16 who were reported for 10 or more offences increased by 20 per cent between 1998 and 2000.

- There are a number of signs from official statistics and self-report studies that the gender gap in offending behaviour is closing, with more girls offending than in previous years.

Key sources:

- Home Office Research and Statistics Division, Scottish Executive Statistical Bulletins, Northern Ireland Statistics and Research Branch

- British Crime Survey, Scottish Crime Survey, Northern Ireland Crime Survey

- Youth Lifestyle Survey and Young Persons' Behaviour and Attitude Survey (Northern Ireland) and Jamieson, J. *et al.* (1999)

Introduction

This chapter reviews research evidence on children, young people and crime. It attempts to assess the degree to which young people are involved in crime, both as offenders and as victims, and examines the known correlates of youth crime. In many ways 'crime' is both a legal and a social construction and this is especially true of youth offending. Different European countries determine that a child may be deemed criminally responsible for a crime at different ages: 10 in England, Wales and Northern Ireland, 8 in Scotland but 16 and 18 in Spain and Belgium respectively. Britain's most widespread crime at the time of the first British Crime Survey in 1982 – theft of bottles of milk from the doorstep – has been eclipsed now that most households buy milk from supermarkets, and other crimes such as those related to cars and mobile phones are related to the growth in their use.

Scotland has its own very distinctive legal and criminal justice system, which often makes comparison with other UK countries difficult. Indeed, it is currently impossible to provide genuine comparative data across the countries of the UK. Despite this, across all countries, it is largely accepted that: crime committed by young people is widespread; that a worryingly high proportion of young people commit a crime at some stage in their lives; that offending behaviour is concentrated within the teenage years; and that youth crime is hugely expensive both to the public and private sectors. Our more exact knowledge about the extent of crime is, however, hugely limited by the unreliability of much of the data.

There are three main sources of our knowledge about crime:

- official statistics of recorded crime
- crime surveys of the victims of crime
- surveys of self-reported criminal behaviour.

Official statistics have played an important role in our understanding of young people's criminal activity as they give exact figures relating to cautions, arrests and convictions of known young offenders. Yet it has long been known that officially recorded crime vastly underestimates the levels of crime revealed from large-scale social surveys. These are of two types. The first are studies of the victims of crime. Here our knowledge has been enhanced by the British Crime Survey (BCS) which, on a biannual basis since 1982, has surveyed large samples of adults (16 and over) living in private households. There are now similar surveys in Northern Ireland and Scotland, with the latter having taken over the Scottish part of the BCS. In Northern Ireland, it is estimated that only one in every two victims of crime reports the crime to the police compared to three out of five victims who report in Britain overall (O'Mahony and Deazley, 2000). In Britain, officially recorded crime in 2000 indicated 5.3 million offences. However, the BCS estimated that there were 12,899,000 offences experienced by adults during the same year. Crime surveys can also point to the experience of various types of offence and who are most likely to be the victims of crime, and in what circumstances. Yet even victims of crime surveys underestimate the true levels of crime. Many offences are not against adults in private households. Some are against corporate bodies or against public property. Other crimes are committed against children under the age of 16. Indeed, the issue of children as victims of crime remains a very much under-researched area.

The third source of evidence is based on surveys of potential offenders rather than victims. Our knowledge of young offenders has been much enhanced by surveys of young people in which they are asked to self-report on offences they have committed. The Youth Lifestyles Survey (YLS), carried out by the Home Office, covers a sample of nearly 5,000 young people aged 12–30 in England

and Wales. The most recent, published in 2000, provides an authoritative insight into self-confessed crimes committed by children and young people in England and Wales (Flood-Page *et al.*, 2000). A similar study has been carried out in Scotland between 1996 and 1999 by a research team at the Social Work Research Centre at Stirling (Jamieson *et al.*, 1999). In Northern Ireland there is a Young Persons' Behaviour and Attitude Survey which is based on a sample of 6,300 11–16-year-olds. This latter survey also reports on young people as the victims of crime. Unfortunately, officially recorded crime statistics, victims surveys and self-report studies sometimes provide contradictory pictures of trends.

Recorded crime

Official crime figures in 2000 for England and Wales indicated that recorded crime had increased to 5.3 million offences, up from 5.1 million offences in 1998–99. Some offences, such as domestic burglary and car-related crime, have been reduced, and there was also a reported reduction of over 10 per cent in drug offences. There have been marked increases in official crime figures for violent offences, with a more than 15 per cent increase in violence against the person, and a 26 per cent increase in robbery (Home Office, 2001). Yet the British Crime Survey indicates a completely opposite trend – a 12 per cent fall in crimes against people in private households between 1999 and 2000 – the third successive fall recorded since 1995. In contrast to recorded crime figures, the 2001 BCS also reports a drop of 19 per cent in violent crime and a 22 per cent decrease in robberies.

In Scotland, police recorded 423,000 crimes in 2000, a decrease of 3 per cent on the previous year's figure and only slightly higher than a 10-year low figure recorded in 1997. Scotland also reports a slight decrease in non-sexual crimes of violence (a 3 per cent decrease in the number of serious assaults) but an increase of 3 per cent in 'handling an offensive weapon'. Recorded cases of vandalism also increased by 5 per cent (Scottish Executive, 2001l). Recorded crime in Northern Ireland has been consistently lower than in England, Wales and Scotland. In 1997 there were 62,222 notifiable offences recorded by the police – around 40 crimes per 1,000. Nor did Northern Ireland see the increases in recorded crime witnessed in England and Wales between 1985 and 1995: Northern Ireland reported only a 3 per cent increase during that period compared to the 30 per cent increase in England and Wales (O'Mahony and Deazley, 2000).

Table 18.1: Offenders found guilty or cautioned in England and Wales for indictable offences by age and sex, 1995–2000

Male offenders by age (1,000s)

	10–11	12–14	15–17	18–20	21+
1995	4.8	31.5	65.4	72.2	238.6
1996	4.1	27.7	65.6	70.5	235.8
1997	4.0	26.0	65.7	73.6	250.5
1998	4.5	27.3	67.2	77.5	259.3
1999	4.2	26.7	63.8	75.4	247.7
2000	3.9	25.1	58.8	70.0	228.3

Female offenders by age (1,000s)

	10–11	12–14	15–17	18–20	21+
1995	1.3	13.7	16.1	11.7	47.9
1996	1.1	10.7	15.2	11.3	48.0
1997	0.9	9.4	14.1	12.0	59.9
1998	1.1	11.4	15.4	13.1	55.2
1999	1.1	10.2	14.5	13.4	54.3
2000	1.1	10.4	14.2	12.7	50.6

Source: Johnson *et al.* (2001) Table 5

Official statistics show that in England and Wales over 196,200 young people under 21 were cautioned or found guilty for an indictable offence in 2000, the vast majority (80 per cent) of whom were male (Johnson *et al.*, 2001). Table 18.1 gives the age breakdown of male and female offenders. This shows that rates of offending rose among 15–20-year-old young men between 1995 and 1998, but has been declining in all age groups since 1998. Offending by young women has also fallen during the same period. The table also indicates that the peak age of offending is slightly lower for female offenders than young men.

It is almost impossible to provide any meaningful comparison of official crime figures for the different countries within the UK. NACRO Wales is attempting to use the annual reports of Youth Offending Teams to provide some picture of youth crime in Wales, but this has not been completed at the time of writing. Nor is a summary account of the reports of Youth Offending Teams available. Moreover, there remains some suspicion about the robustness of the data that they are collecting and doubt about whether it is genuinely comparable.

Table 18.2 is based on data produced for *Regional Trends,* which does indicate that official crime rates for 10–17-year-olds are higher in Wales than in England, although they have been declining in both countries.

Table 18.2: Rates of indictable offences (plus assaults), young persons aged 10–17 found guilty or cautioned, England and Wales

	Young men	Young women
1998 England	3,851 per 100,000	1,173 per 100,000
1999 England	3,706 per 100,000	1,110 per 100,000
1998 Wales	4,519 per 100,000	1,419 per 100,000
1999 Wales	4,347 per 100,000	1,343 per 100,000

Source: Regional Trends 35 and 36

Data for Scotland is produced as rates per 1,000 in each age group who have had a charge proved against them (see Table 18.3). Table18.3 indicates that the peak age of offending among young men and women in Scotland is 18 years.

Table 18.3: Persons with a charge proved per 1,000 population by sex and age in Scotland

	Male offender by age (years)						Female offender by age (years)					
	<16	16	17	18	19	20	<16	16	17	18	19	20
1995	0.7	80	194	247	218	200	0.07	9	18	25	24	24
1996	0.6	79	201	267	234	214	0.05	8	22	28	25	25
1997	0.5	74	194	255	240	210	0.04	8	22	29	27	26
1998	0.5	72	179	227	217	199	0.02	8	21	28	25	25
1999	0.3	62	161	199	201	182	0.02	6	19	26	25	25
2000	0.2	46	139	194	178	171	0.04	6	17	24	23	24

Source: Scottish Executive (2001k) Table 7

Despite the rates for under-16-year-olds being much lower than older year groups, *Scotland's Action Programme to Reduce Youth Crime* reports particular concern about this younger group's offending behaviour. In 1999/2000 it reports that there were 14,000 children referred to the Children's Reporter and that a growing number of these were responsible for a disproportionate number of offences – 890 children with 10 or more offences reported against them – an increase of around 20 per cent since 1998/99 (Scottish Executive 2002).

In England and Wales there are significant differences to be found between male and female offenders in different age groups with regards to the types of offences for which they are cautioned or found guilty. This is shown in Table 18.4. Among female offenders, the overwhelmingly predominant offence is theft and handling stolen goods. Among male offenders, while theft is the most widespread offence, other relatively common offences include violence against the person and, in the older age group, motoring and drugs offences.

Table 18.4: Type of offence of those found guilty or cautioned in 2000 by age and sex, 1,000s

			Male aged:		
	10–11	12–14	15–17	18–20	21+
Violence against the person	0.3	3.1	8.3	7.9	27.4
Sexual offences	0	0.3	0.6	0.4	3.4
Burglary	0.7	3.7	6.8	5.9	13.9
Robbery	0.1	0.6	1.7	1.2	2.3
Theft and handling stolen goods	2.3	13.5	23.6	22.7	79.9
Fraud and forgery	0	0.3	1.3	2.7	13.2
Criminal damage	0.3	1.5	2.2	1.9	6.1
Drug offences	0	1.1	9.6	18.1	47.6
Other (excluding motoring)	0	0.8	4.1	8.0	28.7
Total indictable	3.9	25.1	58.8	70.0	228.3
Summary non-motoring	2.3	14.9	33.6	49.3	326.7
Summary motoring	0	0.6	13.4	55.7	454.2

			Female aged:		
	10–11	12–14	15–17	18–20	21+
Violence against the person	0	1.1	1.8	1.1	4.1
Sexual offences	0	0	0	0	0.1
Burglary	0.1	0.4	0.5	0.3	0.6
Robbery	0	0.1	0.2	0.1	0.2
Theft and handling stolen goods	0.9	8.1	9.4	7.3	27.7
Fraud and forgery	0	0.2	0.6	1.1	5.9
Criminal damage	0	0.2	0.3	1.7	0.7
Drug offences	0	0.1	0.8	1.7	6.6
Other (excluding motoring)	0	0.2	0.6	1.0	4.3
Total indictable	1.1	10.4	14.2	12.7	50.6
Summary non motoring	0.2	3.5	6.6	9.6	130.3
Summary motoring	0	0	0.5	4.7	76.6

Source: Johnson *et al.* (2001) Table 4

Gender difference among known offenders is even more marked in Northern Ireland, where the rate of known male offenders per 10,000 is 400 compared to 48 for young women. This represents a ratio of nine male offenders to each female offender (O'Mahony and Deazley, 2000).

Although official records provide some solid evidence about known and convicted young offenders, only a tiny proportion of all offences committed by young people result in even an arrest. An Audit Commission report in 1996 indicated that, of the seven million offences estimated to have been committed by young people each year, less than one in five were reported to the police and only one in 20 crimes were cleared up by them. Only 3 per cent of offences resulted in an arrest and only 1.3 per cent resulted in a charge or summons (Audit Commission, 1996). Given this, only a very small tip of a very large iceberg is revealed by relying upon the official statistics alone. Only by relying upon what young people themselves tell us about their offending can we begin to appreciate the nature and extent of the criminal activities of children and young people.

Self-reported crime

One of the first major self-report studies of young people and crime in Britain was carried out by Graham and Bowling in 1995. This involved interviews with, and the construction of life histories of, a random national sample of young people aged 14–25. Of this sample, 55 per cent of males and 31 per cent of females admitted ever committing an offence, although the majority of offenders had committed no more than one or two minor offences. Twenty-eight per cent of males and 12 per cent of females said they had committed an offence in the year before the survey was carried out – 1992. Levels and types of offending varied with age and gender. Among males, expressive and violent offences were most prevalent among 14–17-year-olds. Property offences, including fraud and theft from work were most prevalent among 18–21-year-olds, and theft of motor vehicles was most prevalent among 22–25-year-olds. The most common age for young people to start offending was 15 for both males and females (Graham and Bowling, 1995).

The most recent survey in England and Wales, the Youth Lifestyles Survey (YLS), found that 57 per cent of young men and 37 per cent of young women aged 12–30 admitted having committed one or more offences at some time. This indicates that the proportion of young people offending has risen slightly since 1995, although it must be noted that this study included a wider age range of young people and this will have impacted upon the results. Nineteen per cent of the sample admitted committing one or more offence in the past 12 months, showing overall little change since 1992 (Flood-Page et al., 2000, p. 9). However, the survey does report significant increases (of 14 per cent in the proportion of 14–17-year-old boys admitting to an offence, but a decline (of 6 per cent) in offences admitted by 18–25-year-olds. At age 14–15 boys' most common crimes included buying stolen goods, getting into fights, criminal damage and theft. By age 18–21 it was fairly similar, although shoplifting gradually decreased and workplace thefts became more common. For girls, shoplifting and criminal damage were the most common offences among those under 15, whereas the majority of offences committed by women aged 26–30 were either fraud or buying stolen goods (Flood-Page *et al.*, 2000).

A similar self-report study was carried out in Scotland between 1996 and 1999 (Jamieson *et al.*, 1999). This is reported here, as the methodology is largely the same as that used in England and Wales and thus allows for some comparisons to be made. This survey also made an attempt to examine not only the sorts of offences that young people committed, but what behaviours they thought of as being 'serious' and what social patterns were associated with the onset of offending, persistent offending and ceasing to offend. In Scotland, levels of self-reported crime appear to be very significantly higher than in England and Wales, with few convincing explanations as to why this should be. Jamieson found that 94 per cent of boys and 82 per cent of girls in their sample admitted that they had committed one or more offences in the past, with 85 per cent of boys and 67 per cent of girls reporting having offended at least once during the previous 12 months (Jamieson *et al.*, 1999, p. 12). Among boys, only 6 per cent reported never offending, 3 per cent confessed only to minor offences and a further 10 per cent had not offended within the last year. Among girls, 18 per cent said they had committed no offence, 5 per cent only a minor offence and 11 per cent had not offended in the last year. For both boys and girls vandalism, fighting in the street and shoplifting were the three most common offences. Boys outnumbered girls in these and all other categories. Although these gender differences are statistically significant, a majority of girls still reported that they had committed the first of these offences (vandalism or property damage) and 49 per cent reported being involved in street fights. Nearly a half (47 per cent of boys and 41 per cent of girls) reported committing property damage or vandalism within the past year and 34 per cent of boys and 24 per cent of girls also reported shoplifting within the past year. Boys were also more likely to have committed more offences and to have been involved in violent offences. Nearly a half (47 per cent) reported beating someone up and 28 per cent hurting someone with a weapon, compared to 21 per cent and 11 per cent of girls admitting these offences, respectively.

Overall girls have lower rates of self-reported crime. In Scotland, Jamieson found that girls were less likely to have committed all but the least common offences and girls who did offend tended to do so less frequently than boys. In England and Wales, girls were also less likely to have offended than boys, although the differential varied at different ages. Among 12–13-years-olds a similar proportion of girls and boys offended. The peak age of self-reported offending for girls was 14, after which offending declined. The peak age of self-reported offending for boys was 18, starting to decline after age 21. Flood-Page *et al.* argue that as a result of these patterns, over the age of 17, male offenders outnumber females by a ratio of around three to one, supporting the YLS findings that women 'grow out of crime' earlier (Flood-Page *et al.*, 2000).

It is important to note that, although female self-reported crime rates are lower than males, these prevalence figures are much higher than the official statistics on female offenders: very few girls come into contact with the criminal justice system. It has been argued that young female crime rates are rising and that the gap is narrowing between girls and boys. Among the professionals interviewed in Jamieson *et al.*'s research, there was an opinion that relatively few young people were involved in serious offending, but that there was an increase in young women's and girls' involvement in delinquency and crime. This was thought to be linked to an increase in drug misuse among young women and to contemporary cultural influences that encouraged girls' identification with attitudes and behaviour traditionally associated with boys (Jamieson *et al.*, 1999).

In Northern Ireland, one self-report study of 14–21-year-olds in Belfast found that, despite recorded crime levels being very low in Northern Ireland, very high numbers of young people (75 per cent of the sample) admitted to offending. Much of this offending was reported to be relatively trivial, although a half of boys and a quarter of girls admitted to property crimes. The vast majority of self-reported crimes (88 per cent) had gone undetected by the police (O'Mahony and Deazley, 2000). The gender differences in offending behaviour between boys and girls decreased to three to one in this self-report study, compared to the nine to one in officially recorded crime figures, although young men were five times more likely to commit more serious offences (McQuiod, 1994).

Drug and alcohol use was found to be linked to criminal activity among both boys and girls in self-report studies in England, Wales and Scotland (also see Chapter 19). In Scotland around three-quarters of boys and girls in the youngest age group reported having consumed alcohol and almost a third reported having used cannabis. There was an escalation in the frequency and severity of substance use with age. Through their research Jamieson and colleagues classified young people into three bands:

- resisters – young people who had never offended
- desisters – young people who had offended in the past but had not done so in the past 12 months
- persisters – young people who had committed at least one serious offence or several less serious offences in the past six months.

Persisters were most likely to identify a link between their use of drugs and offending (Jamieson *et al.*, 1999). In England and Wales the average amount of money spent on drugs a month among the sample was £13. The more money men spent on drugs, the more likely they were to be offenders: 39 per cent of men who do not spend money on drugs had committed an offence in the previous year, compared with 43 per cent of those who spend under £50 and 53 per cent of those who spend over £50 (Flood-Page *et al.*, 2000).

The self-report studies examined above contain fairly limited data on ethnicity and its relation to youth crime. Flood-Page *et al.* found that white males were more likely than black, Pakistani or Asian men to admit offending in the last year, although the difference was too small to be statistically significant (Flood-Page *et al.*, 2000).

Risk factors and correlates of crime

Over recent years there has been a significant body of research concerned with identifying factors that can explain or predict criminal activity among young people. It has been argued by some that factors such as education, levels of school exclusion and truancy, family background and location can all have an effect on the likelihood of young people offending. A systematic review of evidence conducted by David Farrington in 1996 identified nine significant risk factors of crime and argued that these increased the risk that children and young people will become criminally involved in the future (Farrington, 1996). These were:

- pre-natal and perinatal factors – the children of teenage mothers were especially found to be more likely to be juvenile offenders
- personality
- intelligence and attainment
- parental supervision and discipline
- parental conflict and separation
- socio-economic status

- delinquent friends
- school influences
- community influences.

Findings by Flood-Page *et al.* would appear to support some of these findings. Among their sample they found that those who lived with two parents had lower levels of serious or persistent offending than those living in either lone parent families or stepfamilies. Those who had weak family attachments were more likely to be serious or persistent offenders, and the relationship was stronger for women than for men. Flood-Page *et al.* argue that the degree to which teenagers are supervised by their parents is directly related to the number of evenings that they go out: generally, young teenagers who went out several evenings during the week, or who went to pubs, nightclubs, parties, etc, were more likely to be offenders. This study also found that having delinquent friends was a factor in levels of offending. Boys with friends or relatives who had been in trouble with the police were over three times as likely to be offenders themselves. For girls the figure was six times more likely. A close correlation between educational disaffection (especially truancy and school exclusion), low educational achievement and crime has also been identified. In this study, women who left school at 16 and men who left before the age of 18 were much more likely to be offenders than those who continued into further education. Among men over 16, those without any qualifications were nearly three times more likely to be offenders (Flood-Page *et al.*, 2000). They conclude that: "This current YLS . . . shows that poor parental supervision, having delinquent friends and acquaintances, persistent truanting and exclusion from school are all predictive of offending" (Flood-Page *et al.*, 2000, p. 56). Another significant correlate of crime identified in this study is geographical location. In the YLS, boys living in rural areas were less likely to have committed any offence in the last year. But there was no difference in offending between those living in inner cities and other urban areas. However, there was a clearer relationship to be found between type of area and serious or persistent offending. Twice as many boys living in inner-city areas were serious or persistent offenders compared to those living in rural areas (Flood-Page *et al.*, 2000).

Young people as the victims of crime

Young people are not only the perpetrators of crimes. It is also important to remember that each year a significant number of children and young people become the victims of crime. While much has been done in recent years to collect data systematically on young people who report that they commit crime, this has not been matched by studies of children and young people as the victims of crime. An important exception is an extension to the 1992 British Crime Survey which covered a sub-sample of over 1,000 12–15-year-olds, with a booster sample drawn from minority ethnic groups (Maung, 1995). The sample were asked about six different types of offences they may have experienced in the previous 6–8 months, as well as attitudes to the police and offending behaviour. Of the sample, 60 per cent reported that they had experienced at least one crime, with assaults being reported by 40 per cent of boys and 34 per cent of girls. These were predominantly (seven out of ten) in and around the school. The victim was often with friends, although some 20 per cent of those who were assaulted were on their own. One in ten assaults were reported to be from strangers, although often assaults were regarded as 'just something that happens' rather than a criminal offence – only 12 per cent of those reporting an assault regarded it as being a crime. One in five of the sample also reported 'harassment' – incidents in which they had been threatened, shouted at, stared at or followed. Much of this followed a similar pattern to that of assaults, with much of it being in and around the school. Harassment from adults, on the other hand, was largely on the streets and where the victim was alone rather than with friends. Sexual harassment (restricted to harassment by those estimated to be over the age of 16 in this survey) was reported by 19 per cent of girls. Six out of ten of these involved men unknown to the victim, a third occurred when the victim and the perpetrator were alone and in a third the perpetrator was estimated to be over 30 years old. Other evidence from the survey suggests that property crime against young people is also widespread – including theft of equipment, clothing, books and food. Multiple victimisation was also reported, with the majority of victims reporting that they had been subject to crime more than once. A fifth said they had been a victim 'too many times to say'. Young people from minority ethnic communities, especially African-Caribbean young people, experienced five of the six types of crime more than their white peers – the only exception being in the case of assault.

A number of local studies have been conducted since 1992. In Scotland, the 2000 Scottish Crime Survey has reported that half of all 12–15-year-olds reported that they had been the victim of at least one crime. The most common offence was harassment (22 per cent) followed by bullying (19 per cent), assault (19 per cent) and theft (15 per cent) (Scottish Executive, 2002). In Northern Ireland, the Young Persons' Behaviour and Attitudes Survey conducted towards the end of 2000 reports that around a fifth of 11–16-year-olds think the area in which they live is unsafe. Many report that they have been the victim of crime, including having things stolen from them (47 per cent) or being bullied (43 per cent). Many more (66 per cent) worry about being caught in a bomb explosion and others fear name-calling (32 per cent) or assault (21 per cent) because of their religion (NISRA, 2002). Another report indicates that there were over 1,000 'punishment shootings' by the paramilitaries between 1988 and 2000, that 23 per cent of the victims were under the age of 20 and 6 per cent under the age of 17 (Kennedy, 2001).

In England, the Children and Young People's Unit report that more than one in three 12–15 year olds are assaulted each year (CYPU, 2001a, p. 3). This clearly adds up to a large number of young people and presents a problem that needs to be more systematically addressed. The unit has indicated that measuring the degree to which children and young people are the victims of crime is an important welfare outcome against which to assess whether the government's strategy for them is working (CYPU, 2001b).

Conclusions

This chapter has attempted to distil some of the main 'facts' about youth crime across the UK although many of these are far from robust and often present a confused and confusing picture. Comparison between the different countries within the UK is also extremely difficult as records are kept in different ways. It is also very difficult to compare other countries with Scotland, which has its own distinctive legal and criminal justice system. Yet some general conclusions can be drawn from this review as was indicated in the box at the start of this chapter: youth crime is widespread, predominantly male, most is undetected, and some is highly damaging to victims and communities.

This chapter has not described in any detail the involvement of children and young people in the criminal justice system. But it is not without significance that all countries within the UK have undertaken far-reaching reviews of the approaches taken to youth crime *and* their youth criminal justice systems in the past few years (Home Office, 1997; O'Mahony and Deazley, 2000; Scottish Executive, 2002). Within these reviews there are broad agreements on strategy: to act early, quickly and effectively; to ensure that offenders are aware of the damage and distress they cause; and to assess and confront offending behaviour holistically and though multi-agency teams. What will be important to judge in future years is how these policy developments impact upon the various measures of the extent of youth crime.

19 Smoking, Drinking Alcohol and Drug Use

Bob Coles and Suzanne Maile

Key statistics:

- Around one in five boys and nearly one in four girls smoke cigarettes regularly by the age of 15.
- Drinking alcohol is more prevalent in the UK than many other European countries. The majority of 15-year-olds in the UK (including seven in ten boys in this age group in Wales) report being drunk on two or more occasions.
- By the age of 18 nearly a third of young people will be using cannabis, the overwhelming drug of choice among young people. In England, 16 per cent of girls and 19 per cent of boys are using it at the age of 15, with much higher levels of drug use reported in Scotland and much less in Northern Ireland. The use of other drugs (including heroin) is much less widespread (less than 1 per cent) but is thought to be more prevalent in some regions and some communities.

Key trends:

- Smoking among children increased in the 1990s in Scotland and Wales, with Wales, for instance, moving up in the European League Table from 23rd to 5th.
- The drinking of alcohol by young people is increasing, with some evidence of increasing and widespread drinking to excess, getting drunk and binge drinking.
- Self-report studies of drug use indicate that drug use among children and young people is increasing, although much of this is the use of cannabis only. Some local studies report of the ready availability of hard drugs such as heroin.

Key sources:

- *Health and Health Behaviour among Young People* – a WHO cross-national study
- Department of Health surveys of *Smoking, Drinking and Drug Use amongst Teenagers*
- Northern Ireland *Young Persons' Behaviour and Attitude Survey*
- British Crime Surveys
- The Youth Lifestyle Surveys

Introduction

When young people smoke, drink alcohol or take drugs, it often involves illegal behaviour. It is not strictly illegal for children and young people to consume alcohol, although it is illegal for them to purchase it under the age of 18. It is also illegal for them to buy cigarettes. Concern about teenagers smoking tobacco, however, is also linked to the long-term health consequences of smoking rather than its illegality *per se*. Involvement in drug use, or unsupervised consumption of alcohol at an early age, may also threaten their welfare. Smoking, drinking alcohol and taking drugs are covered together in this chapter, as much of the most reliable data is based on surveys of self-reported use and in recent years survey research has increasingly covered different types of behaviours together.

Main data sources

The study *Health and Health Behaviour among Young People: Health behaviour in school-aged children* (HBSC) is a cross-national study of children aged 11, 13 and 15 drawn from a large number of different countries across Europe and North America. Questionnaires are administered in school classes by teachers to an agreed protocol. The questionnaire asks respondents to self-report on a wide range of behaviours including smoking, drinking alcohol and using drugs. The first of the surveys was carried out in 1985/86 and an increasing number of countries have taken part in the subsequent surveys which have taken place every four years. The latest published survey was carried out in 1997/98 and included all four countries within the UK, with England taking part in the survey for the first time (Currie *et al.*, 2000).

The Department of Health has also carried out biennial surveys of secondary school pupils since 1982. These surveys were originally designed to provide basic information on smoking, but in recent years the surveys have also included questions on alcohol and drug use. Systematic data from these surveys is available for England and Scotland only. Northern Ireland published the results of a large survey of 6,300 11–16-year-olds in autumn 2002 – the *Young Persons' Behaviour and Attitudes Survey*. It is important to stress that there are some differences in sampling procedures, questions asked and the analysis conducted on some of these surveys. This goes some way to explaining some contradictory findings. Numerous other studies will be used within this chapter to provide a more complete and rounded picture.

Children and young people who smoke tobacco

The main baseline data on smoking which allows for comparison across the countries of the UK and Europe is from the HBSC surveys.

Table 19.1 indicates the percentage of each age group who self-report daily smoking and Chart 19.1 provides a wider picture of how the smoking behaviour of UK children compares with other European countries.

Table 19.1 and Chart 19.1 indicate that nearly a quarter of 15-year-olds smoke cigarettes on a daily basis and that rates are higher in the countries of the UK than in many other European and North American countries. As elsewhere in Europe and North America, daily smoking is more prevalent among 15-year-old girls than boys in all the countries of the UK.

This is confirmed by other self-report studies. In Northern Ireland, for

Table 19.1: Daily smoking by age, country and sex, % of each sex cohort by country

Country	Aged 11		Aged 13		Aged 15	
	Boys	Girls	Boys	Girls	Boys	Girls
England	1.0	1.0	7.0	8.0	21.0	24.0
Scotland	1.0	2.0	5.0	8.0	19.0	24.0
Wales	1.0	1.0	6.0	12.0	18.0	23.0
Northern Ireland	1.0	1.0	7.0	10.0	16.0	24.0
Ireland	2.0	2.0	14.0	12.0	25.0	25.0
Germany	0.1	1.0	9.0	9.0	22.0	25.0
France	0.5	1.0	5.0	6.0	20.0	25.0
Sweden	0.3	0.0	2.0	2.0	10.0	16.0
USA	1.0	2.0	5.0	3.0	12.0	13.0
Canada	1.0	1.0	8.0	8.0	17.0	21.0

Source: Based on Currie *et al.* (2000)

Chart 19.1: Daily smoking among 15-year-olds across Europe in 1998

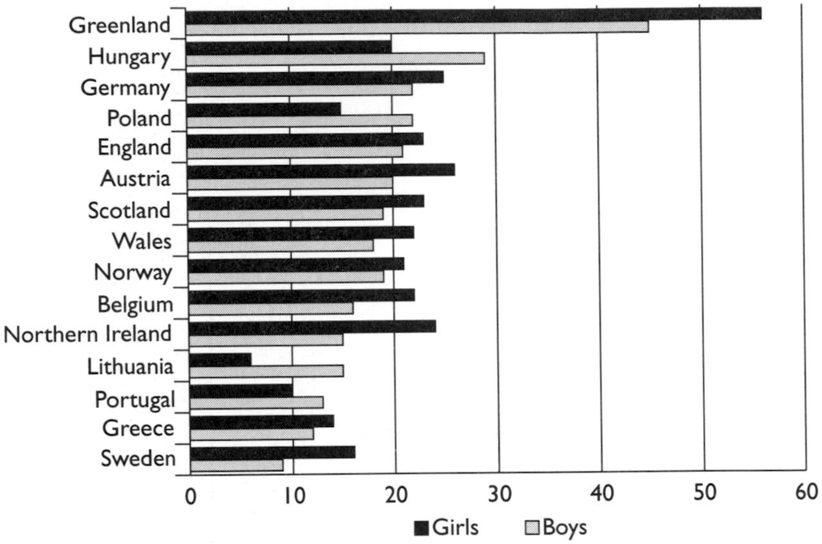

Sources: Based on Currie *et al.* (2000) and Griesbach and Currie (2001)

instance, the *Young Persons' Behaviour and Attitude Survey* reports that a quarter of its sample smoke every day. Yet this survey also indicates there is a widespread acceptance that smoking is harmful to health (95 per cent), causes lung cancer (99 per cent) and that stopping is difficult (93 per cent). The survey does not disaggregate its findings for girls and boys. The HBSC survey indicates that, while the proportion of girls smoking at the age of 15 in Northern Ireland is commensurate with those in other countries of the UK and the Republic of Ireland, smoking among 15-year-old boys in Northern Ireland is markedly less common.

Chart 19.2 is based on the Department of Health (DoH) surveys and indicates that, in both England and Scotland, girls report being regular smokers more than boys, and rates in Scotland are higher for both boys and girls (Goddard and Higgins, 1999a, 1999b).

According to the HBSC survey, the median number of cigarettes smoked per week by 15-year-olds is 30 (Currie *et al.*, 2000). The DoH surveys, however, report that, among regular child smokers in England, the quantity of cigarettes consumed has increased from 50 cigarettes a week in 1992 to 56 a week 1998. This was largely due to an increase in consumption among boys (Goddard and Higgins, 1999a). Thus, although girls are more likely than boys to be regular

Chart 19.2: Regular smoking by age and sex among 11–15-year-olds, England and Scotland

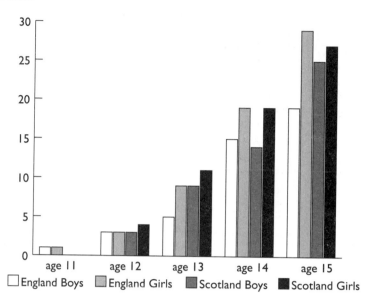

England Boys ☐ England Girls ▨ Scotland Boys ▦ Scotland Girls ■

smokers, among those who do smoke, boys smoke more cigarettes in an average week. As well as simply self-reporting their smoking, the young people in the DoH surveys were asked to keep a 'diary' to record the number of cigarettes they smoked over the course of a week. This suggests heavier levels of smoking than other self-report studies. In England, for instance, the majority of 'regular smokers' (71 per cent) recorded that they smoked more than 20 cigarettes a week in the diary, with a third of pupils recording more than 70 a week (Goddard and Higgins, 1999a). Regular smoking produces addiction; 58 per cent of the 'regular' smokers reported that it would be 'difficult' for them to go without smoking for a week and half said they would find it 'very difficult'. Nor did all of them want to give up; indeed there was a decline in the numbers of 'regular smokers' saying they wanted to give up from 45 per cent in 1996 to 35 per cent in 1998 (Goddard and Higgins, 1999a).

Trends over time

Goddard and Higgins report that, in England, overall patterns of smoking prevalence have, on average, remained fairly stable within the secondary school-aged population over the last two decades (Goddard and Higgins, 1999a). This seems at odds with findings from the HBSC surveys for other countries within the UK (there is no trend data for England within the HBSC surveys). The HBSC study indicates that among 15-year-old school children in Scotland, daily smoking is reported to have increased between 1990 and 1998 from 12.4 per cent to 19.2 per cent for boys and from 12 per cent to 24 per cent for girls (Griesbach and Currie, 2001). Smoking among both girls and boys in Wales has shown marked increases. Its position in the league table has changed from 23rd of 25 in 1993–4 to the seventh highest in 1997/98 (trend data for Wales is to be released by mid-March 2002).

Correlates of smoking

The HBSC survey reports that, although a number of different measures of socio-economic status of the family were collected, this was not related to smoking behaviour. Other surveys have also failed to find strong socio-economic differences in children's smoking behaviour. However, some studies and surveys have consistently found a social class gradient in smoking behaviour among adults and older teenagers. This suggests that socio-economic factors only begin to have a stronger influence in the later teenage years (Botting, 1995).

The Department of Health studies report that one factor which is highly significant in taking up smoking is having other family members who smoke. The 1996 DoH study found that those who lived with two parents, both of whom smoked, were more than twice as likely to smoke as those who lived in households where neither parent smoked: 21 per cent compared with 8 per cent. Children who had at least one brother or sister who smoked were over four times as likely to be smokers themselves as those who said that none of their brothers or sisters smoked (Jarvis, 1997).

Alcohol

Public concern about young people's consumption of alcohol and drinking patterns has mainly been about problematic binge drinking, drunkenness in public places and the associated social disorder issues this has created. Yet much of the research on alcohol use and misuse does not seem to connect with this concern. In a recent review of the evidence, Newburn and Shiner (2001) are critical of the ability of many of the established data sources to provide reliable answers to these important questions.

Prevalence

The HBSC surveys ask a series of questions about the drinking of alcohol by children and young people that allow some comparisons between the countries of the UK and other countries. Table 19.2 indicates the percentage of each age group who report drinking alcohol at least once a week.

In the countries of the UK (and in Wales and England especially) drinking alcohol at least once a week is reported by far higher proportions of 15-year-olds than in other European and North American countries. The table also indicates that the gender difference in terms of smoking is reversed for the regular drinking of alcohol, with boys much more likely to drink it weekly than girls. However,

Table 19.2: Drinking beer, wine or spirits at least weekly by country, age and sex, percentage

Country	Aged 11		Aged 13		Aged 15	
	Boys	Girls	Boys	Girls	Boys	Girls
England	14.0	9.0	22.0	16.0	47.0	36.0
Scotland	8.0	4.0	17.0	11.0	37.0	33.0
Wales	12.0	5.0	24.0	16.0	53.0	36.0
Northern Ireland	5.0	1.0	14.0	6.0	33.0	20.0
Ireland	7.0	1.0	8.0	6.0	27.0	12.0
Germany	2.0	0.3	10.0	5.0	29.0	22.0
France	6.0	3.0	12.0	5.0	31.0	15.0
Sweden	3.0	1.0	6.0	4.0	17.0	11.0
USA	8.0	7.0	10.0	11.0	23.0	15.0
Canada	3.0	2.0	10.0	6.0	22.0	17.0

Source: Based on Currie *et al.* (2000)

Table 19.3: Getting drunk twice or more often by country, age and sex, percentages

Country	Aged 11		Aged 13		Aged 15	
	Boys	Girls	Boys	Girls	Boys	Girls
England	9.0	3.0	25.0	22.0	51.0	52.0
Scotland	10.0	4.0	26.0	21.0	53.0	56.0
Wales	12.0	6.0	38.0	35.0	72.0	63.0
Northern Ireland	6.0	2.0	24.0	17.0	53.0	44.0
Ireland	7.0	1.0	15.0	8.0	42.0	29.0
Germany	2.0	0.4	10.0	7.0	36.0	31.0
France	1.0	0.4	8.0	5.0	29.0	20.0
Sweden	1.0	0.3	8.0	6.0	40.0	40.0
USA	3.0	3.0	12.0	11.0	34.0	28.0
Canada	3.0	2.0	15.0	13.0	42.0	42.0

Source: Based on Currie *et al.* (2000)

the HBSC report makes clear that, of the 28 countries taking part in the 1997/ 98 surveys, the only countries in which girls consumed more wine and spirits than boys at the age of 15 were Scotland (2 per cent for wine and 12 per cent for spirits), England (5 per cent for wine and 7 per cent for spirits) and Wales (8 per cent for wine and 3 per cent for spirits).

Another question asked in the HBSC surveys was whether respondents had became drunk on at least two occasions. Data from the four countries of the UK and other comparison countries is summarised in Table 19.3. Again this indicates that children in the UK countries self-report being drunk much more than in many other countries. Some gender differences are also apparent, with boys reporting being drunk more than girls in Wales and Northern Ireland, but in approximately the same proportions in England and Scotland. Boys aged 15 in Wales are by far the most likely to report having been drunk on at least two occasions compared to other countries. Girls in the same age group in Wales also self-report being drunk much more than either boys or girls in the other UK countries.

Trends over time

Since 1988, the DoH surveys into smoking among young people have been expanded to include alcohol consumption and are also important sources of information on young people's drinking habits. These surveys indicate that, over the full 11–15 age range, there has been some decline in the weekly consumption of alcohol. For instance, in 1998 21 per cent of children aged 11–15 in England in this survey said that they had had an alcoholic drink in the last seven days – a significant decrease since 1996 when 27 per cent had done so (Goddard and Higgins, 1999a, p. 43). In Scotland the figure for 12–15-year-olds was slightly lower at 19 per cent – again a slight decrease from the 1996 figure of 23 per cent (Goddard and Higgins, 1999b, p. 7). Chart 19.3 summarises differences between boys and girls in England and Scotland over time. In England, of those who had drunk alcohol 'in the last week', four in five had done so only on one or two days – usually at weekends.

In England, according to the DoH surveys, although there was a decrease in the proportion of children who said they drank alcohol at least once a week, the average weekly amount among those who did drink was 9.9 units, an increase since 1996 from 8.4 units. Thus, although the proportion of young people drinking in the previous week had fallen in 1998 compared with 1996, those

Chart 19.3: Drinking alcohol in the last week by boys and girls in England and Scotland, 1990–1998

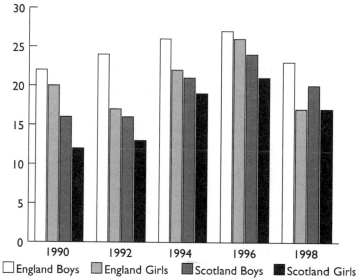

Sources: Based on Goddard and Higgins (1999a and 1999b)

who did drink drank more (Goddard and Higgins, 1999a). These findings are also in line with the 1998 Youth Lifestyles Survey, which indicated increased levels of binge drinking. Approximately 22 per cent of 12–15-years-olds and 63 per cent of 16–17-year-olds reported having felt very drunk in the last year (Harrington, 2000). The amount of alcohol young people drink is also associated with age.

Chart 19.4 shows the average number of units consumed in the last week by boys and girls in England and Scotland. Like smoking, alcohol consumption increases with age and varies between different gender groups. The Youth Lifestyles Survey also reveals some significant differences to be found in drinking behaviour between different ethnic groups. Harrington found that minority ethnic teenagers were less likely than 'whites' to say that they drink alcohol or drink frequently. The majority of 'non-whites' aged 12–17 had either never drunk alcohol or had not done so in the last year; this was compared to 20 per cent of whites (Harrington, 2000). A school-based study in Leicestershire by Denscombe found that 94 per cent of South Asians described themselves as non-drinkers compared with 38 per cent of 'whites'. South Asian pupils also had less favourable attitudes towards drinking (Denscombe, 1995).

Chart 19.4: Mean number of units of alcohol consumed by those who drank in the last week, 1998 surveys in England and Scotland

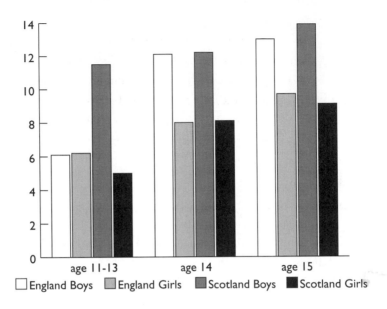

England Boys   England Girls   Scotland Boys   Scotland Girls

Sources: Based on Goddard and Higgins (1999a and 1999b)

Levels of abstinence have also been fairly stable, remaining at about 40 per cent of all 11–15-year-olds since the early 1980s (Newburn and Shiner, 2001, p. 19). On the other hand, we have seen over recent years that those young people who are drinking appear to be doing so with greater frequency and involving larger amounts of alcohol than was previously the case.

Where and with whom do young people drink?

One of the marked features of age-related drinking patterns is what is drunk, with whom and in what circumstances. This is also related to the degree of adult supervision associated with drinking alcohol and whether this is in a public or private place.

According to the DoH surveys, overall the most popular place for drinking by 11–15-year-olds in England and Scotland was at home or at the home of a friend or relative: 58 per cent of pupils claimed to have drunk here. Other locations for young people's drinking included parties (23 per cent), pubs (12 per cent), clubs or discos (10 per cent) and elsewhere (21 per cent) (Goddard and Higgins, 1999a, p. 56). Yet the places where people drank and who they drank with changed over different ages, and the proportion of drinkers who said they drank at home fell from 79 per cent of 11-year-olds to 51 per cent of 15-year-olds. Seven out of ten of the youngest drinkers reported that they usually drank with their parents, while only three in ten 15-year-olds did so, with many more stating that they drank with friends (Goddard and Higgins, 1999a, p. 56). A number of studies have pointed to the 'graduation' from small amounts of supervised drinking in the home, to unsupervised drinking in public places (parks and street corners), to licensed premises (mainly pubs) and finally to clubs with extended hours of license popular amongst young people in their late teens (Coles, 2000; Parker *et al.*, 1998).

Correlates of drinking

In similar ways to research into smoking behaviour, studies of alcohol use among young people have struggled to find many clear links between drinking and socio-economic position. A survey by the Office for National Statistics found no consistent association between children's drinking behaviour and families' socio-economic position. On the one hand, the highest proportions of frequent drinkers were from among the better-off families, but on the other, also from among those with lower educational achievements (Goddard, 1997). There is also some evidence that young people are, or at least regard themselves as being, street-wise about alcohol and drugs (Aldridge *et al.*, 1999). Many young people regard drinking alcohol (especially getting drunk) as potentially more dangerous to their welfare than the use of 'soft' recreational drugs.

Drug use

Much of the data collected on drug use has attempted to reveal the extent of use, with some claims that it is now widespread and part-and-parcel of the lives of the majority of young people, ie, it is 'normal' for young people to take drugs. This 'normalisation' thesis is far from proven, however. Much of the evidence support-ing it is based upon self-report studies of 'ever having used an illegal drug'. This can, of course, include as 'drug users' those who have once tried a single 'experiment', rather than any sustained involvement with drugs.

Prevalence

Over the last few years, surveys of young people's drug use and habits have been carried out by the Home Office and the Department of Health, and further information has been gained through the inclusion of questions on drug use in the British Crime Survey (BCS), Youth Lifestyles Surveys, independent academic studies and other studies supported by the Drugs Prevention Advisory Service. Questions on drugs and drug use have also been added to the Department of Health study of smoking and alcohol use among young people. In this latter survey, pupils are given a list of illegal drugs, including both their correct names and their street names. In England in 1998, 34 per cent of pupils aged 11–15 stated that they had been offered at least one of the drugs listed. However, this high level of access to drugs does not imply a high take-up; only 13 per cent of pupils reported that they had used drugs (Goddard and Higgins, 1999a). In Scotland the figures were considerably higher: 41 per cent of pupils had been offered at least one of the drugs and 18 per cent had ever used them (Goddard and Higgins, 1999b). Yet, as with smoking and drinking alcohol, access to and use of drugs change with age. Table 19.4 and Chart 19.5 use data from the DoH and HBSC surveys of 11–15-year-olds and the BCS self-reporting study of 16–19-year-olds to plot drug use among different age groups of boys and girls. Separate figures for Scotland and England are most easily comparable using the DoH surveys. The figures indicate that the monthly taking of drugs starts at an earlier age in Scotland and is significantly higher than rates in England by the age of 15.

Table 19.4: Self-reported drug use within the past month by boys and girls aged 12–15, percentage of each age group, England, Scotland and Wales

	Age 12	Age 13	Age 14	Age 15
England				
Boys	2	4	10	19
Girls	2	4	9	16
Scotland				
Boys	2	9	14	26
Girls	2	7	14	22
Wales				
Boys				28*
Girls				22*

*Data for Wales is for 1996. 1998 data will be released in mid-March 2002.

Chart 19.5: Regular drug use: the proportion of each age group who had used drugs within the past month

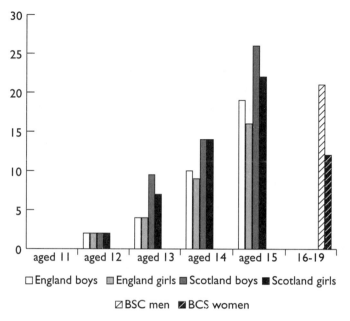

Trend data from the HBSC surveys in Wales indicate that self-reported drug use within the last month increased from 11.6 per cent to 27.9 per cent for boys between 1990 and 1996 and from 9.9 per cent to 21.8 per cent for girls (Health Promotion Agency for Wales, 1997). Other separate national reports from the HBSC surveys are not available at the time of writing.

Some data for Northern Ireland is also available through the Young Persons' Behaviour and Attitude Survey but is presented in a way which is not commensurate with data for England and Scotland and does not indicate drug use by age and sex. However, the aggregate data suggests that drug taking in Northern Ireland is at a considerably lower level than in the three other countries of the UK.

The report indicates that the peak years for first use of cannabis are between 13 and 15 years of age, although 19 per cent of those who have ever used the drug say they first used it at the age of 12 or earlier. Nine per cent of those reporting use of speed were age 8 or under when they first started using it. Around 30 per cent of the whole sample think it would be easy or very easy to get cannabis, but 26 per cent think it would be difficult and 45 per cent don't know.

Table 19.5: Prevalence of drug taking in Northern Ireland, percentage of sample reporting drug use among pupils in (school) years 8–12

Type of drug	Reported use: Ever	Last week	Last month	Last year
Cannabis	13.0	4.0	4.0	3.0
Speed	2.0	0.5	0.4	0.8
LSD	3.0	0.4	0.5	1.0
Ecstasy	4.0	1.0	1.0	1.0
Poppers	5.0	1.0	1.0	2.0
Tranquillisers	2.0	0.3	0.3	0.7
Heroin	1.0	0.2	0.2	0.2
Semeron (Fake Drug)	1.0	0.2	0.2	0.2

The YLS covers young people aged 12 to 30 living in England and Wales. This suggests that the peak ages for drug use are between the ages of 18 and 21 and, as such, are much later than the years covered by the HBSC surveys. According to the YLS, 44 per cent of young people said that they had used drugs within the last year, 26 per cent within the last month and 17 per cent within the last week (Flood-Page *et al.*, 2000).

A study of drug use in 1999 in two regions of northern England distinguishes between four types of relationship to drugs: 'regular users'; 'former triers'; 'abstainers'; and 'in transition' (Aldridge *et al.*, 1999). By the age of 18 just under a third (31 per cent) were current users (they had taken drugs and intended to do so again). A further 30 per cent were 'abstainers' – they had never taken drugs and had no intention of doing so in the future. A smaller group (11 per cent) were 'former triers' – they had used drugs but had stopped and did not intend to take them again in the future. The fourth group (28 per cent) had used drugs in the past, did not identify themselves as current users but remained agnostic about whether they may use them again in the futures. It is the size of this fourth group that perhaps helps explain the disparity in the size of the 'abstainer' group. Based on the BCS evidence the claim is still that around a half of 16–19-year-olds abstain from using drugs (Ramsay and Spiller, 1997).

Types of drugs taken

Surveys have consistently shown that the most popular and widely available type of drug among young people is cannabis. Within the BCS the majority of young drug users were found to consume only one drug – cannabis. Much has also been written about 'gateway drugs', on the assumption that once a child or young person is involved in even the most infrequent use of cannabis, this is the first step down the slippery slope to the use of harder and more addictive drugs. Yet such an assumption flies in the face of evidence from young people themselves, who seem to set clear boundaries about what is 'acceptable' and totally 'unaccept-able' in terms of drug-taking behaviour (Aldridge *et al.*, 1999). Regardless of age group and time frame, consumption of cannabis alone is more common than cannabis combined with any other drug. Consumption of single drugs other than cannabis is also comparatively rare – particularly among young users and those who have used drugs within the last month (Ramsay and Partridge, 1999; Ramsay *et al.*, 2001). The most recent British Crime Survey indicates that, among 16–19-year-olds who had used drugs other than cannabis in the past month, 5 per cent had used Class A drugs. Of these, 5 per cent had used hallucinogens, 3 per cent had used opiates and 2 per cent had used cocaine (Ramsay *et al.*, 2001).

There are worries that particular estates have been flooded with cheap heroin-based drugs, that some young people regard smoking such drugs as unlikely to lead to addiction, and that as young people get older they do cross the line in search of the bigger 'high' being achieved by their older peers (Johnson *et al.*, 2000).

Correlates of drug taking

Research has located some correlates of drug taking among young people. Goddard and Higgins have argued that those 11–15-year-olds who did not think they were going to live up to the expectations others had of them in terms of examination performance, were most likely to have the highest levels of drug use (Goddard and Higgins, 1999a, 1999b). The 2001 report from the BCS also shows that 30 per cent of 16–19-year-olds with no qualifications had taken drugs within the past year, compared with 26 per cent of those who had attained 'intermediate qualifications' (Ramsay *et al.*, 2001). The relationship between drug taking and social class is more complex, with the highest drug use being concentrated at the two extremes of household income groups – the very rich and the poorest. According to the ACORN classification of neighbourhoods, last year and last month drug users, regardless of age, were more likely to live in households located in relatively affluent 'rising' areas, ie, those with a preponder-ance of affluent urbanites, prosperous professionals and better off executive households (Ramsay and Partridge, 1999; Ramsay *et al.*, 2001). The relationship between drug use and unemployment, however, is also clear, with 40 per cent of 16–29-year-olds who were unemployed in the week before the BCS interview reporting using drugs in the previous year – almost double the rate of those with jobs (Ramsay and Partridge, 1999). The Youth Lifestyles Survey for England and Wales reports strong links between drug taking and truancy and school exclusion (see also Chapter 17) and smoking, drinking alcohol and being involved in crime (see also Chapter 18). Boys and girls aged 12–17 who had used drugs in the last year were five times more likely to be offenders than non-drug-users. Of those admitting drug use, 60 per cent reported that they drank alcohol at least once a week, 19 per cent regularly truanted from school and 21 per cent had been excluded from school (Flood-Page *et al.*, 2000).

One large-scale study of over a thousand young people in western Scotland (including Glasgow) examined the relationship between smoking, drinking alcohol, drug taking and other aspects of lifestyle including early sexual experiences (West and Sweeting, 1996). Young women who use drugs before the age of 15 were found to be more than three times as likely to smoke, drink alcohol and have early sexual experiences. This study has also made links between all four 'risk taking' behaviours and family background. It claims that all four behaviours are considered 'normal' by young people living in poor neighbourhoods and that drug taking was 15 times less likely when young men lived in 'intact' families. The authors also report correlations between the experience of death of a parent and 'risk behaviours'.

Conclusions

This chapter has reviewed data on the smoking, drinking and drug-taking behaviour of children and young people in the four countries within the UK and examined how this compares to other countries. It can be concluded that young people in the UK do indulge in what many health experts regard as 'risky' behaviour which can be deleterious to the health and welfare of young people. Yet, while we have a huge array of 'facts' about such behaviours, it is far from clear that this is matched by any profound understanding that could better inform those who seek to intervene in young people's lives for the promotion of welfare.

In the case of drug taking, the vast majority of young people 'using drugs' do not regard themselves as 'mis-using' them. Furthermore, moral panics about the 'normalisation' of drug use seem to fly in the face of the fact that much 'use' is experimental and confined to cannabis. Many young people regard even regular use of cannabis as less harmful than other forms of behaviours, such as drinking alcohol or smoking cigarettes. But smoking cannabis is illegal. The drinking of alcohol by children and young people is not illegal, although it is illegal for those under the 18 to buy it. The chapter has reviewed some data about lifetime use of alcohol and the age at which young people begin to drink it. But perhaps more important is where, and with whom, young people drink, and even more importantly where, and with whom they drink to excess and become intoxicated. Unsupervised drinking to excess is much more likely to cause medical and welfare harm. In the case of smoking, higher proportions of young people in the UK than elsewhere smoke cigarettes regularly, despite evidence that they know perfectly well that it is harmful to their health and is addictive. Despite this knowledge they continue to do it.

It is difficult to resist the conclusion that young people take drugs, drink to excess and smoke because it is thought to be 'cool' to do so and that experimenting in behaviour regarded by authority as being 'wrong' is part of the attraction. But until we have a clearer understanding of the motivations of children and young people we will struggle to be able to offer them help, even in terms of supporting harm reduction.

20 Youth Suicide

Beverley Searle

Key statistics:
- Suicide accounts for a fifth of all deaths of young people.
- Over two young suicides are committed every day.
- In 1998 24,000 adolescents self-harmed, that is one every three hours.
- In 1999, 80 per cent of young suicides were committed by boys.

Key trends:
- The number of suicides of young people in the UK has fallen 16 per cent from 854 in 1989 to 737 in 1999.
- Suicide rates among boys are increasing in Scotland, Wales and Northern Ireland, and among girls are increasing in Northern Ireland.

Key sources:
- Population Trends
- Mortality Statistics
- World Health Organisation, World Health Statistics Annual

Introduction

Suicide and para-suicide is an effectual indication of lack of mental well-being. This chapter explores the extent of youth suicide and attempted suicide in the UK. Five key issues are examined:
- the problems of defining and measuring suicide
- the trends in suicide rates in the countries of the UK
- international comparisons of suicide and self-injury
- trends in preferred methods of suicide and attempted suicide
- a synthesis of the available literature that seeks to explain suicide trends and highlight those most at risk of suicide.

Within each topic, attention is given to gender differences in suicide and attempted suicide. Due to limited data, differences between ethnic groups are not fully explored. Separate chapters address the specific issues of mental health (Chapter 22), unintentional injury (Chapter 6), and child abuse and neglect (Chapter 7). However, a child's desire to take his or her own life is influenced by the many aspects associated with well-being that are examined throughout this volume.

Problem of definition and measurement

Constructing a statistical profile of youth suicide and para-suicide (attempted suicide), as with any statistical profile, is only as reliable as the data available. The recording of youth suicide is a particularly sensitive issue. There are strong pressures on doctors and coroners to avoid a verdict of suicide (Coleman, 1999), particularly for young people below their mid-teens (Madge, 1996). Consequently there is little data available on suicide among those under the age of 15. Historical heritage and cultural beliefs mean there is still a stigma attached to youth suicide in parts of the UK, particularly where this is in conflict with perceived visions of childhood (Hill, 1995; Stillion *et al.*, 1989). In Scotland certification of death is the responsibility of a doctor and is a private issue, whereas in England, Wales and Northern Ireland deaths suspected to be accidents or suicides are referred to a coroner and are subject to public inquest (Griffiths and Fitzpatrick, 2001). Where decisions are made in the presence of bereaved relatives, coroners may justifiably want to spare the feelings of families and record an accidental rather than suicide verdict (Hill, 1995; Madge and Harvey, 1999).

The legal definition of suicide in the UK requires that intention is beyond any doubt, supported by clear evidence that the injury was self-inflicted. This is in contrast with the 'balance of probabilities' approach adopted in other countries such as Hungary or Norway (Madge and Harvey, 1999). In 1968 the introduction in the UK of 'Injury undetermined whether accidentally or purposefully inflicted' became instantly popular in dealing with less clear cases. However, is it widely recognised that they mainly consist of self-inflicted deaths (Hill, 1995). In youth suicide, doubt is often inevitable, with the potential for a misclassification of accidental death or open verdict being recorded (Charlton *et al.*, 1992; Hill, 1995; Madge and Harvey, 1999). This is especially so where there is a preference among young people, particularly females, to use more ambiguous methods such as substance misuse, where intent and evidence may be 'befuddled by alcohol or drugs' (Hill, 1995, p. 15). The discrepancies around determining death by suicide, together with the reluctance of coroners and doctors to pass such a verdict on young people, suggests there is a considerable under-recording of suicides in the UK (Coleman, 1999; Hill, 1995). Therefore any analysis based on officially recorded suicide statistics will be subject to their limitations.

Suicide and undetermined death in the UK

Taking the above reservations into consideration, official statistics for the UK show that overall there has been a reduction in the number of recorded suicides in the late 1990s. This is a reversal of the trend during the early 1990s, when the number of suicides, especially among young men aged 15–24, increased significantly. Statistics available for the last ten years show there has been a 16 per cent reduction in the number of youth suicides and undetermined deaths in the UK from 854 in 1989 to 737 in 1999 (Table 20.1). During this period there has been a greater decrease in the number of female suicides and undetermined deaths (19 per cent) compared to males (15 per cent).

Despite this welcome trend, there is still concern that the incidence of suicide increases with age, and there is still a high rate of youth suicides among the 15–24 age group, particularly among young males. Using government statistics, the Samaritans estimate that suicide accounts for over a fifth of all deaths of young people and there are still over two young suicides every day, 80 per cent of which are by young men (Samaritans, 2001).

Table 20.2 shows that there are differences between the male and female suicide rates of different UK countries. However, actual numbers of suicides are

Table 20.1: Suicide and undetermined death in the UK among 0–24-year-olds, by gender, age group and year

	1989	1990	1991	1992	1993	1994	1995	1996	1997	1998	1999
0–14 years											
Male	11	18	14	19	37	24	17	22	22	18	14
Female	12	4	9	10	13	15	15	9	13	7	8
15–24 years											
Male	667	731	674	690	701	660	601	560	628	571	575
Female	164	142	160	151	142	117	139	149	138	159	140
Total	854	895	857	870	893	816	772	740	801	755	737

Sources: Office for National Statistics; Register General for Scotland; Register General for Northern Ireland

low (for example only eight female suicides per 100,000 population aged 15–24 were recorded in Northern Ireland), therefore the scope for any analysis is limited. What the statistics do show is that while the suicide rate among males aged 15–24 decreased in England from 16 to 13 per 100,000 population aged 15–24 between 1990 and 1999, it rose in the other countries, most notably in Scotland (from 19 per 100,000 in 1989 to 33 per 100,000 in 1999) and in Northern Ireland (which has seen nearly a 100 per cent increase from 13 per 100,000 in 1989 to 25 per 100,000 in 1999) (Table 20.2). Among females aged 15–24, the suicide rate has remained fairly constant in England at 3 to 4 per 100,000. However, there is a marked contrast in the downward trends of Scotland and Wales compared to the 300 per cent increase in Northern Ireland from 3 per 100,000 in 1989 to 8 per 100,000 in 1999.

It is unclear why there should be variations in suicide rates in the UK, most notably the rise in Scotland and Northern Ireland. Individual factors have been identified which characterise those most at risk, including: lower social status, unemployment, mental illness, substance misuse, history of self-harm, physical or sexual abuse, and having been in prison. These individual factors also need to be set in the context of other social factors including: the state of the employment market, accessibility of methods of committing suicide, changing patterns in family composition, public attitudes to and understanding of mental illness, and high risk settings such as certain prisons, local authority care and some schools (Director of Public Health, 2000). Cultural and ethnicity issues may also be a

Table 20.2: Suicide and undetermined deaths in UK among 15–24 year olds, by gender, country, age group and year

	1989	1990	1991	1992	1993	1994	1995	1996	1997	1998	1999
Males											
England		16	15	16	16	15	14	13	15	14	13
Scotland	19	23	20	26	31	28	25	25	30	25	33
Northern Ireland	13	13	17	16	26	23	23	18	20	22	25
Wales		17	16	20	22	20	14	23	22	22	25
Females											
England		3	4	3	4	3	4	4	3	4	4
Scotland	4	4	4	7	6	6	6	9	8	10	6
Northern Ireland	3	5	4	2	3	1	3	2	5	4	8
Wales		1	6	6	2	6	3	5	4	4	2

Rates per 100,000 population aged 15–24

Sources: Office for National Statistics; General Register Office for Scotland; General Register Office for Northern Ireland

factor. Some explanations may arise as a result of the recent consultation on reducing suicide and self-harm in Scotland (Scottish Executive, 2001h).

Suicide and self-injury: international comparisons

Although the latest figures available are for different years, international comparisons of 26 countries by WHO show that the UK had the lowest rate of suicide of under 14s at 0.1 per 100,000 population under 14 for both males and females in 1997. It also had a relatively low rate for 15–24-year-olds (11.1 and 2.3 per 100,000 in 1997 respectively). Russia has the highest rate of suicide and self-inflicted injury among boys in both age groups at 3 per 100,000 for 5–14-year-olds and 53 per 100,000 for 15–24-year-olds in 1997. The highest rate of suicides and self-inflicted injury among girls in both age groups is in New Zealand where in 1996 the rate was 1.5 per 100,000 for 5–14-year-olds and 13.9 per 100,000 for 15–24-year-olds (Chart 20a) (WHO, 2001).

Comparative studies have shown there is a relationship between trends in suicide rates in countries with similar characteristics, suggesting that "suicide rates are determined by persisting cross-national differences, including traditions, customs, religions, social attitudes and climate" (Cantor, 2000). Rapid changes in industrialisation, increases in alcoholism, promiscuity, violence, hopelessness and gender roles have all been associated with differences in suicide trends (Cantor, 2000). Cross-cultural comparisons are problematic due to the different meanings and attitudes associated to suicide within different countries (Charlton et al., 1993). Nevertheless, comparative studies have given cause for concern over recent international trends in the rise in suicide rates in 15–24-year-olds, especially males, which has been most evident in English-speaking nations (Cantor, 2000).

Methods of suicide and suicide behaviour

Most methods of suicide reflect the availability of methods within individual nations. For example, in the USA, suicide by shooting is popular due to the availability of guns. However, this method is less common among Asian nations (Cantor, 2000; Cheng and Lee, 2000). Equally, in urbanised areas suicide by jumping off tall buildings is more prevalent, whereas in rural areas self-poisoning is more popular (Cheng and Lee, 2000). Drug overdoses are common to most

Chart 20.1a: Suicide and self-inflicted injury: 5–14 years

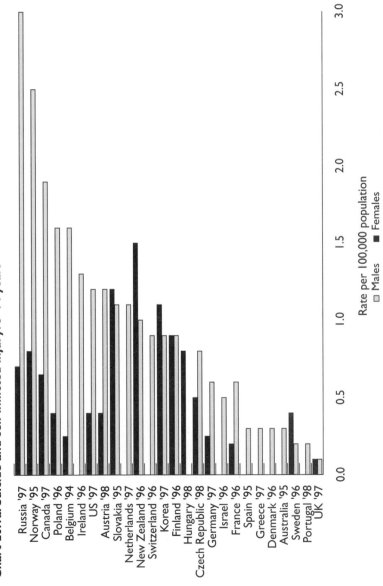

Rate per 100,000 population
□ Males   ■ Females

Chart 20.1b: Suicide and self-inflicted injury: 15–24 years

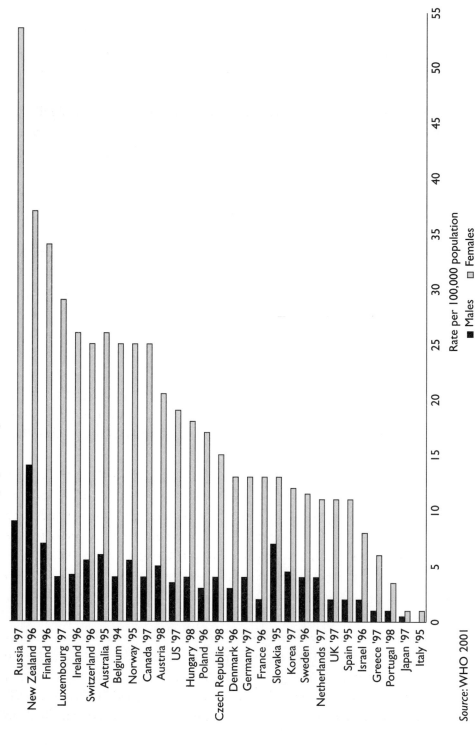

Source: WHO 2001

countries, and hanging is becoming more common (Cantor, 2000). Within the UK, regional variations exist in the prevalence of suicide methods. Drug-related suicide is mostly confined to inner-London, Glasgow and Manchester. Alcohol-related suicide is concentrated in urban areas, though more widespread in Scotland (Griffiths and Fitzpatrick, 2001). No spatial data on the prevalence of hanging is available.

The preference of different methods of suicide could have significant implications for the way that suicide verdicts are recorded, which in turn has implications for the difference in levels of recorded youth suicides of males and females. Between 1968 and 1992 Hill's (1995) research showed that, among young people, male suicides due to overdoses dropped from 31.4 per cent to 14.4 per cent, while suicide by hanging rose from 16.8 per cent to 29.5 per cent during the same period. For young females, although the rate of suicides by overdoses decreased, they still accounted for around half of all suicide and undetermined deaths, falling from 63.7 per cent to 43.7 per cent during 1968 to 1992, with death by hanging increasing from 7.5 per cent to 15.4 per cent during the same period (Hill, 1995, p. 27). More recent analysis of trends in suicide methods suggests that there have been three phases in methods of suicide which can be described as 'epidemics of suicide'. The epidemic of overdosing in the 1970s was followed by a preference of motor vehicle exhaust gas during the 1980s to the mid-1990s. Then, following the introduction of catalytic converters this method declined, leading to the current preferred method of hanging. These trends, though, mainly reflect changes in male suicide methods, rather than female (McClure, 2000, 2001).

Such findings support previous research which shows there are marked gender differences in the methods used to commit, or attempt to commit, suicide. Young men are more likely to resort to more aggressive methods such as hanging or jumping from high places, whereas young women prefer passive methods and tend to overdose on paracetamol (Marttunen *et al.*, 1992; Coles, 2000). Different suicidal methodology allows for different degrees of doubt in recording cause of death and this has consequences for official statistics. Aggressive means such as hanging, favoured by males, show a degree of preparation and therefore intent (Hill, 1995). They are more likely to result in death and are most likely to receive a suicide verdict (Platt *et al.*, 1988). In contrast, overdosing may be regarded as a gamble; it leaves time for intervention and is often associated with ambiguous intentions (Hill, 1995). Deaths by self-poisoning, favoured by females, are less likely to be fatal and are least likely to be classified as suicide (Adelstein and Mardon, 1975). As a result, official statistics show that young males are more likely to commit suicide while young females are more likely to attempt suicide.

Statistics on attempted suicide are more difficult to obtain, and are more likely to be under-recorded than completed suicides because they reflect only the numbers of people seeking medical or other professional help (Carlton and Deane, 2000; Hawton *et al.*, 1999). However, evidence suggests that past suicidal behaviour is a strong risk factor for subsequent suicide, with multiple acts of self-harm increasing the risk of suicide (Hawton *et al.*, 1998; Shaffer *et al.*, 1996). Using government statistics, the Samaritans estimate that 24,000 adolescents self-harmed in 1998, which equates to one every three hours (Samaritans, 2001). Girls are four times more likely to attempt suicide than boys, with their preferred method being self-poisoning (Kerfoot, 1996) reflecting a similar pattern to preferred methods of actual female suicide. The value judgements of professionals, methods of suicide adopted and the lack of knowledge of para-suicides not only suggests that suicide is under-recorded, but also that this may be significantly so in the case of females, as their preferred methods of suicide make it more difficult to judge intent and are therefore more likely to receive an accidental verdict.

Explaining trends in suicide

Although data is available to show trends in suicide behaviour, as explained earlier, finding causal explanations for those trends is a complex process, involving both the individual and their social environment (McClure, 2000; Director of Public Health, 2000). Analysis into suicide faces particular problems since the perpetrator is inevitably unavailable, and therefore it is not possible to be completely sure of the original motives leading to death. Research is always retrospective (Stillion *et al.*, 1989) and based on the, often emotionally charged, opinions of others.

In the UK reducing the suicide rate is used as the proxy to cover the whole of the mental health priority area (DoH, 1998) recognising that suicidal behaviour is a function of mental health (see Chapter 22). The causal relationship between mental illness and suicide is however very complex. Associations have been made between suicidal behaviour and the depressive effects of: experiencing physical or sexual abuse (Kienhorst *et al.*, 1995; see also Chapter 7); youth unemployment (Coles, 2000); being in the prison system (Liebling, 1992; Coles,

2000; Samaritans, 2001; see also Chapter 18); drug and alcohol misuse (Fombonne, 1995, 1998; Shaffer, 1998; see also Chapter 19); bullying and school exclusion (Kaltiala-Heino *et al.*, 1999; Wilkinson, 1994; see also Chapter 17) and as a consequence of social inequality in society generally (Wilkinson, 1994). Young people who have attempted suicide have been shown to have difficulty in maintaining social relationships within their family setting (Asarnow, 1992) and outside of the home, including relationships with peers at school (Hawton and Heeringen, 2000).

Although research has shown that suicidal behaviour has a strong and independent association with symptoms of depression, depression cannot account solely for the rise in suicide in young males, since girls are twice as likely to suffer a depressive disorder than boys (Fombonne, 1995, 1998). This suggests that girls adopt more successful coping methods than boys. Overall, "suicidal children have poor reality testing, are impulsive and have problems in emotional and social problem solving" (Pfeffer *et al.*, 1995). However, despite this evidence it is still unclear why in similar circumstances some young people decide to take their own life, while others do not (Coles, 2000).

Conclusion

Suicide statistics show that youth suicide rates in the UK were comparatively low in an international context and were falling towards the end of the 1990s, although variations exist, most notably in Scotland for males and Northern Ireland for females. This is in marked contrast with the beginning of the decade which had seen an increase in suicide, particularly among young males. Despite the decrease, there is still a significant gender gap, with young women more likely to attempt suicide, and males more likely to succeed. Such statistics, however, need to be treated with caution, particularly in an area as sensitive as child suicide, which is bound up in values and beliefs relating to perceptions of childhood and gender stereotypes.

Although limited, statistics do provide evidence of trends in suicide. What is more difficult to identify is the causal factors associated with suicide and para-suicide. Previous analysis has sought to identify the reasons for increases in the suicide rate in both a social and psychological context. Rises in youth unemployment, prison population, marital breakdown, child abuse and school exclusion have all been linked as possible influences in suicidal behaviour. Mental illness and the prevalence of depression among young people, either as a consequence of imposed life stressors or self-inflicted substance misuse, has also been suggested as increasing the risk of suicide.

However, in the light of changing trends, further research needs to be carried out in order to understand the factors that influence suicidal behaviour. In particular, research is needed into the level of exposure to life stressors and the coping methods adopted by individuals which may in part explain why some children in similar circumstances commit suicide, while others do not.

21 Child Labour

Anwen Jones

Key statistics:
- It has been estimated that between 1.75 and 2 million school children in the UK work at any one time.
- Between two-thirds and three-quarters of these children are thought to be working illegally.

Key findings:
- Research on child labour in developed countries is patchy and under-developed, and the extent and nature of child labour are poorly documented as are children's motivations to work.

Key sources:
- Trades Unions Congress
- British Household Panel Survey

Introduction

This chapter provides an overview of existing research on child labour in the UK. The first part of the chapter considers the recent revival of interest in child employment and discusses some of the difficulties in defining and measuring child employment in the absence of agreed definitions and reliable comparable data. The next section provides a brief summary of the current legislative framework in the UK. The remainder of the chapter is organised around a number of questions to do with the nature and extent of child employment, children's motivation to work and the effects of work on children.

Background

There has been a renewed interest in child labour among academics, policy makers, trade unions and politicians in recent years and there is now conclusive evidence that paid employment of children is an extensive feature of British social life (Campbell *et al.*, 1998; GMB/MPO, 2000; Hobbs and McKechnie, 1998; Leonard, 1999). Mizen *et al.* (2001a) suggest that two factors have been important in the growth in this area of research: first, the political debates around the ineffectiveness of child employment legislation and, second, the increasingly high profile of children's rights issues. The proposal for an EU Directive on the Protection of Young People at Work stimulated political interest, debate and research about the nature and extent of child labour and resulted in a number of quantitative studies, although for the most part these have been small scale and localised. The debates stimulated by the United Nations (UN) Convention on the Rights of the Child and the argument that children's voices should be heard and their views and perceptions given a place in the policy arena have resulted in more qualitative studies. There is now a small but growing qualitative literature that considers children's perspectives of their work. It should also be emphasised that child labour is often regarded as essentially a Third World problem and most research has set out to examine and explain child employment in newly industrialising countries and under-developed countries (Lavalette, 1999).

Defining and measuring child labour

Despite the increased interest in child employment, there remain important gaps in knowledge. None of the UK governments collect data on the employment of children aged younger than 16 and there have not been any large-scale national surveys which would allow for reliable comparisons to be made between, and within, the UK regions or European member states. Data from the research is difficult to compare for two other reasons. First, studies have included children and young people of various ages: some studies only include children of compulsory school age who are legally old enough to work (13 and older in most cases); others have included children as young as 10 years of age and young people as old as 19 or 20. Official definitions of 'child' also vary, which further undermines attempts to compare data. For example, under the European Directive, a child is any young person of less than 15 years of age or who is still subject to compulsory full-time schooling under national law (Commission of the European Communities, 2000). In Britain, by contrast, a child is any young person aged less than 16, while the UN Convention on the Rights of the Child defines a child as any person under the age of 18. Second, researchers have also varied in the way they have defined employment (Hobbs and McKechnie, 1997). Employment can take many forms including paid and unpaid work, work within and outside the home (see Chapter 10 on children as carers), work for family members and friends and illegal economic activity. Some researchers disregard work done for other family members, babysitting and unpaid work that are considered 'grey areas' (Pettit, 1998). However, McKechnie and Hobbs (2001) argue that to exclude babysitting would underestimate the extent of female work, as many girls report this activity as their employment. The exclusion of work for family members and unpaid work similarly underestimates the extent of employment among children working in a wide variety of occupations. Some of these occupations might involve working long hours and/or be physically demanding and dangerous, for example farming and construction work. There is now fairly extensive evidence of the extent of child prostitution in the UK (Lee and O'Brien, 1995; Melrose *et al.*, 1999) but this, like other forms of economic activity such as drug running and shoplifting, are not generally considered in the child labour research. Such omissions disregard some of the most exploitative and dangerous forms of work children undertake.

Child employment legislation

The employment of children in the UK is governed by the Children (Protection at Work) Regulations 1998, which amended pre-war legislation in order that the UK could conform to the European Commission Directive on the Protection of Young People at Work (94/93/EC) (Newman, 2000). The UK is also a signatory to the UN Convention on the Rights of the Child (United Nations, 1989). This states that nations must protect children from "economic exploitation and from performing any work that is likely to be hazardous or to interfere with the child's education, or to be harmful to the child's health or physical, mental, spiritual, moral or social development". The UK law defines the age at which a child can be legally employed, the hours during which a child can work and the occupations that children are not allowed to work in. As a rule of thumb, work under the age of 13 is illegal (there are exceptions, for example, modelling, acting and working under direct parental supervision in horticulture or light agricultural tasks). There are also restrictions on the hours that young people can work, on the number of hours they can work during term time, on school days and during holidays (these vary depending on age). These regulations are amended by a variety of local authority byelaws. Employers are obliged to register employees under the minimum school leaving age with the local authority and it is the duty of the local education authority to police this system and to ensure that children are properly registered and protected under the legislation. Research suggests, however, that most children do not possess an employment permit and that child employment is poorly policed by overstretched education welfare officers. Only 15 local authorities in the UK employed child employment officers in 1996, and most of these worked part time (Heptinstall *et al.*, 1997).

The extent of children's employment

An NCH report (Ruxton, 1996) found that all countries in Europe agreed that children were involved in economic roles, but hard evidence was lacking as child employment has been poorly documented and inadequately researched. Obtaining comprehensive, comparable and current data across countries is extremely difficult, particularly in the case of children under 16 years of age (Heptinstall *et al.*, 1997). In the UK for example, the Labour Force Survey collects data on the employment of people aged 16 and older only. Most data on employment before the age of 16 is based on a variety of sources, for example the number of work permits issued, indirect sources such as reported accidents at work or cases of illegal child employment, small-scale research studies and expert opinion. As Table 21.1 demonstrates official sources suggest that a relatively small proportion of very young people are working across Europe and that recognised employment is concentrated in a few countries, notably the UK and Denmark.

Although the UK figures for child employment are high relative to those of other European countries, survey evidence suggests that employment levels may be as much as double the official figures presented in Table 21.1. The main tool utilised by the authorities to monitor child labour is the issuing of employment permits but, as Table 21.2 demonstrates, few children possess permits. Survey evidence, as demonstrated in Table 21.2, suggests that 1.75 to 2 million children were employed in Britain (Pond and Searle, 1991). McKechnie and Hobbs (2001) suggest that reviews of more recent research show considerable consistency of results between different investigations. It is also important to remember that children move in and out of jobs and any true estimate of the numbers of children who work should include those who are not working at the time of the study. On the basis of their research McKechnie and Hobbs estimate that the number of children who have had experience of employment outside the family before the age of 16 is between 2.2 and 2.6 million (Heptinstall *et al.*, 1997).

Table 21.1: Employment of 13–17-year-olds as proportion of population and of those in education, percentages

	Belgium	Denmark	France	Germany	Greece	Ireland	Italy	Luxem-bourg	Nether-lands	Portugal	Spain	UK	Eur 12
As proportion of total													
All employment	1	44	5	12	8	7	8	*	16	25	9	43	15
Self employed	*	*	*	0	1	*	0	*	1	1	0	0	0
Family workers	*	*	*	*	3	*	1	*	1	5	1	–	–
Employees													
(13)	*	18	*	*	*	*	1	*	2	5	1	29	6
14	(*)	(28)	*	(*)	3	*	2	(*)	5	9	(2)	(33)	(7)
15	*	41	1	2	3	*	6	*	14	18	(5)	(31)	(10)
16	*	53	8	15	4	10	11	*	19	29	11	46	19
As proportion of those in education													
All employment	*	39	0	1	1	2	1	*	15	3	1	35	7
Self employed	*	*	*	*	*	*	*	*	1	*	*	0	0
Family workers	*	*	*	*	*	*	*	*	1	*	0	–	0
Employees													
(13)	*	18	*	*	*	*	*	*	2	*	*	29	5
14	(*)	(28)	*	(*)	*	*	*	(*)	5	*	*	(33)	(6)
15	*	41	*	*	*	*	1	*	13	*	*	(31)	(7)
16	*	53	*	2	*	*	–	*	18	5	*	36	9

Key:
* Nil or negligible
(*) Expert estimate
Note: Portugal's minimum school leaving age was 14 years old
Source: Heptinstall et al. (1997) based on data from: Proposal for a Council Directive on the protection of young people at work, CEC, 1992, 1989 EC Labour Force Survey supplemented by national expert estimates (in parenthesis)

Table 21.2: Surveys of young people's employment in the UK

Source	Year	Coverage	Survey size	Age range	% Young people working	% with work permit/legally employed
The Hidden Army: Children at Work in the 1990s	1990	Birmingham	1,827	10–16	43%	26%
Young People at Work Survey	1992	UK	1,663	13–18	52% 13–15 66% 13–18	Not surveyed
Part-Time Employment in North Tyneside	1992	North Tyneside	281	15–16	46.2%	10%
Child Employment in Cumbria	1992	Cumbria	490	14–15*	50.4%	12%
Child Employment in Dumfries and Galloway	1993	Dumfries & Galloway	259	8–16**	34.7%	29%
Child Employment in Greenwich	1995	Greenwich	1,600	10–16	41%	21.3%
TUC Survey: Working Classes	1997	England and Wales	4,295	11–16	38%	36% had worked before 7am/after 7pm 23% were 11/12 years old so working illegally
TUC Survey: Class Struggles	2001	England and Wales	2,475	11–16	34%***	45% had worked after 8pm and 23% had worked before 6am so working illegally

* Year 10 children were asked if they were working at the time of the survey
** Year 4 children were asked if they had worked any time in the past.
*** approximate
Source: Heptinstall et al. (1997) and TUC (2001)

What sort of work do children do?

McKechnie and Hobbs (2001) argue that the idea of 'children's jobs', that is, specific forms of work suitable for, and within the abilities of, children which can be combined with education and provide pocket money, is a myth. Contrary to popular belief, many working children in the UK occupy jobs more commonly associated with part-time adult employment, although it is unclear whether

Table 21.3: Term-time jobs

Type of job	All	Male	Female	10–11	12	13	14	15–16
Paper round	39%	51%	26%	39%	39%	48%	38%	35%
Babysitting	38%	22%	55%	31%	33%	39%	42%	39%
Shop work	15%	14%	17%	20%	17%	9%	14%	18%
Cleaning	14%	15%	13%	18%	27%	14%	7%	12%
Catering	13%	7%	19%	7%	5%	9%	12%	21%
Gardening	8%	10%	4%	9%	9%	9%	8%	5%
Office work	6%	5%	7%	4%	7%	3%	8%	4%
Market stall/ street stand	4%	4%	3%	5%	8%	2%	2%	3%
Farm work	4%	6%	2%	13%	2%	4%	2%	3%
Milk delivery	3%	4%	1%	4%	6%	2%	–	3%
Factory work	2%	1%	2%	–	2%	4%	1%	1%
Other	21%	23%	19%	25%	30%	17%	20%	20%
Not stated	4%	5%	4%	13%	4%	4%	3%	2%

Source: TUC (2001)

Table 21.4: Summer jobs

Type of job	All	Male	Female	10–11	12	13	14	15–16
Babysitting	39%	18%	62%	33%	42%	36%	41%	39%
Paper round	29%	35%	21%	23%	36%	34%	31%	23%
Cleaning	23%	19%	27%	32%	34%	25%	16%	18%
Shop work	17%	18%	15%	23%	12%	11%	14%	22%
Gardening	13%	14%	11%	15%	19%	22%	9%	6%
Catering	12%	9%	16%	13%	14%	11%	10%	13%
Market stall/ street stand	6%	7%	6%	13%	10%	5%	5%	3%
Farm work	6%	7%	4%	5%	3%	9%	8%	4%
Office work	6%	6%	5%	6%	1%	3%	8%	8%
Factory work	2%	4%	1%	–	1%	4%	2%	4%
Milk delivery	2%	3%	*	3%	5%	1%	1%	1%
Other	17%	17%	16%	13%	21%	13%	16%	19%
Not stated	7%	10%	3%	15%	7%	4%	7%	4%

Source: TUC (2001)

children perform the same task as adult workers. A TUC (2001) survey of 2,475 schoolchildren aged between 11 and 16 in England and Wales found that babysitting and paper rounds were the most common jobs. However, as Tables 21.3 and 21.4 show, children are engaged in a wide variety of occupations.

Research conducted by the European Forum for Child Welfare (1998) suggests that in western European countries forms of unacceptable child labour exist and include commercial sexual exploitation and employment of children. Children in Europe work in a wide range of jobs including, tourism, prostitution, car washing, begging, loading and unloading goods, factory and construction work, agriculture and fishing (McKechnie and Hobbs, 1998a).

How many hours do children work?

The TUC (2001) survey found that almost two-thirds of school children work at least one day during the school week and as many as a quarter work for four or five days; this includes children aged 13 or younger. Analysis of the British Household Panel Survey (Bradshaw and Williams, 2001) shows that the mean hours worked by children aged 11–15 was just over six hours a week. Table 21.5 shows the number of days worked by children during term time.

Table 21.5: Number of days worked during term time

Days worked	All	Male	Female	Age (years) 10–11	12	13	14	15–16
1 day	24%	21%	27%	27%	31%	23%	21%	21%
2 days	24%	18%	30%	11%	29%	19%	28%	25%
3 days	10%	7%	14%	6%	9%	15%	10%	10%
4 days	5%	6%	4%	3%	3%	6%	6%	6%
5 days	8%	8%	8%	14%	8%	7%	8%	5%
6 days	9%	12%	5%	8%	4%	10%	10%	9%
7 days	12%	19%	3%	9%	8%	14%	9%	16%
2 or 3 weekdays	19%	16%	23%	18%	17%	22%	22%	17%
4 or 5 weekdays	26%	37%	13%	22%	19%	31%	25%	28%
At least 1 weekday	65%	66%	62%	46%	66%	77%	64%	63%
Weekdays only	16%	14%	19%	10%	21%	25%	18%	9%
Saturday or Sunday	75%	77%	73%	68%	71%	69%	75%	83%
Both Saturday and Sunday	30%	37%	21%	26%	19%	32%	25%	37%
Weekends only	27%	25%	29%	32%	27%	17%	28%	29%

Source: TUC (2001)

Table 21.6: Hours worked during summer holidays

Hours worked	All	Male	Female	Age (years) 10–11	12	13	14	15–16
Under 5 hours	28%	30%	26%	22%	35%	42%	29%	18%
5 to 10 hours	30%	30%	31%	31%	29%	28%	34%	28%
11–20 hours	14%	11%	18%	18%	11%	7%	13%	20%
21–30 hours	7%	7%	8%	5%	2%	10%	4%	12%
31–35 hours	3%	4%	3%	–	2%	4%	5%	5%
36–40 hours	1%	2%	1%	–	1%	1%	2%	2%
Over 41 hours	4%	5%	1%	4%	2%	–	5%	8%
Don't know	5%	4%	7%	6%	9%	5%	1%	3%
Not stated	7%	8%	6%	14%	9%	4%	7%	4%

Source: TUC (2001)

Of children who work on weekdays, 30 per cent work for more than two hours a day (the legal maximum) and one in ten works for more than five hours a day. Of those aged 10 to 13 years who work on weekdays, 40 per cent work for more than two hours a day. Boys are significantly more likely than girls to work on more days of the week. This in part reflects the fact that boys are more likely to have a paper round with the hours spread over the week.

Summer holiday working is generally regarded as less damaging, both to children's school work and to their well-being. According to the law, 15-year-olds are allowed to work for up to 35 hours a week during holidays, but, as can be seen in Table 21.6, one in ten actually work longer than this. Children aged 14, and those aged 13 who are allowed to work, cannot work for more than 25 hours a week, yet the study found children exceeding these time limits, not just among 13- and 14-year-olds but among 10–12-year-olds as well.

Table 21.6 shows that there is no tendency for working hours to rise with age. In fact, whereas 13 per cent of 14-year-olds work between 11 and 20 hours a week, this is exceeded by the proportion of 10- and 11-year-olds in that category (18 per cent). The UK legislation states that children are not allowed to work between 19:00hrs and 07:00hrs and European Laws state that children cannot work before 06:00hrs and after 20:00hrs. The TUC survey (2001) found that almost a quarter of school-age workers have worked before 06:00hrs and nearly half have worked after 20:00hrs. Almost a third of 10- and 11-year-olds said that they had worked before 06:00hrs during term time.

Why do children work?

There are a number of important motivations behind the decision of children to take up paid work. These include the desire for access to new forms of sociability and for 'something to do'. Children also see paid employment as a means of establishing independence. However, studies in the UK and other European countries suggest that the key motivation for children taking employment is money (Ingenhorst, 2001; Mizen *et al.,* 2001; Mansurov, 2001). Nevertheless, the way in which earned income is used varies. Ingenhorst (2001) suggests that two-thirds of German children regarded money as the single most important reason for working. "Money earned from working is regarded as the key to the consumer world of adults; it opens up to them the possibility of purchasing brand-name clothing, televisions, computers, mountain bikes and other desirable items" (Ingenhorst, 2001, p. 141). A study of young workers in Belfast (Leonard, 1999) also found money to be the main motivation for children to work and found that children spent their earnings on a wide range of consumer items. The most common items were goods for immediate consumption such as sweets, food, cigarettes and alcohol. In other countries and among socially excluded groups it is often poverty and privation, rather than consumerism, which compel children to work. Mansurov quotes a young Russian worker. "I dress myself; I buy myself and my younger brother shoes and clothes; I give my mother some money too" (Mansurov, 2001, p. 160). Similarly, many European Roma families need their older children to assist in the family trade or to help care for younger children while the parents work (Van der Stoel, 2000).

Contribution to the household income

There is little systematic data upon which to explore the impact of material deprivation on children's work. Research has not proved a conclusive link between poverty and child employment in the UK (see Higate, 2001; Middleton and Shropshire, 1998; Mizen *et al.,* 2001). Indeed, one of the most significant changes to have taken place within the child labour market during the 20th century, according to Lavalette (1998), was that children from more affluent working and middle-class homes started to take jobs. However, studies do suggest that motivations to work and the use of children's earned income are to some degree dependent on their material circumstances. UK studies have found that working children make a significant contribution to their families' living standards (Middleton and Loumidis, 2001; Middleton and Shropshire, 1998; Leonard, 1998). Leonard (1998) found that a substantial number of children stated that they spent some of their earnings on clothes, thus indirectly subsidising family income. There is also evidence to suggest that children contribute directly towards the household income. Leonard (1998) interviewed 122 Belfast school pupils between the ages of 14 and 17 and found there was some evidence of children giving money to their family: 24 per cent of the children gave some of their wages to their parents. These children were more likely to live in unemployed households and to attend secondary school, indicating that household poverty may be a factor influencing the employment of some children. Similarly, an earlier study of child employment in North Tyneside (O'Donnell and White, 1998) found that one child in 15 gave some of their earnings to their parents and one in ten children who had a part-time job was the only member of their household in employment.

Bradshaw and Williams (2001) found that the proportion of young people employed was lower (21 per cent) among families receiving Income Support/Job Seekers Allowance than among those who were not (33 per cent). Young people in families with two parents in employment are more likely to be employed than those in families with no parents in employment. One possible explanation of this is that many children living in unemployed households might want to work, but local labour markets provide few opportunities for them to do so.

How much do children earn?

It is generally assumed that children work for pocket money and that this notion, and the fact that children are excluded under the Minimum Wage legislation, serves to legitimise children's low pay and encourages the exploitation of children (GMB/MPO, 2000). Previous studies have found extremely low rates of pay among child workers. Bradshaw and William's analysis of the British Household Panel Survey found the average hourly rate of pay for 11–15-year-olds was £2.17. The TUC (2001) survey found a wide variation in the amount children earned, with 14 per cent of children earning over £5 an hour, 18 per cent earning £2 to £2.15 an hour and 17 per cent of children earning less than £2 an hour. During term time 66 per cent of boys earned £4 or less an hour compared with 70 per cent of girls, but during the summer holidays this gap widens with 52 per cent of boys earning £4 or less compared with 66 per cent of girls. The findings of Bradshaw and Williams (2001) show that boys earn more than girls and that rates of pay increase with age, as do hours of work. About half the children employed in babysitting and paper delivery earn less than £3.20 an hour and over half the children employed in the service sector work earned less than £3.20 an hour.

Interestingly, Bradshaw and Williams (2001) found there was no trade-off between pocket money and working. Ninety-one per cent of young people in the British Household Panel Survey received pocket money from their parents, the average amount being £9.15 per week. There was no variation in the percentage receiving pocket money by age or gender, but the amount of pocket money increased with age from £5.50 on average at 11 to £12.64 on average at 15. Those in employment were just as likely to receive pocket money as those who did not work.

Is employment bad for children?

McKechnie and Hobbs (2001) raise the question of whether it is possible to decide whether work has a positive or negative effect on children's education and others have questioned the effect of paid employment on other aspects of children's development and well-being. In the USA, a number of commissions set up in the 1980s highlighted the benefits to children from gaining some form of employment. Work was viewed as a positive contribution to the individual's development (see Mizen *et al.,* 2001; Pettit, 1998). The dominant view in the USA and in Britain appears to be that combining part-time employment with full-time compulsory education is acceptable. Myers and Boyden (1998) suggest that the part-time work that most children typically do, if it allows time for rest and education, might have a positive developmental influence, even if some negative aspects are present. Appropriate work can help build children's social and economic skills, self-esteem and confidence and children, for the most part, report such positive benefits. Nevertheless, surveys also report tiredness and stress among working children struggling to cope with the demands of full-time education and part-time work (Allatt and Dixon, 2001; Barry, 2001; Bell, 2001). The TUC (2001) survey found that 29 per cent of children reported being too tired to do their homework and 10 per cent played truant in order to work.

Accidents at work

One of the arguments against child labour, especially in developing countries, is that certain forms of employment are dangerous for young children. In developed countries, child employment legislation has formally excluded children from a range of hazardous occupations, for example, working with chemicals and factory work (although the TUC survey found that 2 per cent of children worked in factories). Childhood accidents are discussed in detail in Chapter 6, but in considering the well-being of children who work it is necessary to briefly consider the available data on children's accidents at work. There is very little detailed information published about accidents and injuries to children who work and there are no European statistics on accidents to working children aged less than16 years old. However, research in the USA suggests that many working children risk accidents and other hazards to health and, although the evidence in the UK is limited, there is enough to indicate that the matter requires more attention (McKechnie and Hobbs, 1998b). The official source of information on injuries at work in the UK is reports from employers to the Health and Safety

Table 21.7: Reported injuries to employees under 16 years old

	Fatal	Major	Resulting in over 3 days absence	
1993/94	1	16	17	34
1994/95	1	15	20	36
1995/96	0	12	25	37
1996/97	1	14	24	39
1997/98	1	19	26	46

Source: Heptinstall (1998)

Table 21.8: Self-reported accidents and injuries to boys and girls under 16 years old while at work

Q: Have you ever had an accident or injured yourself at work?

	All (%)	Boys (%)	Girls (%)
Yes	19	24	13
No	75	69	82
Don't know	3	3	2
Not stated	4	4	3

Source: TUC (1997)

Executive under the Reporting of Injuries, Diseases and Dangerous Occurrences Regulations 1985 (O'Donnell and White, 1999). Tables 21.7 and 21.8 detail reported injuries to child workers between 1993 and 1998.

There are a number of problems associated with these data. It is acknowledged that official statistics under-report all injuries in the workplace, but under-reporting is thought to be especially high in sectors where children are employed. Furthermore, official definitions of reportable accidents are often inapplicable to the casual and part-time nature of children's employment. Accidents may not be reported to the authorities because the employment is illegal, or the accident is not recorded as having happened at work. This is particularly true of data recorded at hospital accident and emergency departments (Heptinstall *et al.*, 1997). The official statistics also exclude all accidents that are regarded as minor. This, as Heptinstall *et al.* (1997) note, is a cause of concern for two important reasons: first, accidents should not cause children to miss even one day of school; second, the Child Accident Prevention Trust has found that even minor physical accidents can cause lasting emotional distress in children and young people. The under-reporting of accidents to children at work is borne out in the findings of a number of studies (see Heptinstall *et al.*, 1997). The 1997 TUC study found that 19 per cent of children questioned had had an accident or injured themselves at work, but other studies have reported accident rates of about a third. These studies provide few details about the nature or severity of the injuries or the type of work they were associated with. However, there is some evidence to suggest that boys are twice as likely to have accidents at work as girls and that 27 per cent of children injured at work required medical attention (Heptinstall *et al.*, 1997).

Conclusion

This chapter has demonstrated that children's employment is a widespread phenomenon in the UK and Europe, that employment legislation is confusing and ineffective and that many children work illegally, often for low rates of pay. There are, however, significant gaps in knowledge. There is a lack of comparable national or regional data on the extent and nature of children's work and there is very little evidence currently available of gender and ethnic differences in child employment. A forthcoming report for the International Labour Office will provide a comprehensive review of the literature on child employment in Europe, but there is also a need for new primary research. Very little is known about the effects of employment on children's physical and emotional well-being or on their educational achievement. Studies suggest that employment can have both positive and negative effects but it is not clear what these are nor what types of work or length of working hours are more or less detrimental or beneficial. In order to understand fully the effect of employment on children and to tackle those forms of employment found to be harmful, large-scale longitudinal quantitative and qualitative research studies would be required. These would have to take into account a range of indicators in addition to measuring the extent and nature of child employment: these would include educational attainment and physical and mental well-being. Similarly, little is known about children's motivations to work, the relationship between child employment and material deprivation and whether some children feel compelled to work. Further, if suitable employment has beneficial effects as studies suggest, then it is important for children who wish to work to have the opportunity to find suitable employment.

22 The Mental Health of Children

Deborah Quilgars

Key findings:

- Age and gender are highly associated with mental health. Older children experience more mental health problems; boys are more likely to experience conduct and hyperkinetic disorders; girls, emotional disorders and lower levels of happiness. However, there is a lack of data on the link between ethnicity and children's mental health.

- The quality of family relationships and levels of parental stress were linked to children's mental health. Family type was also sometimes found to be significant.

- The link between social class and income of the family and children's mental health was inconsistent. There appeared to be a link on clinical measures but not on broader measures of mental health. There was, however, a link between mental health and young people's own socio-economic status.

- Most young people in the Western world report relatively high levels of happiness. Studies show little variation between levels of mental health disorders across the UK, though one study suggested lowest levels of self-reported 'happiness' in Scotland, followed by Northern Ireland then England and Wales.

Key trends:

- Available data suggested a rise in mental health disorders among children and young people in the post-war period. Time trend data, however, was weak.

Key sources:

- The British Household Panel Survey

- The ONS Survey of Children's Mental Health in England, Scotland and Wales
- The Annual Health Survey of England
- International WHO Health Behaviour Survey
- School Health Education Unit Health Related Behaviour Questionnaire

Introduction

This chapter critically reviews the evidence on the nature of the mental health of children in the UK. The chapter begins by discussing definitional issues and data sources, before examining links between mental health and age, gender, ethnicity, family set-up and poverty. Variations by geographical area, between countries in the UK, and international and time trends are also reviewed. A separate chapter (Chapter 20) examines suicide among young people.

Definitions and data sources

There are no easy definitions of 'mental health'. The Western medical or clinical model tends to focus on 'mental disorders', or illnesses, in which clinicians diagnose a specific problem that is usually associated with considerable distress and interference with the child's everyday life (Meltzer *et al.*, 2000). Table 22.1 gives some examples of 'mental disorders'. Many commentators, however, stress the importance of adopting a more positive and holistic definition of 'mental health'. The Mental Health Foundation (1999) has stressed the importance of children being 'mentally healthy' – being able to develop and enjoy life fully.

We believe that children who are mentally healthy will have the ability to:
- develop psychologically, emotionally, creatively, intellectually and physically
- initiate, develop and sustain mutually satisfying personal relationships
- use and enjoy solitude
- become aware of others and empathise with them
- play and learn
- develop a sense of right and wrong
- resolve (face) problems and setbacks and learn from them.

Source: Mental Health Foundation (1999), p. 6.

In this definition, levels of general happiness and overall satisfaction with life, rather than just the absence of clinical disorders, are given precedence; some commentators refer to this as 'emotional well-being' (eg, Currie *et al.*, 2000).

Table 22.1: Examples of 'mental disorders'

Emotional disorders	eg phobias, anxiety states and depression
Conduct disorders	eg fire-setting and anti-social behaviour
Hyperkinetic disorders	eg Attention Deficit Disorder
Developmental disorders	eg delay in acquiring certain skills such as speech, social ability or bladder control
Eating disorders	eg pre-school eating problems, anorexia nervosa and bulimia nervosa
Habit disorders	eg tics, sleeping problems and soiling
Post-traumatic syndromes	eg post-traumatic stress disorder
Somatic disorders	eg chronic fatigue syndrome
Psychotic disorders	eg schizophrenia, drug-induced psychosis

Source: Kurtz (1996), p. 10

Key data sources

Measuring mental health is beset with difficulties. Medical records record only those people who use services and focus on narrow clinical definitions. The best data sources use specially designed questionnaires to collect data from the general population. However, even here, the use of different measures can result in varying estimates of levels of mental health. For example, many commentators agree that at any one time up to one in five children and young people experience some form of psychological problem (Mental Health Foundation, 1999; Kurtz, 1996). However, the recent ONS survey, using strict clinical measures, reported that one in ten children and young people suffered from mental disorders (Meltzer *et al.*, 2000). It is therefore important to be clear about what 'measure' of mental health is being used in any survey. As the following list of key available data sources show, most surveys focus on mental health disorders or psychological 'problems' rather than general levels of happiness.

ONS Survey of the Mental Health of Children and Young People

In 1999, the Office for National Statistics carried out the first specially commissioned survey of the mental health of children (aged 5–15), covering

England, Scotland and Wales (Meltzer *et al.*, 2000). The study focused on mental 'disorders'. The study used:

- a range of clinical measures used to diagnose mental illness, including the International Classification of Diseases
- the General Health Questionnaire (GHQ12), a self-completion question-naire asking about general levels of happiness, depressive feelings, anxiety and sleep disturbance in the last month (detects non-psychotic disorders in a community setting)
- the Strengths and Difficulties Questionnaire (SDQ), filled out by parents, focusing on emotional and behavioural problems.

In total, 10,438 interviews were completed with children. Follow-up interviews are scheduled for 2002.

The British Household Panel Survey (BHPS)

Since 1993, the BHPS (which covers England, Scotland, Wales and Northern Ireland) has included interviews with young people aged 11–15. The survey uses measures of psychological health based on the GHQ12, giving measures of 'sadness' (how unhappy or depressed people were); 'worry' (loss of sleep, worrying); 'happiness' (feelings about school, family, friends, etc); and 'image' (whether people feel they have good qualities, feel useless, etc). Brynin and Scott (1996) and Scott (1996) have examined one year ('wave') of the BHPS, Bergman and Scott (2001) four years and Clarke *et al.* (1999) and Johnson *et al.* (2001) five years.

Annual Health Survey of England

The Annual Health Survey of England has included questions about children's mental health since 1995 (Prescott-Clarke and Primatesta, 1998). Young people aged 13–24 complete the GHQ12, and parents complete the Strengths and Difficulties Questionnaire for 5–15-year-olds. Obviously, data from this study only relates to England.

International WHO Health Behaviour Survey of School-aged Children (HBSC)

The WHO Health Behaviour Survey of School-aged Children is the only international dataset that covers mental health issues. The survey, begun in 1982, is carried out every four years; the 1997/98 survey involved 26 countries/

regions in Europe, Canada and USA. WHO produces international reports and the respective countries publish findings (see Haselden *et al.*, 1999; Health Promotion Agency for Northern Ireland, 2001a). The questionnaire is based on non-clinical measures of self-reported feelings of being 'happy' and 'low'. The 1997/98 survey included 20,000 children in school years 7–11 across England, Scotland, Wales and Northern Ireland.

The School Health Education Unit Health Related Behaviour Questionnaire (HRBQ)

The School Health Education Unit has surveyed young people since 1980. Recently a specific report was published on the 'worries' of young people, including data from 122 secondary schools, throughout the UK, for 16,732 12–15-year-olds (Balding *et al.*, 1998). The main worry question, 'How much do you worry about the problems listed . . .', has been asked since 1991, and is non-clinical in nature.

Other national or regional studies

A number of other national or regional studies examine mental health. For example, the West of Scotland Twenty-07 Study, a longitudinal health study of 1,000 adults in Glasgow (including 15-year-olds) from 1987/88 has investigated the mental health of young people using the GHQ12 (West *et al.*, 1990; West and Sweeting, 1996).

Age

Older children are more likely to experience mental health problems than younger children. Looking at mental disorders (Meltzer *et al.*, 2000), 8 per cent of children aged 5–10-years-old suffered from a mental disorder, compared to 11 per cent of children aged 11–15 (Table 22.2). The odds of having a disorder were 50 per cent higher for older children (Table 22.3). The differences were particularly pronounced for emotional disorders. Looking at the older age range, the Annual Health Survey of England (Prescott-Clarke and Primatesta, 1998) reported that while only 6 per cent of boys aged 13–15 had a high score on the GHQ12, 10 per cent of young men aged 16–19 did. This compared to 14 per cent of girls aged 13–15 and 21 per cent of young women aged 16–19. However, slight decreases were found over the age range 4–15 on the SDQ measure. Using broader measures of mental health, the HRBQ (Balding *et al.*, 1998) also found

Table 22.2: Prevalence of mental disorders, by age and sex, England, Wales and Scotland

	5–10-year-olds (%)			11–15-year-olds (%)			All children (%)		
	Boys	Girls	All	Boys	Girls	All	Boys	Girls	All
Emotional disorders	3	3	3	5	6	7	4	5	4
Conduct disorders	7	3	5	9	4	6	7	3	5
Hyperkinetic disorders	3	*	2	2	I	I	2	*	I
Less common disorders	I	*	I	*	I	I	I	*	I
Any disorder	10	6	8	13	10	11	11	8	10
Base	2,909	2,921	5,830	2,310	2,299	4,609	5,219	5,219	10,438

Source: Meltzer et al. (2000), Table 4.1, p. 33

that older pupils worried more than younger ones, and the WHO HBSC studies also revealed age variations (Currie *et al.*, 2000; Haselden *et al.*, 1999; Health Promotion Agency for Northern Ireland, 2001a).

Gender

Most studies have found pronounced differences in mental health by gender, although effects differ by type of disorder (and age of children). The ONS study (Meltzer *et al.*, 2000) of mental disorders found that 11 per cent of boys suffered from mental disorders compared to 8 per cent of girls (Table 22.2). The rates of conduct and hyperkinetic disorders, in particular, were much higher for boys. Overall, the odds of having a mental disorder increased by 50 per cent for boys compared to girls (Table 22.3). The Annual Health Survey of England (Prescott-Clarke and Primatesta, 1998) also found that boys had higher SDQ scores (see Table 22.7) of a similar order of difference to the ONS study (12 per cent for boys compared to 8 per cent for girls).

However, the ONS study found few differences for emotional disorders between genders, and the Annual Health Survey of England found that girls had higher GHQ12 scores than boys (Table 22.4). The likelihood of girls, particularly older girls, having lower rates of emotional well-being was also found in other studies. The BHPS (Bergman and Scott, 2001) showed that boys reported higher positive self-esteem, lower negative self-image, less unhappiness and fewer past worries than girls. The HBSC survey (Currie *et al.*, 2000; Haselden *et al.*, 1999; Health Promotion Agency for Northern Ireland, 2001a) also found that girls

Table 22.3: Odds ratios for correlates of mental disorders, England, Wales and Scotland

Variable	Conduct disorders Adjusted odds ratio	Emotional disorders Adjusted odds ratio	Hyperkinetic disorders Adjusted odds ratio	Any disorder Adjusted odds ratio
Age				
5–10	1.00	1.00	1.00	1.00
11–15	***1.45	***1.84	0.96	***1.48
Sex				
Female	1.00	1.00	1.00	1.00
Male	***2.42	0.89	***5.56	***1.58
Number of children				
1	1.00	1.00	1.00	1.00
2	1.05	0.96	0.92	0.94
3	1.11	1.13	0.79	0.98
4	***1.80	1.23	0.65	*1.32
5	***2.23	1.43	0.71	**1.63
Family type				
Two parents	1.00	1.00	1.00	1.00
Lone parents	***1.68	***1.55	1.42	**1.57
ACORN Group				
Thriving	1.00	1.00	1.00	1.00
Expanding	1.27	1.40	1.61	*1.39
Rising	*1.84	1.48	*3.00	**1.72
Settling	**1.68	1.34	**2.47	***1.58
Aspiring	***2.48	1.33	**2.78	***1.85
Striving	***2.45	**1.73	*2.41	***1.96
Family's employment				
Both parents working	1.00	1.00	1.00	1.00
One parent working	1.14	**1.44	*1.73	**1.30
Neither working	***1.90	***1.82	**2.13	***1.94

*** $p<0.001$; ** $p<0.01$; * $p<0.05$
Source: Meltzer et al. (2000), Table 4.15, p. 60

Table 22.4: General Health Questionnaire 12 score (4 or above on scale), by age and sex, England

	Age 13–15 (%)	Age 16–19 (%)	Age 20–24 (%)	Age 13–24 (%)
Males	6	10	14	10
Females	14	21	23	19
Base * (males)	830	795	1,049	2,674
Base *(females)	813	892	1,242	2,947

* Base number is weighted data. 1995 and 1997 data combined.
Source: Prescott-Clarke and Primatesta (1998), Table 10.1

(particularly older girls) were less likely to score highly on 'happiness' indicators than boys. In the Northern Ireland study, 10 per cent more boys than girls in school year 12 reported being happy and twice as many girls as boys reported feeling low on a weekly basis. The English study also reported that boys felt more confident, as well as happier, than girls. The HRBQ (Balding *et al.*, 1998) study revealed that girls worried more than boys.

Ethnicity

There is very little research on mental health of children and ethnicity. The ONS study (Meltzer *et al.*, 2000) found some differences between ethnic groups (Table 22.5), suggesting higher rates for black children, but small numbers made interpretation difficult and ethnicity was not significant in logistic regression analysis. Studies have found much higher rates of medically diagnosed mental illness (eg, schizophrenia) and psychiatric admissions among African-Caribbean adults (see Smaje, 1995); while some studies show lower rates (but not consistently) of diagnosed mental illness among Asian communities (Raleigh, 1995). Eating disorders appear to be more prevalent among white (female) children, but are higher for upwardly mobile minority ethnic groups (Fombonne, 1995). Mental health organisations believe that differences by ethnicity are likely to reflect socio-economic factors and cultural bias within the mental health system, rather than any inherent susceptibility to mental illness amongst different ethnic groups (Mental Health Foundation, 1997). Clearly, however, more research is needed in this area.

Table 22.5: Prevalence of mental disorders, by ethnicity, England, Wales and Scotland

	White	Black	Indian	Ethnic Group Pakistani & Bangladeshi	Other	All
		Percentage of children with each disorder				
Emotional disorders	4	3	3	6	6	4
Conduct disorders	5	9	2	3	4	5
Hyperkinetic disorders	2	<1	-	-	<1	1
Less common disorders	1	<1	-	-	1	1
Any disorder	10	12	4	8	10	10
Base	9,474	271	224	196	265	10,430

Source: Meltzer *et al.* (2000), Table 4.2, p. 35

Family type, relationships and stress

A number of studies suggest that family type, the nature of family relationships and stress levels of family members, may affect children's mental health.

Family type

In the ONS study (Meltzer *et al.*, 2000), 16 per cent of children of lone parents were defined as having a mental disorder, compared to 8 per cent of children of couples. (Logistic regression analysis showed increased odds of about 50 per cent for children from lone parents having a mental disorder (Table 22.3).) Mental health problems were also more common (15 per cent of children) in reconstituted families (where step-children were present), as well as in larger households (18 per cent for a 5-child family). The Health Survey of England (Prescott-Clarke and Primatesta, 1998) also found that children in lone parent families were statistically more likely to have worse SDQ scores for behaviour. Young men in lone parent households also had statistically significant higher GHQ12 scores; these were higher but not statistically significant for girls in lone parent households.

Analysis of the British Household Panel Survey by Bergman and Scott (2001) found that children were more likely to report past worries if they came from lone parent or 'other family' households. This effect was greater for boys, and unhappiness and self-esteem levels were only affected for boys but not girls. Johnson *et al.* (2001) also found that changes in maternal marital status and employment were associated with poorer self-esteem, sadness, more worry and less happiness among children (however, the study did not test for statistical significance). Earlier analysis of the BHPS by Scott (1996) found that children of lone parents were no less likely to be unhappy than those in two-adult families. However, Brynin and Scott (1996) found that young (but not older) children with one parent, and more so those with a step-parent, were statistically less likely to be self-confident.

Family relationships

The ONS study (Meltzer *et al.*, 2000) explored the nature of family relationships, utilising the General Functioning Scale of the MacMaster Family Activity Device, asking parents to agree or disagree with a series of statements (eg, 'We don't get along well together' and 'We confide in each other'). The study found that children in families defined as 'unhealthy' (where parents stated there was poor communication and low levels of support within the family) were much more likely to have a mental disorder than children in other families (18 per cent compared to 7 per cent).

Examining family relations more generally, Sweeting and West (1996) using the West of Scotland Twenty-07 study found that young people aged 15 who reported more conflict with parents were also more likely to have health problems (both physical and psychological health) and lower self-esteem at age 18. This relationship was strongest for young women. A study by Glendinning et al. (2000) of young people (aged 11–16) in rural Scotland and rural Sweden found positive parental support and accepting and uncritical parenting associated with higher levels of self-esteem, and lower levels of depression and anxiety.

Parental mental health

The ONS study (Meltzer et al., 2000) assessed the mental health of the interviewed parent (usually the mother) using the GHQ12. Parents who were assessed as having a neurotic disorder using the GHQ12 were more likely to have children with mental disorders than children of parents with better GHQ12 scores (18 per cent of children compared to 8 per cent, respectively). It was not possible to assess cause and effect (ie, whether parental mental ill health made it more likely for a child to have a mental health problem, or vice versa).

The Annual Health Survey of England also reported a significant relationship, particularly strong for girls, between SDQ scores and both parents' scores on the GHQ. Young women's GHQ scores were also found to be associated with their mothers' GHQ scores (though no relationship was found for boys, or to the fathers' GHQ scores for either gender). Brynin and Scott (1996) also found a close relationship with life satisfaction (happy scales) of children, particularly for girls, with their mothers' GHQ scores (although not with the father's GHQ score).

Children's stressful experiences

The ONS study (Meltzer et al., 2000) found that 31 per cent of children with mental disorders had experienced three or more stressful life events (such as illness, death of a family member) compared to only 13 per cent of those with none. A number of studies have also found a significant relationship between mental health and bullying. A study of 904 pupils aged 12–17 in two different schools (Salmon *et al.*, 1998) found high levels of anxiety (as well as school and gender) to be associated with bullying. They also found low levels of anxiety, but high levels of depression, associated with bullying others.

Social class and poverty

The link between social class/poverty and the mental health of children appears to differ by type of disorder and method of measurement. The ONS study (Meltzer *et al.*, 2000) found a clear relationship between social class and mental health, with nearly three times as many children in Social Class V families having a mental disorder compared to children in Social Class I families (Table 22.6). In particular, 10 per cent of children in Social Class V families suffered a conduct disorder, compared to only 2 per cent of children from Social Class I families. In addition, 16 per cent of children in families with a gross weekly household income of under £100 had a mental disorder, compared to only 6 per cent of children in families earning £500 a week or more.

The Annual Health Survey of England (Prescott-Clarke and Primatesta, 1998) found a relationship between social class of head of household and income and SDQ conduct/ behaviour scores. Five per cent of boys and 2 per cent of girls in Class 1 had high SDQ scores compared to 20 per cent of boys and 14 per cent of girls in Class V (Table 22.7). Six per cent of boys and 4 per cent of girls in the top quintile (household income over £24,381 per annum) compared to 20 per

Table 22.6: Prevalence of mental disorders, by social class, England, Wales and Scotland

	I	II	IIIN	IIIM	IV	V	Never worked	All*
				Percentage of children with each disorder				
Emotional disorders	2	3	5	5	6	6	9	4
Conduct disorders	3	3	6	5	8	10	16	5
Hyperkinetic disorders	1	1	2	2	2	1	3	1
Less common disorders	1	1	1	*	1	1	1	1
Any disorder	5	7	12	9	12	15	21	10
Base	777	3,199	1,225	2,586	1,548	511	201	10,438

* No answers, members of the Armed Forces and full-time students are excluded from the six social class categories but included in the *All* category.
Source: Meltzer et al. (2000), Table 4.10, p. 51

Table 22.7: SDQ score, ages 4–15, by social class of head of household and gender, England

High deviance score of 17–40	I %	II %	IIIN %	IIIM %	IV %	V %	All classes** %
Males	5	6	9	13	18	20	12
Females	2	4	5	8	13	14	8
Bases (weighted*):							
Males	119	501	200	529	356	95	1,878
Females	136	520	217	536	304	75	1,874

* unweighted base figures were 2,843 (males) and 2,862 (females)
** *All classes* includes all responses, not only those with a social class I–V categorisation.
Source: Prescott-Clarke and Primatesta (1998), p. 355

cent and 15 per cent in the bottom quintile (up to £6,500) exhibited high SDQ scores. However, no clear relationship was found between GHQ12 score and social class or income.

Clarke *et al.* (2000), looking at the BHPS (1993–97), also found little evidence of a link between poverty and well-being at age 11–15. They examined equivalent income (less than 50 per cent of average income), receipt of means-tested benefits and household assets. The only association they found was that children living in families receiving means-tested benefits were found to have a lower self-image. Scott (1996) also found a correlation between self-image and economic circumstances, and a weak relationship between happiness and family resources for boys, but Brynin and Scott (1996) found no relationship between children's life satisfaction or self-confidence and the social class of their parents. Bergman and Scott (2001) also found no discernible link between occupational status of father, or income levels, and well-being.

Haselden *et al.* (1999), reporting on the 1997/98 English HBSC survey, found little difference between ABC1 and C2DE households on mental health measures (92 per cent of ABC1 self-reported as very or quite happy, compared to 91 per cent of C2DE households), although 70 per cent of ABC1 children said they never or rarely felt helpless compared to only 62 per cent of C2DE children. The West of Scotland Twenty-07 Study (West *et al.*, 1990) found no evidence for differences by social class for psychological well-being among young people aged 15.

Employment status of parents

The ONS survey (Meltzer *et al.*, 2000) found that the odds of a child having a mental disorder in a family where both parents were unemployed was nearly twice that of the odds of a child in a family where both adults in the family were employed (Table 22.3). A few studies also seem to have found links between employment status of parents and children's well-being, where social class and income variables show no clear link. Clarke *et al.* (2000) found that some children whose father was unemployed appeared to have lower well-being scores. By contrast, Scott (1996) reported that boys were much less happy if their mother was working full-time.

Young people's own socio-economic status

Glendinning *et al.* (1992), using the Scottish Young People's Leisure and Lifestyle Study of people aged 17–22, found no significant relationship between mental health and social class of parents. However, they reported that young men and women on training schemes, unemployed young people and women at home were more likely to report psychological stress. West and Sweeting's (1996) examination of the West of Scotland Twenty-07 Study revealed similar findings. While there was very little difference between the mental health of young people aged 15, or aged 18, by parental social class, on almost all mental health measures, unemployed young people were in much poorer health. After controlling for other factors, the odds of GHQ scores of clinical significance at age 18 increased twofold or more among unemployed young people compared to those

Table 22.8: SDQ score, ages 4–15, by ACORN category and gender, England, 1997

SDQ Total Deviance score	ACORN category						Total
	A %	B %	C %	D %	E %	F %	%
Males							
17–40	7	7	10	11	12	20	12
Females							
17–40	3	2	7	7	8	15	8
Bases (weighted *):							
Males	366	257	107	429	234	480	1,878
Females	354	262	85	475	245	452	1,874

* unweighted. Base figures were 2,843 (males) and 2,862 (females).
Source: Prescott-Clarke and Primatesta (1998)

at work/on YTS (rising to threefold by the age of 21) and the odds of attempted suicide increased by a factor of six.

Differences by type of area

Only two studies have examined whether the mental health of children varies between localities. Both studies (Prescott-Clarke and Primatesta, 1998; Meltzer *et al.*, 2000) used ACORN, a classification which combines geographical and demographic characteristics into six categories: A-F, or thriving; expanding; rising; settling; aspiring; and striving. The ONS study found that 13 per cent of children in the 'striving' category had a mental disorder, compared to only 5 per cent of children in the 'thriving' category. Children in striving families had nearly double the odds of having a mental disorder compared to children in 'thriving' households (Table 22.3). In the Annual Health Survey of England, there was also a strong relationship between SDQ score and ACORN Category (Table 22.8), However, there was not a significant relationship between the categories and GHQ12 scores.

The two studies also examined mental health by regions. The ONS study reported no differences between metropolitan and non-metropolitan areas of England. There were also no clear trends in GHQ12, and little variation for SDQ score, by region within England for the Annual Health Survey. However, the Glendinning *et al.* (2000) study in Scotland and Sweden did find social class variations in well-being among rural youth (for self-esteem and general health, though not depression), suggesting that those from disadvantaged backgrounds may be more disadvantaged in rural areas.

International and inter-UK differences

The WHO survey on health behaviour in school-aged children represents the only ongoing international (though Western world) data source on the psycho-social health of young people. The studies (see Currie *et al.*, 2000) report that the vast majority of children included in the survey feel happy. However, some differences were found by country as to the levels of young people feeling happy (or quite happy). The least happy students were from Israel (62 per cent feeling happy), with Scandinavian students reporting the highest scores (eg, Sweden 94 per cent), though many northern European countries followed close behind, including England (92 per cent) and Northern Ireland (90 per cent). Similar

Table 22.9: The WHO HBSC survey, 1997/98, students who report feeling low at least once a week during the last 6 months

	Female %	Male %	Rank*	Base
11-year-olds				
England	27	27	11	2,279
Wales	33	25	7	1,539
Northern Ireland	24	24	14	1,068
Scotland	20	14	24	2,092
13-year-olds				
England	33	25	10	222
Wales	33	24	11	1,571
Northern Ireland	31	21	16	1,197
Scotland	26	13	23	1,813
15-year-olds				
England	40	24	12	1,872
Wales	41	26	10	1,427
Northern Ireland	38	18	17	1,081
Scotland	28	13	26	1,727

* Rank represents country position out of the 28 participating country and regions. The lower the score the greater the proportion of children who reported 'feeling low'.
Source: Currie et al. (2000), Figure 3.1, p. 26

findings were found for the percentage of young people who reported feeling low at least once a week in the past six months. The average percentage of students feeling low on a weekly basis was over 25 per cent, but the highest rates of feeling low (over 40 per cent) were found in Greece, Israel and Hungary. In Glendinning et al.'s (2000) rural study of young people, young Swedes also reported better self-esteem and emotional well-being than young Scots.

Table 22.9 shows that there were also some differences by country within the UK, with England and Wales being consistently in the top half of the countries with high rates of young people 'feeling low'. Northern Ireland's young people had about average, or slightly above average, scores for feeling low, while Scotland appeared to have lowest rates of young people feeling low. For example, 40 per cent of young women aged 15 in England reported feeling low at least once a week in the last six months, compared to only 28 per cent of young women aged 15 in Scotland. However, in contrast, the ONS study (Meltzer et al., 2000) found no significant differences for prevalence of mental disorders in children between England, Scotland and Wales.

A number of studies have examined the particular issue of young people growing up in Northern Ireland and the effects of the Troubles on their health.

A recent Omnibus study of 414 16–24-year-olds explored the worries of young people (Health Promotion Agency for Northern Ireland, 2001b). While it found that only 2 per cent of young people, unprompted, mentioned the Troubles as a common worry, when prompted about half (52 per cent) of young people said they did worry about a 'return to the Troubles'. Trew (1995), reviewing the evidence in this area, concluded that although the majority of children might not have experienced mental health problems as a result of the Troubles, a minority of children and young people would have suffered mentally. A detailed study of the Troubles (Smyth, 1998) found that a quarter of those killed in the Troubles since 1969 had been aged between 18 and 23, and interviews with young people in areas with high Troubles-related deaths in Belfast revealed how children had been affected emotionally by Trouble-related bereavements, as well as by rioting and difficult relations between community members.

Trends over time

Rutter and Smith (1995) undertook an international review of the mental health of children and young people and concluded that mental health problems had become more prevalent in Western societies in the post-war period. Other commentators concur with this finding (eg, Mental Health Foundation, 1999; NHS Health Advisory Service, 1995). However, time trend data is limited. Most studies are small scale, usually focusing on a particular type of mental disorder. Three surveys include a time dimension: the British Household Panel Study (1992 onwards); the School Health Education Unit HRBQ survey (from 1991); and WHO HBSC data (since 1982). However, much of this data is unanalysed and/or unpublished. It is acknowledged that better national and international indicators need to be developed (Rutter and Smith, 1995).

Balding *et al.* (1998) reviewed HRBQ data on young people's worries between 1991 and 1997. They found that the top three worries had been fairly consistent: 'family', 'the way you look', and for boys, 'drugs' and for girls, 'friends'. Increasing worries appeared to have been drugs, family, friends and possibly (to some extent) school, whereas decreasing worries were HIV/AIDS and gambling.

Fombonne (1995) reviewed a number of, mainly US, studies which indicate that depressive disorders and eating disorders may have increased since the war. The number of young people diagnosed with mental health problems and/or admitted to hospital increased over the 1980s (Scottish Community Education Council, 1994). However, some of this increase is likely to have been accounted for by more young people presenting problems to professional services and/or changing approaches to treatment. Lewis and Wilkinson (1993) compared a 1977 study and a 1985 study, and found 'cases' of psychological morbidity increased from 22 to 31 per cent (including young people aged 16–24). Hawton *et al.* (1996) found an upward trend in deliberate self-poisoning and self-injury in under-16-year-olds in Oxford over the period 1976 to 1993. Controversy sometimes surrounds particular conditions. For example, Attention Deficit Hyperactivity Disorder (ADHD), a conduct disorder associated with poor attention span, has received considerable media and medical coverage, that makes it difficult to disentangle any perceived rise in prevalence from increased publicity and discussion of the condition.

Rutter and Smith (1995) concluded that the most likely reasons for any rise in disorders include increased family problems and break-up, lack of parental support, increasing expectations on young people and possibly the growth of youth cultures and markets leading to increased peer pressure and isolation from older age groups. Changes in socio-economic conditions were not seen as a major factor.

Conclusions

Definitional issues, and the complexity of the nature of mental health, mean that the data available on the mental health of children is not always consistent. In particular, different trends can be examined for different disorders. Nonetheless, the review of available evidence suggests that age and gender (though not ethnicity) and family-related factors are extremely important in explaining the mental health of children and young people. Evidence for the role of environmental factors is less clear-cut. Evidence is quite strong for a link between childhood poverty and some mental disorders, especially conduct disorders, but much weaker for emotional problems and general levels of happiness (though demographic/geographical ACORN category and young people's own independent emerging socio-economic status does show an association). Most young people in the Western world report reasonably high levels of happiness, though there appeared to be some differences within the UK. Data is weak on time trends, though experts agree that there is no evidence for improved mental health among children and young people and possibly some suggestion of worsening mental health among young people over time. Improved prevalence data is required at both UK and international levels in order to monitor trends over time.

23 Conclusion

Jonathan Bradshaw

Introduction

This has been the first attempt to produce a report on the well-being of children in the UK. In this concluding chapter we start by reviewing the approach that we have taken and acknowledging some of the gaps and weaknesses that might be dealt with in future reports. Then we attempt a summary review of the well-being of children paying attention to two particular topics – evidence of variation within the countries that make up the UK and evidence of change over time. Finally, we conclude with a recommendation for improvements in the data, which would enable us to do the job better in the future.

Review of the approach taken

This report grew out of the work undertaken for *Poverty: the outcomes for children* (Bradshaw 2001a). It employed some of the same authors and, though in this report the focus was not entirely on poverty, we have followed the same approach to the task. Thus:

- Well-being has been understood and represented in physical, cognitive, behavioural and mental/emotional domains.
- We have not sought to identify a selection of key or representative indicators of well-being such as those published by the Department for Work and Pensions in the *Opportunity for All* reports (DWP 2001b) or the Policy Research Institute in its reports (Rahman *et al.* 2001) or the comparative indicators that the *International Comparative Study of Child Well-being* is seeking to produce. However, it maybe that this review will assist the governments throughout the UK as they develop their work to monitor the well-being of children and evaluate public policy as it affects children and young people.
- The main focus has been on *outcomes* for children. We eschewed as far as

possible the description of policy inputs or the evaluation of services. However, some of the topics included here have covered service provision. For example, we have presented data on the level of Income Support for families with children, the number of children receiving benefits, children looked after by local authorities and childcare provision. The justification for this is that data on the use of these benefits or services are either an indication of the outcomes of other processes or they are, arguably, a measure of child well-being in their own right.

- The work has consisted of a critical, scholarly review of the evidence. The evidence consists of:
  - administrative statistics
  - the findings of surveys, both academic and official
  - more qualitative studies of children.

These reviews have not had all the components of a formal *systematic review* in the sense of one which includes an explicit search strategy, with clear criteria for inclusion and exclusion, quality assessment of all relevant studies, data extraction and a meta analysis (NHS Centre for Reviews and Dissemination, 2001). We do not consider that that formal approach is appropriate for the task we were set. Nevertheless, our strategy was to search for evidence on the well-being of children in the UK, how it varied over time, how it varied between the countries in the UK and between the UK and other countries, and how it varied by social class, income, gender, ethnicity and other socio-economic circumstances of families.

- We have tried to be critical of the evidence. Thus, for example, the only evidence on the numbers of children maltreated over time is that derived from social services department registers. Those greedy for evidence on whether child maltreatment is increasing or decreasing are forced to rely on this source, but it presents a flawed picture, one that has more to do with administrative practice, legislative categories and fashion than the reality of maltreatment of children. We have tried not to reject such evidence but to give warnings about its reliability and validity.
- While there is a considerable body of evidence on the well-being of children, readers will be as frustrated as we are at our failure to be able to reveal trends in well-being, make reliable comparisons by country and region, and describe the associations of outcomes – how they vary by socio-economic status. Too often the data is just not there. That is why at the end of this conclusion we

briefly argue for a purpose-built survey of the well-being of children, which would go some way to filling the gap in evidence that exists.

- Then there are challenges to be made about the balance and coverage of different elements of well-being.
  - *About balance.* Authors were given word limits for their topic and there is some variation in the length of chapters. However, there is scope to reconsider the balance of space devoted to different topics.
  - *About coverage.* There are gaps that we recognise – for example, there is very little on learning difficulties in this report. There are other topics that we sought to cover but found very little material on. Thus, for example, child refugees and asylum seekers are clearly some of the most deprived children in the UK, not even eligible for the minimum income standard that other children are entitled to, badly housed, undernourished and possibly traumatised. Of course agencies working with these children, including Save the Children, have a good deal of *intelligence* about their well-being, and we are aware that there is empirical research in progress. However, there is very little of it published. The same arguments hold for Gypsy and Traveller children.

For all these reasons it is important to recognise that this is not the last word on the well-being of UK children. Indeed to some extent it is the first word. We would welcome criticisms, suggestions for improvement and references to material that we have missed (jrb1@york.ac.uk).

Country variations in child well-being

Save the Children is an organisation with offices based in each country within the UK. Thus they are as interested in the state of well-being of children in their country as they are in children in the UK as a whole. This was the reason that special efforts were made to report country and regional level differences where the data was available. While there is usually data available at country level, it is very commonly not comparable. Indeed it may be that one of the costs of devolved government in the UK is that the way each country measures the well-being of its children will increase in variation. In each of the chapters we have reported county data where we have found it. In Table 23.1 we have bought together data, which is comparable and enables comparisons to be made between countries. Only one variable has been selected to represent a domain.

The first thing to note is that there are some domains where there are no comparable data. Thus, for example, there are no adequate comparable data on young people leaving care and going missing, children as carers, the environment of children, child homelessness, youth crime, child labour and the mental health of children. Some of the comparable data presented in the table representing a given domain leaves much to be desired – for example, children on the child protection register. Perhaps it is particularly surprising how little comparable data there is on child health. It is also interesting to note how reliant we are in this table on the WHO *Health Behaviour of School-Aged Children* (HBSC) survey – because it is almost unique in having samples in each country of the UK (though they are probably not representative).

From the results in Table 23.1 it is not possible to claim a consistent relative level of well-being for children in a particular country. For example, Northern Ireland almost certainly has the highest child poverty rate, and it has the highest infant mortality rate, but it has low teenage fertility, and probably the best educational attainment levels. Children in Scotland appear to have the worst diets and the highest youth suicide rate, but the smallest proportion feeling low. Wales has a high child poverty rate, the highest rate of infant mortality and teenage pregnancies and the worst problems of alcohol and drugs. So considering all the indicators there is a mixed picture.

Is the well-being of children improving or deteriorating in the UK?

This is perhaps the key question arising out of this review. The answer is more complicated. As we have seen, well-being varies by country and region and here we are making an overall judgement about the UK as a whole. Many indicators of well-being also vary by age of child, gender, family type, ethnicity and socio-economic level. Well-being may be improving overall but becoming more diverse – for example the gap between poor children and better-off children may be growing. Making a judgement on trends in overall well-being commonly involves a judgement based on conflicting evidence and/or selecting one indicator, or a few indicators, from a range that have been presented in the chapters above. Also we could find no adequate trend data on young people leaving care and going missing, children as carers, child labour and the mental health of children.

It can be seen in Table 23.2 that in the majority of respects the well-being of

Table 23.1: Comparative summary of child well-being in the countries of the UK

Indicator	England	Wales	Scotland	N. Ireland
Child poverty rates (income <50% average before housing costs) % 2000/01	20	24	26	—
Child poverty rates (income <50% average after housing costs) % 2000/01	30	33	30	—
Infant mortality rates 1999	5.7	6.1	5.0	6.4
Diet and nutrition				
Rank order of poor diets (out of 19 countries) 1997/8	15	16	19	17
Child health:				
MMR uptake % 2000	87.6	87.2	92.8	91.9
Breastfeeding % all births 2000	70 in E & W		63	54
Child road fatal and severe accident rates 1999 per 1,000	0.47 in E & W		0.62	—
Children on the child protection register rate per 1,000 in 2000	2.7	3.6	2.0	3.2
Children looked after per 1,000 in 2000	5.1	4.9	(10.0)	5.3
% of those looked after in foster placements	65	75	(27)	66
Reported rates or running away %	10	8.5	10	9
Estimated % of children attending early education 2001	90	79	88	—
Under 20 age specific fertility rate per 1,000 2000	28.8	35.2	29.1	26.1
% achieving 5 or more A*–C	49.2	49.1	58.3	56.9
% achieving 2 or more A levels	30.0	27.2	31.4	37.7
% achieving Key Stage 2 in English	70	70	—	71
% achieving Key Stage 2 in Maths	72	71	—	75
% achieving Key Stage 2 in Science	79	78	—	—
% 11–16 exercising at least 4 hours per week outside school 1998	22	26	33	31
% boys aged 15 smoking daily 2000	21	18	19	16
% girls aged 15 smoking daily 2000	24	23	24	24
% boys aged 15 drinking alcohol at least weekly 2000	47	53	37	33
% girls aged 15 drinking alcohol at least weekly 2000	36	36	33	20
% boys aged 15 using drugs in the last month 1998	19	28	26	
% girls aged 15 using drugs in the last month 1998	16	22	22	
Suicides 15–24 per 100,000 in 1999, males	13	25	33	25
Suicides 15–24 per 100,000 in 1999, females	4	2	6	8
% of 15-year-olds who report feeling low at least once a week in the last 6 months				
males	24	26	13	18
females	40	41	28	38

children is improving. Thus child poverty is now falling (in Britain), infant mortality continues to decline, breastfeeding is increasing, survival rates for cancer and cystic fibrosis are up, fewer children are entering care, childcare is improving, teenage conception rates are down, housing conditions are improving, educational attainment is improving, school exclusions are down, sporting participation is increasing and youth suicide has fallen.

However, associated with these improvements there may have been an increased dispersion – a growing gap between poor and better-off children. This is probably true of the spatial dispersion of child poverty, of the adequacy of diet and nutrition and the prevalence of accidental injuries. There is some evidence of a narrowing of differentials in relation to infant mortality and educational attainment.

Then there are the domains where there is evidence of a deterioration: an increase in obesity; immunisation rates down; self-reported morbidity up; an increase in diabetes, asthma, HIV and sexually transmitted infections; longer stays in care; more competition between traffic and space to play; and a fall in free play.

Finally, there are those domains where there is evidence over time which indicates no change: diet and nutritional standards, child homicides, recent Key Stage 2 scores and recorded crime all look stable.

Of course in order to evaluate these trends, account needs to be taken of the rate of increase and decrease and the base from which it has occurred. Thus, for example, the diets of UK children have not improved, and from what appears to be a very inadequate level absolutely and one which also appears to be low comparatively. The infant mortality rate is falling slowly, but it is still high compared with most other rich countries – we would be saving many thousands of children's lives if we achieved the rate of Sweden. The same is true of the teenage conception rate – probably going down, but from the highest level in Europe. Our child accidental death rates are still falling despite the fact that we have one of the lowest accidental death rates in the world (and there are worries about whether we are overprotecting our children).

Also account needs to be taken of how robust the trends are. For example, the decline in the teenage conception rate is very recent and only in England and Wales. The decline in youth suicides is also recent and not shared throughout the UK.

The need for more and better evidence on child well-being

There is no doubt that the evidence base on child well-being has been improving in recent years. For example, the Family Resources Survey now provides robust data on child poverty, provides it more quickly and will provide it for all UK countries in the future. Administrative data now gives us excellent information on the spatial distribution of child poverty within the UK. International comparative studies of child poverty, though not very up to date, are much improved. The English Health Survey is going to become a very valuable resource for monitoring the health of children over time. Among the other useful new sources of evidence are *Child Maltreatment in the UK* (Cawson *et al.*, 2000) (especially if it is repeated), PRILIF (Lone Parent Cohort), SoLIF/SoF (Survey of Low Income Families/ Families with Children), and ALSPAC (the Avon Cohort). The British Household Panel Survey has had national booster samples to enhance its usefulness in Scotland and Wales. There are other national surveys coming on stream, including the Scottish Household Survey and a Northern Ireland Panel Survey.

Also, more could be made of the secondary analysis of existing data, especially the youth questionnaire in the British Household Panel Survey. There is also huge scope for developing the use of administrative data and linking administrative data to survey data.

However, together, all these sources leave big gaps. In order to monitor the well-being of children better there needs to be a new sample survey of children, ideally covering the whole of the UK. This is not the place to outline in detail the design of such a survey. However, there would be advantages in a split-age cohort design that enabled different age samples of children to be followed over time, but at the same time produce useful results more quickly than the birth cohorts are able to. The children do not need to be interviewed every year, perhaps every two or three years. Children would be the unit of analysis, but it would give added value if the sampling strategy enabled data to be collected on their family, their school and their neighbourhood, so that the impact of families, schools and neighbourhoods on child well-being can be better understood. The most important element in the survey would be to hear from children themselves – about what they think and feel – about their living standards, diet, health, time, leisure, play, space, schooling, behaviour, relationships with friends and family, and what they have to say about their beliefs, fears, joys, self-esteem, aspirations and hopes.

Table 23.2: Assessment of trends in child well-being

Well-being improving	Well-being deteriorating
Child poverty began to decline after 1999/00 in Britain	
Infant and child mortality trend slowly down over the 1990s	
	% of overweight and obese children has increased % immunised for measles fell 1995–1999
% breastfeeding increased 1995–00	
	Increase in % of parents reporting longstanding illness especially among boys
	Increasing prevalence of diabetes, asthma in young adults, HIV/AIDS and some sexually transmitted infections
Improved survival rates for cancer & cystic fibrosis	
Child injury death rates are internationally low and falling	
Fall in the number of children entering care over 20 years	But they are staying longer
Increase in daycare nursery, out-of-school clubs and holiday play schemes	
Teenage conception rate high comparatively but declining	
Housing conditions improved overall	
	Traffic volumes increased and children's use of public space has fallen
	The number of homeless households has increased (again) and the numbers in England in temporary accommodation are at record level
More young people are achieving better qualifications and the post-16 staying on rate has increased	
Sporting participation is increasing	But free play is decreasing
Official rates of permanent exclusion from school have been declining	
	Smoking (at least in Scotland and Wales), drinking of alcohol and drug use are all increasing
The number of suicides among young people fell between 1993 and 1999	

No change in in well-being	*Evidence on dispersion*
	Probable increase in dispersion spatially
	Reduction is social class differences between mid-1970s & mid-1990s
No improvement in diet and nutrition in the last two decades	
	Socio-economic differences in mortality as a result of injuries have increased
Child homicide stable in 1980 & 1990s in England and Wales	
Recent slight rise in the numbers entering care	
	Social class gaps in teenage birth rate probably growing
	Children in lone parent and minority ethnic families more likely to be poorly housed
	Differences in attainment by social class increased in the 1990s but may have begun to narrow
Improvements in Key Stage 2 scores were not sustained in the last two years	
Recorded crime has reached a plateau and may be in decline	

It is amazing that this country does not have such a survey and that the nearest thing to it is an international study – the WHO survey of school children which, as we have seen in this report, in the absence of any and better data, is an extremely useful resource. However, it does not and cannot provide what a purpose-built survey of all children could provide.

References

Abrahams, C. and Mungall, R. (1992) *Young Runaways: Exploding the myths*, London: NCH Action for Children.

Acheson, D. (Chair) (1998) *Independent Inquiry into Inequalities in Health*, London: The Stationery Office.

Adams, E. and Ingham, S. (1998) *Changing Places: Children's participation in environmental planning*, London: The Children's Society.

Adelman, L. and Bradshaw, J. (1998) *Children in Poverty in Britain: An analysis of the Family Resources Survey 1994/95*, York: Social Policy Research Unit, University of York.

Adelstein, A. and Mardon, C. (1975) 'Suicides 1961–74', *Population Trends*, 2, 13–18, in Hill, K. (1995) *The Long Sleep: Young people and suicide*, London: Virago Press.

Ahmad, O.B., Lopez, A.D. and Inoue, M. (2000) 'The decline in child mortality: a reappraisal', *Bulletin of the World Health Organisation*, 78: 1175–1191.

Aldgate, J., Colton, M., Ghate, D. and Heath, A. (1992) 'Educational attainment and stability in long-term foster care', *Children and Society*, 6, 91–103.

Aldridge, J. and Becker, S. (1998) *The National Handbook of Young Carers Projects*, London: Carers National Association.

Aldridge, J., Parker, H. and Measham, F. (1999) *Drug Trying and Drug Use Across Adolescence*, DPAS Paper 1, London: Home Office.

Allatt, P. and Dixon, C. (2001) 'Learning to Labour: how 17 year old A-level students manage part-time jobs, full time study and other forms of work in times of rapid social change', *Youth, Citizenship and Social Change Newsletter*, 4, Winter, 3–6, ESRC.

Allison, M., Coalter, F. and Taylor, J. (1999) *Youth Sport in Scotland: Young people and sport*, Edinburgh: The Scottish Sports Council.

Anderson, I. and Tulloch, D. (2000) *Pathways through Homelessness: A review of the research evidence*, Edinburgh: Scottish Homes.

Anderson, I., Kemp, P. and Quilgars, D. (1993) *Single Homeless People*, London: HMSO.

Andrews, B. (1994) 'Family violence in a social context: factors relating to male abuse of children', in J. Archer (ed.) *Male Violence*, London: Routledge.

Armstrong, N., Balding, T., Gentle, P. and Kirby, B. (1990) 'Patterns of physical activity among 11–16 year old British children', *British Medical Journal*, 301, 203–05.

Asarnow, J.A. (1992) 'Suicidal ideation and attempts during middle childhood: associations with perceived family stress and depression among child psychiatric inpatients', *Journal of Clinical Child Psychology*, 21, 34–40.

Atkinson, T., Cantillon, B., Marlier, E. and Nolan, B. (2001) *Indicators for Social Exclusion in the European Union*, EU Subgroup on Social Protection.

Audit Commission (1993) *Unfinished Business: Full time educational courses for 16–19 year olds*, London: OFSTED, HMSO.

Audit Commission (1996) *Misspent Youth: Young people and crime*, London: Audit Commission.

Audit Commission (1999) *Missing Out: LEA management of school attendance and exclusion*, Abingdon: Audit Commission Publications.

Backett-Milburn, K., Cunningham-Burley, S. and Kemmer, D. (2001) *Caring and Providing: Lone and partnered working mothers in Scotland*, London: Family Policy Studies Centre.

Bagilhole, B. and Byrne, P. (2000) 'From hard to soft law and from equality to reconciliation in the United Kingdom', in L. Hantrais (ed.) *Gendered Policies in Europe: Reconciling employment and family life*, London: Macmillan.

Baird, D. (1980) 'Environment and reproduction', *British Journal of Obstetrics and Gynaecology*, 87: 1057–1067.

Balding, J., Regis, D. and Wise, A. (1998) *No Worries? Young people and mental health*, Exeter: Schools Health Education Unit.

Bambamg, S., Spencer, N.J., Logan, S. and Gill, L. (2000) 'Cause-specific perinatal death rates, birth weight and deprivation in the West Midlands', *Child: Care, Health and Development*, 26: 73–82.

Barclay, G., Tavares, C. and Siddique, A. (2001) *International Comparisons of Criminal Justice Statistics 1999*, Home Office Statistical Bulletin, Issue 6/01.

Bardsley, M. and Morgan, D. (2000) 'Measuring inequalities in the health of mothers and children, Briefing Paper 1', in *Inequalities in Maternal and Early Child Health Resource Pack*, London: Health of Londoners Project.

Barn, R. (1993) *Black Children in the Public Care System*, London: Batsford.

Barn, R., Sinclair, R. and Ferdinand, D. (1997) *Acting on Principal: An examination of race and ethnicity in social services provision to children and families*, London: BAAF.

Barry, M. (2001) *Challenging Transitions: Young people's views and experiences of growing up*, London: Save the Children.

Bassuk, E.L. and Perloff, J.N. (2001) 'Multiply homeless families: the insidious impact of violence', *Housing Policy Debate*, 12, 2.

Bates, J. (1999) 'Spare the code and spoil the child', Paper delivered at *Staying Power* Conference, Warwick University, 22–23 September 1999.

Bebbington, A. and Miles, J. (1989) 'The background of children who enter local authority care', *British Journal of Social Work*, 19, 5, 349–68.

Becker, S. (ed.) (1995) *Young Carers in Europe: An exploratory cross-national study in Britain, France, Sweden and Germany*, Loughborough: Loughborough University.

Becker, S., Aldridge, J. and Dearden, C. (1998) *Young Carers and Their Families*, Oxford: Blackwell.

Becker, S., Dearden, C. and Aldridge, J. (2000) 'Young carers in the UK: research policy and practice', *Research, Policy and Planning*, 18, 2, 13–21.

Bell, R. (2001) 'Finding and "managing" part-time work: young people, social networks and family support', *Youth, Citizenship and Social Change Newsletter*, 4, Winter, 7–8, ESRC.

Bergman, M.M. and Scott, J. (2001) 'Young adolescents' well-being and health-risk behaviours: gender and socio-economic differences', *Journal of Adolescence*, 24, 183–97.

Berridge, D. (1985) *Children's Homes*, Oxford: Blackwell.

Berridge, D. and Brodie, I. (1998) *Children's Homes Revisited*, London: Jessica Kingsley.

Berthoud, R. (2001) 'Teenage births to ethnic minority women', *Population Trends 104*, London: The Stationery Office.

Berthoud, R. and Robson, K. (2001) 'The outcomes of teenage motherhood in Europe', EPAG Working Paper 22, University of Essex.

Bertram, T. and Pascal, C. (2001) *Early Excellence Centre Pilot Programme Annual Evaluation Report 2000*, DfEE Research Report 258, Nottingham: DfEE Publications.

Biehal, N., Clayden, J., Stein, M. and Wade J. (1995) *Moving On: Young people and leaving care schemes*, London: HMSO.

Biehal, N., Clayden, J., Stein, M. and Wade, J. (1992) *Prepared for Living? A survey of young people leaving the care of three local authorities*, London: National Children's Bureau.

Bifulco, A. and Moran, P. (1998) *Wednesday's Child: Research into women's experience of neglect and abuse in childhood and adult depression*, London: Routledge.

Blair, P.S., Fleming, P.J., Bensley, D., Smith, I., Bacon, C., Taylor, E., Berry, J., Golding, J. and Tripp, J. (1996) 'Smoking and sudden infant death syndrome: results from the 1993–5 case-control study for confidential inquiry into stillbirths and deaths in infancy', *British Medical Journal*, 313: 195–198.

Blake, M., Finch, S., McKernan, A. and Hinds, K. (2001) *Fourth Survey of Parents of Three and Four Year Old Children and their Use of Early Years Services*, Department for Education and Employment Research Report, 247. Nottingham: DfEE Publications.

Blyth, E. and Milner, J. (1997) *Social Work with Children: The educational perspective*, London: Longman.

Botting, B (ed.) (1995) *The Health of our Children, The Register General's decennial supplement for England and Wales*, London: HMSO.

Botting, B. (1997) 'Mortality in childhood', in F. Drever and M. Whitehead (eds) *Health Inequalities: decennial supplement*, Series DS No. 15. London: The Stationery Office.

Botting, B. and Cooper, J. (1993) 'Analysing fertility and infant mortality by mother's social class as defined by occupation –Part II', *Population Trends*, 74: 27–33.

Botting, B. and Crawley, R. (1995) 'Trends and patterns in childhood mortality and morbidity', in B. Botting (ed.) *The Health of our Children, The Registrar General's decennial supplement for England and Wales*, London: HMSO.

Botting, B. *et al.* (1996) *Health of Children*, London: HMSO.

Braben, B., Smith, M., Milligan, P., Benjamin, C., Dunne, E. and Pearson, M. (1994) 'Respiratory morbidity in Merseyside school children exposed to coal dust and air pollution', *Archives of Disease in Childhood*, 70, 305–12.

Bradbury, B. and Jantti, M. (1999) *Child Poverty Across Industrialised Countries*, Innocenti Occasional Paper, Economic and Social Policy Series, No. 71, Florence: UNICEF International Child Development Centre.

Bradbury, B., Jenkins, S.P. and Micklewright, J. (2001) 'Child poverty dynamics in seven nations', in B. Bradbury, S.P. Jenkins and J. Micklewright (eds) *The Dynamics of Child Poverty in Industrialised Countries*, Cambridge University Press.

Bradshaw, J. (1990) *Child Poverty and Deprivation in the UK*, National Children's Bureau.

Bradshaw, J. (1997a) 'Child welfare in the United Kingdom: rising poverty, falling priorities for children', in G. Cornia and S. Danziger (eds) *Child Poverty and Deprivation in the Industrialised Countries 1945–1995*, Oxford: Oxford University Press.

Bradshaw, J. (1997b) 'Children in poverty', Paper presented at the launch of Breadline Britain in the 1990s, at the House of Commons, 22 July 1997, University of York, Social Policy Research Unit.

Bradshaw, J. (1999) 'Child poverty in comparative perspective', *Journal of European Social Security*, 1/4, 383–404.

Bradshaw, J. (2001a) (ed.) *Poverty: The outcomes for children*, London: Family Policy Studies Centre/National Children's Bureau.

Bradshaw, J. (2001b) 'Child poverty in comparative perspective', in D. Gordon and P. Townsend (eds) *Breadline Europe: The measurement of poverty*, Bristol: Policy Press, pp 223–50.

Bradshaw, J. (2001c) 'Child poverty under Labour', in G. Fimister (ed.) *Tackling Child Poverty in the UK: An end in sight?* London: Child Poverty Action Group.

Bradshaw, J. (2001d) 'Child poverty and child health: international comparisons', Paper presented at the Eighth International Research Seminar of FISS, Issues in Social Security, Support for children and their parents: whys, ways, effects and policy options, Sweden, June 2001.

Bradshaw, J. (ed.) (1993) *Budget Standards for the United Kingdom*, Aldershot: Ashgate.

Bradshaw, J. and Williams, J. (2001) *Earnings and Pocket Money: Analysis of the British Household Panel Survey*, York: Social Policy Research Unit, University of York.

Bradshaw, J., Ditch, J., Holmes, H. and Whiteford, P. (1993) *Support for Children: A comparison of arrangements in fifteen countries*, Department of Social Security Research Report 21, London: HMSO.

Bradshaw, J., Kennedy, S., Kilkey, M., Hutton, S., Corden, A., Eardley, T., Holmes, H. and Neale, J. (1996) *Policy and the Employment of Lone Parents in 20 Countries*, London: HMSO.

Brennan, T., Huizinga, D. and Elliot, D. (1978) *The Social Psychology of Runaways*, New York: Lexington Books.

Brewer, M., Clark, T. and Goodman, A. (2002) 'The government's child poverty target: How much progress has been made?', IFS Commentary 87, London: Institute for Fiscal Studies.

Briggs, C.M. and Cutright, P. (1994) 'Structural and cultural determinants of child homicide: a cross-national analysis', *Violence and Victims*, 9, 1, 3–16.

Britton, L., Chatrik, B., Coles, B., Craig, G., Hylton, C. and Mumtaz, S. (2002) *Missing Connexions: The career dynamics and welfare needs of black and minority ethnic young people at the margins*, Bristol: Policy Press.

Broad, B. (1998) *Young People Leaving Care: Life after the Children Act 1989*, London: Jessica Kingsley.

Brodie, I. and Berridge, D. (1996) *School Exclusion Research Themes and Issues*, Luton: University of Luton Press.

Brooke, O.G., Anderson, H.R., Bland, J.M., Peacock, J.L. and Stewart, C.M. (1989) 'Effects on birth weight of smoking, alcohol, caffeine, socio-economic factors, and psychosocial stress', *British Medical Journal*, 298: 795–801.

Brown, K., McLiveen, H. and Strugnell, C. (2000) 'Young consumers' food preferences within selected sectors of the Hospitality Spectrum', *Journal of Consumer Studies and Home Economics*, 24, 2104–12.

Bruegel, I. and Smith, J. (1999) *Taking Risks: An analysis of the risks of homelessness for young people in London*, London: Safe in the City.

Brynin, M. and Scott, J. (1996) *Young People, Health and the Family*, London: Health Education Authority.

Budd, T. and Mattinson, J. (2000) *Stalking: Findings from the 1998 BCS*, Research Findings No. 129, London: Home Office.

Bullock, R., Little, M. and Millham, S. (1993) *Going Home: The return of children separated from their families*, London: Dartmouth.

Burr, M. (1995) 'Pollution: does it cause asthma?', *Archives of Disease in Childhood*, 72, 377–79.

Burridge, R. and Ormandy, D. (1993) *Unhealthy housing: research, remedies and reform*, London: Spon Press.

Burrows, R. and Rhodes, D. (1998) *Unpopular places? Area disadvantage and the geography of misery in England*, Bristol: Policy Press/Joseph Rowntree Foundation.

Callender, C. (2000) *The Barriers to Childcare Provision*, DfEE Research Report RR231, Nottingham: DfEE Publications.

Campbell, R., Cunningham, C., Mooney, S., Nevison, C., Pettit, B. and Rodgers,

P. (1998) 'Children's perspectives on work', in B. Pettit (ed.) *Children and Work in the UK*, London: Save the Children.

Cantor, C.H. (2000) 'Suicide in the Western world', in K. Hawton and K. Heeringen (eds) *The International Handbook of Suicide and Attempted Suicide*, Chichester: John Wiley & Sons.

CAPT (2000a) *Child Injury Facts and Figures – 1999,* Child Accident Prevention Trust Factsheet.

CAPT (2000b) *Pedestrian Deaths and Injuries*, Child Accident Prevention Trust Focus on Injury, No. 3, August 2000.

Carlton, P.A. and Deane, F.P. (2000) 'Impact of attitudes and suicidal ideation on adolescents. Intentions to seek professional psychological help', *Journal of Adolescence*, 23, 1, 35–45.

Carr Hill, R., Dixon, P., Mannion, R., Rice, N., Rudat, K., Sinclair, R. and Smith, P. (1997) *A Model of the Determinants of Expenditure on Children's Personal Social Services*, York: Centre for Health Economics, University of York.

Carstairs, V. and Morris, R. (1991) *Deprivation and Health in Scotland,* Aberdeen: Aberdeen University Press.

Cawson, P., Wattam, C., Brooker, S. and Kelly, C. (2000) *Child Maltreatment in the United Kingdom: A study of the prevalence of child abuse and neglect*, London: National Society for the Prevention of Cruelty to Children.

Central Health Monitoring Unit (1995) *Asthma: An epidemiological overview*, London: HMSO.

Central Statistical Office (1981) *Regional Trends 16: 1981,* London: HMSO.

Central Statistical Office (1994) *Social Focus on Children*, London: HMSO.

Centrepoint (1998) *The Young Face of Homelessness (Youth Affairs Briefing)*, London: Centrepoint.

Chahal, K. and Julienne, L. (1999) *"We can't all be white!": Racist victimisation in the UK*, York: York Publishing Services/JRF.

Charlton, J., Kelly, S., Dunnell, K., Evans, B. and Jenkins, R. (1993) 'Suicide deaths in England and Wales: trends in factors associated with suicide deaths', in OPCS, *Population Trends*, No. 71, Spring, London: HMSO.

Charlton, J., Kelly, S., Dunnell, K., Evans, B., Jenkins, R. and Wallis, R. (1992) 'Trends in suicide deaths in England and Wales', in OPCS, *Population Trends*, No. 69, Autumn, London: HMSO.

Cheng, A.T.A. and Lee, C. (2000) 'Suicide in Asia and the Far East', in K.

Hawton and K. Heeringen (eds) *The International Handbook of Suicide and Attempted Suicide*, Chichester: John Wiley & Sons.

Cheung, Y. and Buchanan, A. (1997) 'Malaise score in adulthood of children and young people who have been in care', *Journal of Child Psychology and Psychiatry*, 38, 5, 575–80.

Cheung, Y. and Heath, A. (1994) 'After care: the education and occupation of adults who have been in care', *Oxford Review of Education*, 20, 3, 351–437.

Childcare Commission Report (2001) *Looking to the Future for Children and Families*, London: Kids' Clubs Network.

Childline (1998) *Children Calling from Northern Ireland*, London: Childline.

Chinn, S. and Rona, R. (2001) 'Prevalence and trends in overweight and obesity in three cross sectional studies of British children, 1974–94', *British Medical Journal*, 322, 24–26.

CIPFA (2001) *Personal Social Services Statistics 1999–2000 Actuals*, London: Chartered Institute of Public Finance and Accountancy.

Clarke, L., Bradshaw, J. and Williams, J. (2000) *Family Diversity and Poverty and the Mental Well-being of Young People*, Unpublished paper, London School of Hygiene and Tropical Medicine and University of York.

Cliffe, D. with Berridge, D. (1991). *Closing Children's Homes: An End to Residential Childcare?* London: National Children's Bureau.

Cm 3805 (1998) *New Ambitions for Our Country: A new contract for welfare*, London: The Stationery Office.

Cm 4101 (1998) *A New Contract for Welfare: Principles into practice*, London: The Stationery Office.

Cole, T J., Bellizzi, Flegal, K.M. and Dietz, W.H. (2000) 'Establishing a standard definition of overweight and obesity worldwide: international survey', *British Medical Journal*, 320, 1240.

Cole-Hamilton, I. (2001) *The State of Play: A survey of play professionals in England*, London: The Children's Play Council.

Coleman, J. (1999) *Key Data on Adolescence*, Brighton: Trust for the Study of Adolescence.

Coleman, M.P., Babb. P., Damiekcki, P., Grosclaude, P., Honjo, S., Jones, J., Knerer, G., Pitard, A., Quinn, MJ., Sloggett, A. and De Stavola, B.L. (1999) 'Cancer survival trends in England and Wales, 1971–1995. deprivation and NHS region', *Studies on Medical and Population Subjects No. 61*, London: TSO.

Coles, B. (2000) *Joined-Up Youth Research, Policy and Practice: A new agenda for change?* Leicester: Youth Work Press.

Coles, B., England, J. and Rugg, J. (1998) *Working with Young People on Estates: The role of housing professionals in multi-agency work*, Coventry: The Chartered Institute of Housing.

Colton, M. and Heath, A. (1994) 'Attainment and behaviour of children in care and at home', *Oxford Review of Education*, 20, 3, 317–27.

Commission of the European Communities (2000) *Report from the Commission on the effects of the transitional period granted to the United Kingdom concerning certain provisions of Council Directive 94/33/EC on the protection of young people at work*, Brussels: COM.

COMPASS (1999) *A Project Seeking the Co-ordinated Monitoring of Participation in Sports in Europe*, London: UK Sport.

Cornia, G. and Danziger, S. (eds) (1997) *Child Poverty and Deprivation in the Industrialised Countries 1994–1995*, Oxford: Clarendon Press.

Craig, T. and Hodson, S. (1998) 'Homeless youth in London: childhood antecedents and psychiatric disorder', *Psychological Medicine*, 28, 1379–88.

Creighton, S. and Russell, N. (1995) *Voices from Childhood*, London: National Society for the Prevention of Cruelty to Children.

Crown Prosecution Service (1998), *The Inspectorate's Report on Cases Involving Child Witnesses*, London: Crown Prosecution Service.

Croxford, L. (2000) *Inequality in Attainment at Age 16: A "home international" comparison*, Edinburgh: Centre for Educational Sociology Briefing No. 19.

Cullingford, C. (1999) 'The relationship between delinquency and non-attendance at school', in E. Blyth and J. Milner (eds) *Improving School Attendance*, London: Routledge.

Currie, C., Hurrleman, K., Settertobulte, W., Smith, R. and Todd, J. (2000) *Health and Health Behaviour among Young People: Health behaviour in school-aged children: A WHO Cross-National Study (HBSC) International Report*, Copenhagen: World Health Organization, Regional Office for Europe.

CYPU (2001a) *Tomorrow's Future: Building a strategy for children and young people*, London: Children and Young People's Unit.

CYPU (2001b) *Building a Strategy for Children and Young People: Consultation document*, London: The Stationery Office.

Dale, A., Williams, M. and Dodgeon, B. (1996) *Housing Deprivation and Social Change*, London: HMSO.

Dattani, N. (2001) 'Are unascertained deaths the same as sudden infant deaths?', *Health Statistics Quarterly*, 10: 20–24.

Davey, T.L. (1998) 'Homeless children and stress: an empirical study', *Journal of Social Distress and the Homeless*, 7, 1.

Davies, B., Barton, A. and McMillan, I. (1972) *Variations in Children's Services among British Urban Authorities*, London: Bell.

Davies, C., Downey, A. and Murphy, H. (1996) *School-age Mothers: Access to education*, Belfast: Save the Children.

Davies, G.M., Wilson, C., Mitchell, R. and Milsom, J. (1995), *Videotaping Children's Evidence: An evaluation*, London: Home Office

Davis, R.M. and Pless, B. (2001) 'BMJ bans "accidents": accidents are not unpredictable', *British Medical Journal*, 322, 1320–21.

Dawson, N. (2000) 'Education and Occupational Training for Teenage Mothers in Europe', University of Sheffield. www.shef.ac.uk/uni/projects/tme/

Daycare Trust (1999) 'Childcare gaps', Briefing Paper 1 in *Childcare Now, The Next Steps* series, London: Daycare Trust.

Daycare Trust (2001) 'All our futures: putting childcare at the centre of every neighbourhood', Issue 1 of *Thinking Big: Childcare for All*, policy series, London: Daycare Trust.

Dearden, C. and Becker, S. (1995) *Young Carers: The facts*, Loughborough: Loughborough University.

Dearden, C. and Becker, S. (1998) *Young Carers in the United Kingdom: A profile*, London: Carers National Association.

Dearden, C. and Becker, S. (2000) *Growing Up Caring: Vulnerability and transition to adulthood – young carers' experiences*, York: Joseph Rowntree Foundation.

Demie, F. (2001) 'Ethnic and gender differences in educational achievement and implications for school improvement strategies', *Educational Research*, 43, 1, 91–106.

Denscombe, M. (1995) 'Ethnic group and alcohol consumption: the case of 15–16 year olds in Leicester', *Public Health*, 109, 133–42.

Department for Culture, Media and Sport (2000) *A Sporting Future for All*, London: Department for Culture, Media and Sport.

Department of Health Committee on the Medical Effects of Air Pollutants (1998) *Quantification of the Effects of Air Pollution on Health in the United Kingdom*, London: The Stationery Office.

DETR (1998) *English House Condition Survey 1996*, Department of Environment, Transport and Regions, London: The Stationery Office.

DETR (2000) *Tomorrow's Roads: Safer for everyone: The Government's road safety strategy and casualty reduction targets for 2010,* London: Department of the Environment, Transport and the Regions.

DETR, Scottish Executive, National Assembly for Wales (2000) *Road Accidents Great Britain 1999 – The Casualty Report.*

DfE (1995) *National Survey of Local Education Authorities' Policies and Procedures for the Identification of, and Provision for, Children who are out of School by Reason of Exclusion or Otherwise,* London: Department for Education.

DfEE (1998a) *Meeting the Childcare Challenge: Green Paper,* London: HMSO.

DfEE (1998b) *Pupils Under Five years of Age in Schools In England – January 1998,* London: The Stationery Office.

DfEE (1999a) *Circular No 10/99 – Social Inclusion: Pupil support,* London: Department for Education and Employment.

DfEE (1999b) *Circular No 11/99 – Social Inclusion: The LEA role in pupil support,* London: Department for Education and Employment.

DfEE (1999c) *Early Years Education Provision for Four Year Old Children in England January 1999,* London: Department for Education and Employment.

DfEE (1999d) *Learning to Succeed,* Cm 4392, London: The Stationery Office.

DfEE (1999e) *Pupils Under Five Years of Age in Maintained Schools In England - January 1999,* London: Department for Education and Employment.

DfEE (1999f) *Tackling Truancy Together: A strategy document,* London: Department for Education and Employment.

DfEE (2000a) *National Statistics Bulletin Issue No 13/00 Statistics of Education: Pupil absence and truancy, from schools in England, 1999/2000,* Department for Education and Employment, http:www.dfes.gov.uk/statistics/DB/SBU/b0223/sb13–2000.pdf – accessed 9 August 2001.

DfEE (2000b) *National Statistics Bulletin Issue No 10/00 Statistics of Education: Permanent Exclusions from Maintained Schools in England.* Department for Education and Employment, http:www.dfes.gov.uk/statistics/DB/SBU/b0209/sb10–2000.pdf – accessed 9 August 2001.

DfES (2001a) *Permanent Exclusions from Schools, England 1999/2000,* Department for Education and Skills http://www.dfes.gov.uk/statistics/DB/SFR/s0275/sfr32–2001.pdf – accessed 9 August 2001.

DfES (2001b), Press Release 26 January 2001.

DfES (2001c), Press Release 27 February 2001.

DfES (2001d) *Provision for Children under 5 years of age in England: January 2001 (Provisional Estimates),* London: Department for Education and Skills.

DfES (2001e), Press Release 24 July 2001.

DfES (2002a) *14–19 Extending Opportunities, Raising Standards, Consultation Document*, London: The Stationery Office.

DfES (2002b) *Press Release 24.1.02: Revised Draft Guidance on School Exclusions.*

DHSSPS (1996) *Health and Well-being: Into the next millennium regional strategy for health and social well being 1997–2002*, Belfast: Department for Health, Social Services and Public Safety.

DHSSPS (2000a) *Myths and Reality: Teenage pregnancy and parenthood*, Belfast: Department for Health, Social Services and Public Safety.

DHSSPS (2000b), Press Release 10 November 2000, 'Today's Children are Tomorrow's Future, says Minister'. www.ni-executive.gov.uk/press/hss/001110f-hss.htm

DHSSPS (2001) *Teenage Pregnancy Statistics,* Belfast: Department for Health, Social Services and Public Safety.

Dietz, W.H. (2001) 'The obesity epidemic in young children', *British Medical Journal*, 322, 313–14.

Director of Public Health (2000) 'Section 9.7 Suicide Prevention', *Annual Report of the Director of Public Health 2000* – www.show.scot.nhs.uk

Ditch, J., Barnes, H. and Bradshaw, J. (1996) *A Synthesis of National Family Policies 1995* (Volume 1), York: European Observatory on National Family Policies, Social Policy Research Unit, University of York.

Ditch, J., Barnes, H., Bradshaw, J. and Kilkey, M. (1998) *A Synthesis of National Family Policies*, York: European Observatory on National Family Policies, EC/University of York.

Ditch, J., Barnes, H., Bradshaw, J., Commaille, J. and Eardley, T. (1995) *A Synthesis of National Family Policies 1994* (Volume 1), York: European Observatory on National Family Policies, Social Policy Research Unit, University of York.

Dixon, J. and Stein, M. (2002) *Research Findings, Still a Bairn? A study of throughcare and aftercare service in Scotland*, Edinburgh: Scottish Executive.

Dobson, B., Beardsorth, A., Keil, T. and Walker, R. (1994) 'Diet, choice and poverty: social cultural and nutritional aspects of food consumption among low-income families', *Findings: Social Policy Research 66*, York: Joseph Rowntree Foundation.

Dodge, J.A., Morison, S., Lewis, P.A., Coles, E.C., Geddes, D., Russell, G., Littlewood, J.M. and Scott, M.T. (1997) 'Incidence, population and survival of cystic fibrosis in the UK, 1968–95', *Archives of Disease in Childhood*, 77, 493–96.

DoH (1980) *Children in Care of Local Authorities 31 March 1979 England*, Department of Health, London: Government Statistical Service.

DoH (1989) *The Diets of British School Children 1983*, Department of Health, London: HMSO.

DoH (1991) *Dietary Reference Values for Food Energy and Nutrients for the United Kingdom*, Department of Health, Report on Health and Social Subjects, 41, London: HMSO.

DoH (1992a) *Children Looked After by Local Authorities Year Ending 31 March 1991 England*, London: Government Statistical Service.

DoH (1992b) *Health of the Nation*, London: HMSO.

DoH (1995a) *Child Protection: Messages from research*, Department of Health, London: HMSO.

DoH (1995b) *Young Carers: Something to think about*, Report of four SSI workshops, May-July 1995, London.

DoH (1996) *The Health of the Nation: Low income, food, nutrition and health: strategies for improvement*, A report by the Low Income Project Team for the Nutrition Task Force, Department of Health.

DoH (1998) *Our Healthier Nation*, London: The Stationery Office.

DoH (1999) *Saving Lives: Our Healthier Nation*, Department of Health, Cm 4386, London: The Stationery Office.

DoH (2001a) *Children and young people on child protection registers, year ending 31.3.01, England*, Department of Health.

DoH (2001b) *Children Looked After in England: 2000/2001*, London: Department of Health.

DoH (2001c) *Children Looked After by Local Authorities Year Ending 31 March 2000 England*, Department of Health, London: Government Statistical Service.

DoH (2001d) *Infant Feeding Survey 2000*, Statistical press release, Results from the first stage of the 2000 Infant Feeding Survey.

DoH (2001e) 'Next phase of pilots giving free fruit to infants announced after first year study shows scheme is success', Department of Health Press Release, 2001/0565, www.ccta.gov.uk/doh/intpress – accessed 27 November 2001.

DoH (2001f) *The Children Act Report 2000*, London: Department of Health.

DoH (2001g) *The Children's National Service Framework*, London: Department Of Health.

DoH (2001h) *The National School Fruit Scheme*, Department of Health, www.doh.gov.uk/schoolfruitscheme/childrenshealth.htm – accessed 21 November 2001.

DoH (2002) *Children Accommodated in Secure Units, Year ending 31 March 2001: England and Wales*, Department of Health: www.doh.gov.uk/public/sb0117.htm

Dolton, P., Makepeace, G., Hutton, S. and Audas, R. (1999) *Making the Grade: Education, the labour market and young people*, York: YPS for the Joseph Rowntree Foundation.

Donovan, N. and Kenway, P. (1998) 'Introduction', in N. Donovan (ed.) *Second Chances: Exclusion from school and equality of opportunity*, London: New Policy Institute.

Dore, M. and Alexander, L. (1996) 'Preserving families at risk of child-abuse and neglect – the role of the helping alliance, *Child Abuse and Neglect*, 20, 4, 349–61.

Dowler, E. and Leather, S. (2000) 'Spare some change for a bite to eat? From primary poverty to social exclusion: the role of nutrition and food', in J. Bradshaw and R. Sainsbury (eds) *Experiencing Poverty*, Aldershot: Ashgate.

Doyle, C. (1997) 'Emotional abuse of children: issues for intervention', *Child Abuse Review*, 6, 330–42.

Doyle, P. (1996) 'The outcome of multiple pregnancy', *Human Reproduction*, 11: Suppl 4110–4117.

Drewett, A., Olsen, R. and Parker, G. (1999) *Community Care and Informal Carers*, University of Leicester, Nuffield Community Care Studies Unit.

DSS (1999) *Opportunity for All: Tackling poverty and social exclusion*, Department of Social Security, Cm 4445, London: The Stationery Office.

DSS (2000) *Opportunity for All: Second report on tackling poverty and social exclusion*, Department of Social Security, London: Stationery Office.

DSS (2001) *Households Below Average Income 1994/95–1999/00*, Department of Social Security, Leeds: Corporate Document Services.

DTI (1999) *Research on the Pattern and Trends in Home Accidents*, URN 99/858, Consumer Affairs Directorate, Department of Trade and Industry.

DTI (2000) *Drowning Accidents in the Garden Involving Children Under Five*, URN 00/906, Consumer Affairs Directorate, Department of Trade and Industry.

DTLR (2001) *Road Accident Involvement of Children from Ethnic Minorities: A literature review*, Road Safety Research Report No. 19, Department for Transport, Local Government and the Regions.

Duncan, R.D. *et al.* (1996) 'Childhood physical assault as a risk factor for PTSD, depression and substance abuse: findings from a national survey', *American Journal of Orthopsychiatry*, 66, 3, 437–48.

Dunn, A. and Macfarlane, A. (1996) 'Recent trends in the incidence of multiple births and associated mortality in England and Wales', *Archives of Disease in Childhood. Fetal and Neonatal Edition*, 75: F10–19.

DWP (2001a) *Income Support Statistics: May 2001*, Department for Work and Pensions, Newcastle: Analytical Services Division.

DWP (2001b) *Opportunity for All – Making Progress: Third Annual Report 2001*, Department for Work and Pensions, London: The Stationery Office.

DWP (2002) *Households Below Average Income 1994/5–2000/1*, Leeds: Corporate Document Services.

Dyck, N. (2000) *Games Sports and Cultures*, Oxford: Berg.

Edwards, E.H. (2001) Personal communication with the five Northern Ireland Education and Library Boards in 2001/02.

Edwards, E.H. (2002) Personal communication with the Pupil Support Division, Welsh Assembly in 2002.

Edwards, H. (1973) *Sociology of Sport*, St Louis: Mosby.

Edwards, J., Walters, S. and Griffiths, R.K. (1994) 'Hospital admissions for asthma in preschool children: relationship to major roads in Birmingham', *Archives of Environmental Health*, 49, 223–27.

Environment Agency (2000) *Environment 2000 and Beyond*, http://www.environment-agency.gov.uk

Environment Agency (2001) *Environment 2000 and Beyond: The Regional Picture* www.environment-agency.gov.uk accessed on 7/11/2001.

Erens, B., Primatesta, P. and Prior, G. (eds) (2001) *The Health of Minority Ethnic Groups 1999*, London: The Stationery Office.

Ermisch, J. and Francesconi, M. (2001) *The Effects of Parents' Employment on Children's Live*, London: Published for the Joseph Rowntree Foundation by the Family Policy Studies Centre.

Esping-Anderson, G., Gallie, D., Hemerijck, A. and Myles, J. (2001) *A New Welfare Architecture for Europe*, Report submitted to the Belgian presidency of the European Union.

Essen, J., Lambert, L. and Head, J. (1976) 'School attainment of children who have been in care', *Child Care, Health and Development*, 2, 339–51.

EURODIAB ACE Study Group (2000) 'Variation and trends in incidence of childhood diabetes in Europe', *The Lancet*, 355, 873–76.

European Forum for Child Welfare (1998) *Children and Work in Europe*, Brussels: European Forum for Child Welfare.

European Union (2001) Draft Report on Social Inclusion, Results of the European Community Household Panel Survey 1998, Mimeo.

EUROSTAT (2000) *Key data on health 2000*, Luxembourg: Eurostat.

Fairplay (2000) *Celebration 2000: Out of school childcare clubs in Wales*, Report for Young Voice Caerphilly, Wales: Youth Agency.

Farmer, E. and Parker, R. (1991) *Trials and Tribulations,* London: HMSO.

Farrington, D. (1996) *Understanding and Preventing Youth Crime*, York: York Publishing Services.

FEANTSA (1998) *Europe against Exclusion: Housing for all*, Brussels: European Federation of National Organisations Working with the Homeless.

Fear, N.T., Roman, E. and Reeves, G. (1999) 'Father's occupation and childhood mortality: analysis of routinely collected data', *Health Statistics Quarterly*, 2: 7–15.

Ferguson, M., Hutchinson, J., Judge, H. and Magowan, J. (1999) *An Evaluation of PlayCare in Northern Ireland*, Leeds: Policy Research Institute.

Fergusson, D.M. *et al.* (1996) 'Childhood sexual abuse and psychiatric disorder in young adulthood: prevalence of sexual abuse and factors associated with sexual abuse', *Journal of American Academy of Child and Adolescent Psychiatry*, 34, 10, 1355–64.

Fiala, R. and LaFree, G. (1988) 'Cross-national determinants of child homicide', *American Sociological Review*, 53, 432–45.

Finch, H. and Gloyer, M. (2000) *Lone Parents and Childcare: A further look at evaluation data on the New Deal for Lone Parents*, DSS Research Report 68, London: Corporate Document Services.

Finch, N., Lawton, D., Williams, J. and Sloper, P. (2001) *Disability Survey 2000: Survey of young people with a disability and sport*, London: Sport England.

Finkelhor, D., Hotaling, G., Lewis, I.A. and Smith, C. (1990) 'Sexual abuse in a national survey of adult men and women: prevalence, characteristics, and risk factors', *Child Abuse and Neglect*, 14, 19–28.

Fisher, M., Marsh, P., Phillips, D. and Sainsbury, E. (1986) *In and Out of Care*, London: British Agencies for Adoption and Fostering.

Flood-Page, C., Cambell, S., Harrington, V. and Miller, J. (2000) *Youth Crime: Findings from the 1998/1999 Youth Lifestyles Survey*, London: Home Office.

Fombonne, E. (1995) 'Depressive disorders: time trends and possible explanatory mechanisms', and 'Eating Disorders', in M. Rutter and D.J. Smith (eds) *Psychosocial Disorders of Youth*, New York: John Wiley & Sons.

Fombonne, E. (1998) 'Suicidal behaviours in vulnerable adolescents: time, trends and their correlates', *British Journal of Psychiatry*, 173, 154–59.

Frank, J., Tatum, C. and Tucker, S. (1999) *On Small Shoulders: Learning from the experiences of former young carers*, London: The Children's Society.

Friends of the Earth, *Poisoning our children: The dangers of exposure to untested and toxic chemicals* www.foe.co.uk

Garnett, L. (1992) *Leaving Care and After*, London: National Children's Bureau.

Garrett, P.M. (1999) 'The pretence of normality: intra-family violence and the response of state agencies in Northern Ireland', *Critical Social Policy*, 58, 31–57.

Garvie, D. (2001) *Far from Home: The housing of asylum seekers in private rented accommodation*, London: Shelter.

GCCNI (2001) *Hungry for Change – Community Action to tackle Food Poverty*, The Price of Being Poor Report 1, General Consumer Council, Northern Ireland.

Gelles, R.J. (1987) *Family Violence,* London: Sage.

Gelles, R.J. and Straus, M.A. (1988) *Intimate Violence*, New York: Simon and Schuster.

General Register Office for Scotland (2000) *Annual Report of the Registrar General for Scotland*, Edinburgh: Scottish Executive Information Directorate.

General Register Office for Scotland (2001) *Registrar General for Scotland, Annual Report 2000*, Edinburgh: Scottish Executive Information Directorate.

Geraghty, T. (1999) *Getting it Right? The state of children's rights in Northern Ireland at the end of the 20th century*, Belfast: The Children's Law Centre and Save the Children.

Ghate, D. and Daniels, A. (1997) *Talking about My Generation: A survey of 8–15 year olds growing up in the 1990s*, London: National Society for the Prevention of Cruelty for Children.

Gibbons, J., Conroy, S. and Bell, C. (1995) *Operating the Child Protection System: A study of child protection practices in English local authorities*, London: HMSO.

Gillborn, D. and Mirza, H.S. (2000) *Educational Inequality: Mapping race, class and gender, a synthesis of research evidence*, London: Office for Standards in Education.

Gillham, B. *et al.* (1998) 'Unemployment rates, single parent density and indices of child poverty: their relationship to different categories of child abuse and neglect', *Child Abuse and Neglect*, 22, 2, 79–90.

Ginns, S.E. and Gatrell, A.C. (1996) 'Respiratory health effects of industrial air pollution: a study in East Lancashire, UK', *Journal of Epidemiology and Community Health*, 50, 6, 631–35.

GLA (2001a) *Homelessness in London*, *28*, Greater London Authority Housing and Homelessness Team, www.london.gov.uk

GLA (2001b) *Homelessness in London*, *30*, Greater London Authority Housing and Homelessness Team, www.london.gov.uk

Gledhill, J., Rangel, L. and Garralda, E. (2000) 'Surviving chronic physical illness: psychosocial outcome in adult life', *Archives of Disease in Childhood*, 83, 104–10.

Glendinning, A., Kloep, M. and Hendry, L.B. (2000) 'Parenting practices and wellbeing in youth: family life in rural Scotland and Sweden', in H. Ryan and J. Bull (eds) *Changing Families, Changing Communities: Researching health and wellbeing among children and young people*, London: Health Development Agency.

Glendinning, A., Love, J.G., Hendry, L.B. and Shucksmith, J. (1992) 'Adolescence and health inequalities: extensions to Macintyre and West', *Social Science and Medicine*, 35, 5, 679–87.

Glendinning, C., Kirk, S., Guiffrida, A. and Lawton, D. (1999) *The Community-Based Care of Technology-Dependent Children in the UK: Definitions, numbers and costs*, Research Report commissioned by the Social Care Group, Department of Health, Manchester: National Primary Care Research and Development Centre, University of Manchester.

GMB/MPO (2000) *UK School Children at Work: Why local authorities must enforce the law*, http://www.gmb.org.uk/docs/

Goddard, E. (1997) *Young Teenagers and Alcohol in 1996*, Volume 1, England, ONS, London: The Stationery Office.

Goddard, E. and Higgins, V. (1999a) *Smoking, Drinking and Drug Use amongst Teenagers in 1998: England*, Volume 1, London: The Stationery Office.

Goddard, E. and Higgins, V. (1999b) *Smoking, Drinking and Drug Use amongst Teenagers in 1998: Scotland*, Volume 1, London: The Stationery Office.

Godfrey, C., Hutton, S., Bradshaw, J., Coles, B., Craig, G. and Johnson, J. (2001) *Costs of Social Exclusion Among Young People Aged 16–18: Costing estimates*, London: DfEE.

Godfrey, R. and Parsons, C. (1999) 'The correlates of school exclusion', in C. Parsons (1999) *Education, Exclusion and Citizenship*, London: Routledge.

Gordon, D., Parker, R. and Loughran, F. with Heslop, P. (2000) *Disabled Children in Britain: A re-analysis of the OPCS Disability Surveys*, London: The Stationery Office.

Gough, D.A. (1993) *Child Abuse Interventions: A review of the research literature*, London: HMSO.

Graham, J. and Bowling, B. (1995) *Young People and Crime: Self-reported offending amongst 14–25 year olds in England and Wales. Home Office Research Study 145*, London: Home Office.

Gray, J., Jesson, D. and Tranmer, M. (1993) *Boosting Post-16 Participation in Full-Time Education: A study of some key factors. Youth Cohort Study No. 20*, London: Department of Employment.

Greater East Belfast Youth Strategy Group (2001) *Report of the 'Big Brother-Wee Brother' youth conference*, Belfast 31 March 2001, Belfast.

Greene, J.M. and Ringwalt, C.L. (1998) 'Pregnancy among three national samples of runaway and homeless youth', *Journal of Adolescent Health*, 23, 6.

Gregory, J., Colins, D.L., Davies, P.S.W., Hughes, J.M. and Clarke, P.C. (1995) *National Diet and Nutrition Survey: Children aged 1½ to 4½ years*, London: HMSO.

Gregory, J. and Lowe, S. (2000) *National Diets and Nutrition Survey: Young people aged 4–18 years, Volume 1: Report of the diet and nutrition survey*, London: HMSO.

Gregory, J., Foster, K., Tyler, H. and Wiseman, M. (1990) *The Dietary and Nutritional Survey of British Adults*, London: HMSO.

Griesbach, D. and Currie, C. (2001) *Health Behaviours of Scottish Schoolchildren: Report 7*, Edinburgh: Child and Adolescent Health Research Unit, University of Edinburgh.

Griffiths, C. and Fitzpatrick, J. (eds) (2001) *Geographic Variations in Health*, London: The Stationery Office.

Griffiths, C. and Kirby, L. (2000) 'Geographic variations in conceptions to women aged under 18 in Great Britain during the 1990s', *Population Trends 102*, London: The Stationery Office.

Grundy, E., Ahlburg, D., Mohamed, A., Breeze, E. and Sloggett, A. (1999) *Disability in Great Britain: Results from the 1996/97 disability follow-up to the Family Resources Survey*, Department of Social Security Research Report No. 94, Leeds: Corporate Document Services.

Guildea, Z.E., Fone, D.L., Dunstan, F.D., Sibert, J.R. and Cartlidge, P.H. (2001) 'Social deprivation and the causes of stillbirth and infant mortality', *Archives of Disease in Childhood*, 84: 307–310.

Hague, G. and Mallos, E. (1999) 'Homeless children and domestic violence', in P. Vostanis and S. Cumella (eds) *Homeless Children: Problems and needs*, London: Jessica Kingsley.

Hall, S., Powney, J. and Davidson, P. (2000) *The Impact of Homelessness on Families*, Edinburgh: Scottish Council for Research in Education.

Harker, L. (2000) 'The provision of childcare: the shifting public/private boundaries', *New Economy*, September, 7, 3, 172–75 (4).

Harrington, V. (2000) *Underage Drinking: Findings from the 1998–9 Youth Lifestyles Survey*, Research Findings, No. 125, London: Home Office.

Harris, N. and Eden, K. with Blair, A. (2000) *Challenges to School Exclusion: Exclusion, appeals and the law*, London: Routledge Falmer.

Haselden, L., Angle, H. and Hickman, M. (1999) *Young People and Health: Health behaviour in school-aged children*, London: Health Education Authority.

Hawton, K. and Heeringen, K. (eds) (2000) *The International Handbook of Suicide and Attempted Suicide*, Chichester: John Wiley & Sons.

Hawton, K., Arensman, E. and Townsend, E. *et al.* (1998) 'Deliberate self-harm: systematic review of efficacy of psychosocial and pharmacological treatments in preventing repetition', *British Medical Journal*, 317, 441–47.

Hawton, K., Fagg, J. and Simkin, S. (1996) 'Deliberate self-poisoning and self-injury in children and adolescents under 16 years of age in Oxford, 1976–1993', *British Journal of Psychiatry*, 169, 202–08.

Hawton, K., Houston, K. and Shepperd, R. (1999) 'Suicide in young people. Study of 174 cases, aged under 25 years, based on coroners' and medical records', *British Journal of Psychiatry*, 175, 271–76.

Hayden, C. (1997) *Children Excluded from Primary School: Debates, evidence, responses*, Buckingham: Open University Press.

Hayden, C. (2000) 'Exclusion from school in England: The generation and maintenance of social exclusion', in G. Walraven, C. Parsons, D. van Veen and C. Day (eds) *Combating Social Exclusion Through Education: Laissez-faire, Authoritarianism or Third Way?* Leuvan-Apeldoorn: Garant and European Educational Research Association.

HEA (1997) *Young People and Health: Health behaviour in school-aged children: A report of the 1995 survey*, London: Health Education Authority.

HEA (1998) *Young and Active? A policy framework of young people and health-enhancing physical activity*, London: Health Education Authority.

HEA (1999) *Young People and Health: Health behaviour in school-aged children: A report of the 1997 findings*, J. London: Health Education Authority.

Health Education Board for Scotland Research Centre (2000) *Teenage Sexuality in Scotland 1989–1998*.

Health Promotion Agency for Northern Ireland (1994) *The Health Behaviour of School children in Northern Ireland: A report on the 1992 survey*, Northern Ireland: The Health Promotion Agency.

Health Promotion Agency for Northern Ireland (1995) *The Health Behaviour of School children in Northern Ireland: A report on the 1992 survey*, Northern Ireland: The Health Promotion Agency.

Health Promotion Agency for Northern Ireland (2001a) *Minds Matter: Exploring the mental well-being of young people in Northern Ireland*, Health Promotion Agency for Northern Ireland.

Health Promotion Agency for Northern Ireland (2001b) *Design for Living: Research to support young people's mental health and well-being*, Health Promotion Agency for Northern Ireland.

Health Promotion Agency for Wales (1997) *Young People in Wales: Lifestyle changes 1986–1996*, Cardiff: Health Promotion Wales, Technical Report 24.

Hendessi, M. (1992) *4 in 10. Report on young women who become homeless as a result of sexual abuse*, London: CHAR.

Hensey, D., Williams, J. and Rosenbloom, L. (1983) 'Intervention in child abuse: experience in Liverpool', *Developmental Medicine and Child Neurology*, 25, 606–11.

Heptinstall, E. (1998) 'Children at work: healthy or harmful?' in B. Pettit (ed.) *Children and Work in the UK*, London: Save the Children.

Heptinstall, E., Jewitt, K. and Sherriff, C. (1997) *Young Workers and their Accidents*, London: Child Accident Prevention Trust.

Higate, P. (2001) 'Child labour', in J. Bradshaw (ed.) (2000) *Poverty: The outcomes for children*, London: Family Policies Study Centre.

Hill, K. (1995) *The Long Sleep: Young people and suicide*, London: Virago Press.

Hill, M. and Jenkins, S. (2001) 'Poverty among British children: chronic or transitory?' in B. Bradbury, S. Jenkins and J. Micklewright (eds) *The Dynamics of Child Poverty in industrialised Countries*, Cambridge.

Hillier, L., Harrison, L. and Warr, D. (1998) ' "When you carry condoms all the boys think you want it": negotiating competing discourses about safe sex', *Journal of Adolescence*, 21, 15–29.

Hillman, M. (1999) 'The impact of transport policy on children's development', Paper presented at Canterbury Christ Church University College, 29th May 1999.

HMSO (2001) *For Scotland's Children*, J. http://www.scotland.gov.uk/library3/education.

Hobbs, S. and McKechnie, J. (1997) *Child Employment in Britain*, London: The Stationery Office.

Hobbs, S. and McKechnie, J. (1998) 'Children and work in the UK: the evidence', in (ed.) B. Pettit, *Children and Work in the UK*, London: Save the Children.

Hobcraft, J. and Kiernan, K. (1999) *Childhood Poverty, Early Motherhood and Adult Social Exclusion*, Case Paper 28, Centre for Analysis of Social Exclusion, London: LSE.

Hoffman, S. (1996) *Against the Odds: Youth homelessness in Wales*, Swansea: Shelter Cymru.

Holden, C. and MacDonald, A. (2000) *Nutrition and Child Health*, London: Harcourt:

Home Office (1997) *No More Excuses: A new approach to tackling youth crime in England and Wales*, Cmnd. 3809, London: The Stationery Office.

Home Office (2001) *2001 British Crime Survey*, London: Home Office, Research and Statistics Division.

Hood, S. (2001) *The State of London's Children Report*, Office of the Children's Rights Commissioner for London.

Horgan, G. (2001) *A Sense of Purpose: The views and experiences of young mothers in Northern Ireland about growing up*, Belfast: Save the Children.

Housing Today, 31 January 2002.

Howarth, R. (1999) *'If we don't play now, when can we?'* London: Hopscotch Asian Women's Centre.

Howarth, C., Kenway, P., Palmer, G. and Miorelli, R. (1999a) *Monitoring Poverty and Social Exclusion 1999*, Place: New Policy Institute/Joseph Rowntree Foundation.

Howarth, C., Kenway, P., Palmer, G. and Street, C. (1999b) *Monitoring Poverty and Social Exclusion: Labour's inheritance*, Place: New Policy Institute/Joseph Rowntree Foundation.

HPA (2001) *Eating for Health? A survey of eating habits among children and young people in Northern Ireland*, Belfast: The Health Promotion Agency for Northern Ireland.

Hupkens, C., Kibbe, R., Van Otterloo, A. and Drop, M. (1998) 'Class difference in the food rules mothers impose on their children: a cross-national study', *Social Science and Medicine*, 47, 9, 1331–39.

Hutson, S. (1997) *Supported Housing: The experience of care leavers*, Ilford: Barnardo's.

HVA and GMSC (1988) *Homeless Families and their Health*, London: Health Visitors Association and General Medical Services Committee.

Imich, A.J. (1994) 'Exclusions from school: current trends and issues', *Educational Research*, 36, 1, 3–11.

Ince, L. (1998) *Making it Alone: A study of the care experiences of young black people*, London: BAAF

Information and Statistics Division Scotland (2001) *Scottish health statistics 2000*, Edinburgh: ISD.

Ingenhorst, H. (2001) 'Child labour in Germany', in P. Mizen, C. Pole and A. Bolton (eds) *Hidden Hands: International perspectives on children's work and labour*, London: Routledge Falmer.

Inland Revenue (2000) *Working Families' Tax Credit Statistics: Quarterly Enquiry, UK, August 2000*, London: National Statistics.

ISD (2001) *Scottish Health Statistics 2000*, Edinburgh: Information and Statistics Division Scotland.

Istance, D. and Rees, G. (1997*) Status 0: A socio-economic study of young people on the margin*, Belfast: NIERC.

Jamieson, J., McIvor, G. and Murray, C. (1999) *Understanding Offending among Young People*, Edinburgh: The Stationery Office.

Jarvis, L. (1997) *Teenage Smoking Attitudes in 1996: An enquiry carried out by the Social Survey Division of the ONS on behalf of the HEA*, London: The Stationery Office.

Jarvis, M., Goddard, E., Higgins, V., Feyerbend, C. and Bryant, A. (2000) 'Children's exposure to passive smoking in England since the 1980s: Cotinine evidence from population surveys', *British Medical Journal*, 321, 343–45.

Jarvis, S., Towner, E. and Walsh, S. (1995) 'Accidents', in B. Botting (ed.), *The Health of our Children. Decennial supplement*, London: HMSO.

Johnson, A. and King, R. (1999) 'Can routine information systems be used to monitor serious disability?' *Archives of Disease in Childhood*, 80, 63–6.

Johnson, J., Bradshaw, J. and Burrows, R. (2001) 'The impact of life events on the well-being of young people: A secondary analysis of the British Household Panel Survey', Presented at the 2001 British Household Panel Survey Conference, The Embassy Suite Conference Centre, Colchester, Essex, 5–7 July.

Johnson, K. and colleagues (2001) *Cautions, Court Proceedings and Sentencing: England and Wales, 2000*, London: Home Office, Research and Statistics Division.

Johnston, L., MacDonald, R., Mason, P., Ridley, L. and Webster, C. (2000) *Snakes and Ladders: Young people, transitions and social exclusion*, Bristol: Policy Press.

Jones, A. (1999) *Out of Sight, Out of Mind? Homeless women speak out*, London: Crisis.

Jones, A., Pleace, N. and Quilgars, D. (2002) *An Evaluation of Homeless to Home*, London: Shelter.

Jones, A., Quilgars, D. and Wallace, A. (2001) *Life Skills Training for Homeless People: A review of the evidence*, Edinburgh: Scottish Homes.

Kaltiala-Heino, R., Rimpela, M., Marttunen, M., Rimpela, A. and Rantanen, P. (1999) 'Bullying, depression, and suicidal ideation in Finnish adolescents: schools survey', *British Medical Journal*, 319, 348–51.

Kane, R. and Wellings, K. (1999*) Reducing the Rate of Teenage Conceptions: Data from Europe,* London: Health Education Authority.

Karn, V., Mian, S., Dale, A. and Brown, M. (2001) *Tradition, change and diversity: Understanding the housing needs of minority ethnic groups in Manchester. (Insight Research Report no.37)* London: The Housing Corporation.

Kearns, A. and Parkes, A. (2001) *Neighbourhood perceptions and residential behaviour: findings from the Scottish House Condition Survey 1991–1996*, Edinburgh: Scottish Homes.

Kelly, L., Regan, L. and Burton, S. (1991) *An exploratory study of sexual abuse in a sample of 16–21 year olds*, ESRC end of award report.

Kempe Children's Center (1998) *World Perspectives on Child Abuse*, Denver: University of Colorado.

Kennedy, H. (1997) *Learning Works: Widening participation in further education*, Coventry: Further Education Funding Council.

Kennedy, L. (2001) *They Shoot Children, Don't They? An analysis of the age and gender of paramilitary "punishments" in Northern Ireland*, Belfast: Queens University unpublished paper.

Kenwright, H. (1997) *Holding Out the Safety Net: Final report of the North Yorkshire Retention Project*, York: York College of Further and Higher Education.

Kerfoot, M. (1996) 'Suicide and deliberate self-harm in children and adolescents', *Children and Society*, 10, 236–41, in J. Coleman (ed.) (1997) *Key Data on Adolescence*, Brighton: Trust for the Study of Adolescence.

Kienhorst, W.M., DeWilde, E.J. and Diekstra, R.F.W. (1995) 'Suicidal behaviour in adolescents', *Archives in Suicide Research*, 1, 185–209.

Kiernan, K. (1995) *Transition to Parenthood: Young mothers, young fathers – associated factors and later life experiences*, WSP Discussion Paper 113, Welfare State Programme Suntory-Toyota International Centre for Economics and Related Disciplines, London: LSE.

Kilkey, M. (2000) *Lone Mothers between Paid Work and Care: The policy regime in 20 countries*, Ashgate: Aldershot.

Kilpatrick, R., Barr, A. and Wylie, C. (1999) *The 1996/97 Northern Ireland Suspension and Expulsion Study*, DENI Research Report Series No. 12, Belfast: Department of Education Northern Ireland.

King, J. and Taitz, L. (1985) 'Catch-up growth following abuse', *Archives of Disease in Childhood*, 60, 1152–54.

Kirk, S. (1998) 'Families' experiences of caring at home for a technology-dependent child: a review of the literature', *Child: Care, Health and Development*, 24, 101–14.

Koprowska, J. and Stein, M. (2000) 'The mental health of looked after young people', in P. Aggleton, J. Hurry and I. Warwick (eds) *Young People and Mental Health*, Chichester: Wiley.

Kremer, J., Trew, K. and Ogle, S. (eds) (1997) *Young People's Involvement in Sport*, London: Routledge.

Kumar, V. (1995) *Poverty and Inequality in the UK: The effects on children*, London: National Children's Bureau.

Kurtz, Z. (1996) *Treating Children Well*, London: Mental Health Foundation.

La Valle, I., Finch, S., Nove, A. and Lewin, C. (2000) *Parents' Demand for Childcare*, DfEE Research Report 176, Nottingham: DfEE Publications.

LaGreca, A.M., Siegel, L.J., Wallander, J.L. and Walker, C.E. (1992) *Stress and Coping in Child Health*, New York: The Guilford Press.

Land, H. (1999) 'New Labour New Families?', in H. Dean and R. Woods (eds) *Social Policy Review 11*, SPA, Luton: Critical Social Policy article on Family Policy.

Lansdown, G. (2000) 'Implementing children's rights and health', *Archives of Disease in Childhood*, 83, 286–88.

Lavalette, M. (1998) 'Child labour: Historical, legislative and policy context', in B. Pettit (ed.) *Children and Work in the UK*, London: Save the Children.

Lavalette, M. (ed.) (1999) *A Thing of the Past? Child labour in Britain in the Nineteenth and Twentieth Centuries*, Liverpool: Liverpool University Press.

Leach, P. (1999) *The Physical Punishment of Children. Some input from recent research*, London: National Society for the Prevention of Cruelty for Children.

Leather, P. and Morrison, T. (1997) *The State of UK Housing: A factfile on dwelling conditions*, Bristol: Policy Press.

Leather, S. (1997) 'Food poverty: The making of modern malnutrition', *Health Visitor*, 20, 21–24.

Leather, S. (2000) 'Poverty and food: will the Food Standards Agency make a difference?', *Poverty*, Child Poverty Action Group 107, 11–13.

Lee, M. and O'Brien, R. (1995) *The Game's Up: Redefining child prostitution*, London: The Children's Society.

Lee, P. and Murie, A. (1997) *Poverty, Housing Tenure and Social Exclusion*, Bristol: Policy Press/Joseph Rowntree Foundation.

Lemos and Crane (2001) *Mediation and Homelessness: A review of the literature and the views of service providers in Scotland*, Edinburgh: Scottish Homes.

Leonard, M. (1998) 'Children's contribution to the household income', in B. Pettit (ed.) *Children and Work in the UK*, London: Child Poverty Action Group.

Leonard, M. (1999) *Play Fair with Working Children*, Belfast: Save the Children.

Leonard, M. and Davey, C. (2001) *Thoughts on the 11 Plus: A research report examining children's experiences of the transfer test*, Belfast: Save the Children.

Lewis, G. and Wilkinson, G. (1993) 'Another British disease? A recent increase in the prevalence of psychiatric morbidity', *Journal of Epidemiology and Community Health*, 47, 5, 358–61.

Liebling, A. (1992) *Suicides in Prisons*, London: Routledge.

Lightfoot, J., Mukherjee, S. and Sloper, P. (1999) 'Supporting pupils in mainstream school with an illness or disability', *Child: care, health and development*, 25, 4, 267–83.

Lindsey, D. and Trocme, N. (1994) 'Have child protection efforts reduced child homicides? An examination of data from Britain and North America', *British Journal of Social Work*, 24, 714–32.

Lloyd, G., Stead, J. and Kendrick, A. (2001) *Hanging on in there: A study of inter-agency work to prevent school exclusion in three local authorities*, London: National Children's Bureau.

Lobstein, T. (1997) ' "If they don't eat a healthy diet it's their own fault." Myths about Food and low income', National Food Alliance in GCCNI (2001) *Hungry for Change – Community Action to tackle Food Poverty*, The Price of Being Poor Report 1, General Consumer Council Northern Ireland.

Local Authority Caterers Association (2000) 'New nutrition guidelines published by the DfEE' – www.laca.co.uk/news.htm – accessed 21 November 2001.

London Research Centre (1997) *Atmospheric Emissions Inventories for Four Urban areas*, London: DETR.

Lumey, L.H. (1992) 'Decreased birthweights in infants after maternal *in utero* exposure to the Dutch famine', *Paediatric and Perinatal Epidemiology*, 6: 240–253.

Lynch, J.W., Kaplan, G.A. and Salonen, J.T. (1997) 'Why do poor people behave poorly? Variation in adult health behaviours and psychosocial characteristics by stages of the socio-economic lifecourse', *Social Science and Medicine*, 44, 6, 809–19.

Maclean (2000) 'McLean Researchers Document Brain Damage Linked to Child Abuse and Neglect', www.mclean.harvard.edu/PublicAffairs/2000 1214_child_abuse.htm

Madge, N. (1996) 'Suicide behaviour in children and young people', *Highlight*, No. 144, London: National Children's Bureau and Barnardo's.

Madge, N. and Harvey, J.G. (1999) 'Suicide among the young –the size of the problem', *Journal of Adolescence*, 22, 145–55.

Mahon, A. and Higgins, J. (1995) *A Life of Our Own: An Evaluation of Three RHA Funded Projects in Merseyside*, Manchester: University of Manchester.

Mansurov, V. (2001) 'Child labour in Russia', in C. Pole and A. Bolton (eds) *Hidden Hands: International perspectives on children's work and labour*, London: Routledge Falmer.

Mapstone, E. (1969) 'Children in care', *Concern*, 3, 23–28.

Marsh, A. and Kennett, P. (1999) 'Exploring the new terrain', in P. Kennett and A. Marsh (eds) *Homelessness: Exploring the new terrain*, Bristol: Policy Press.

Marsh, A., Gordon, D., Pantazis, C. and Heslop, P. (1999) *Home Sweet Home? The Impact of Poor Housing on Health*, Bristol: Policy Press.

Martin, I. and Coalter, F. (2000) *Sports Participation in Scotland, 1999*, Edinburgh: Sports Scotland.

Martinez, P. and Munday, F. (1998) *9,000 Voices: Student persistence and drop out in further education*, London: Further Education Development Agency.

Marttunen, M.J., Hillevi, M. and Lonnqvist, J.K. (1992) 'Adolescent suicide: endpoint of long-term difficulties', *Journal of the American Academy of Child and Adolescent Psychiatry*, 31, 649–54.

Matthews, M., Taylor, M., Percy-Smith, B. and Limb, M. (2001) 'The unacceptable *flaneur*: The shopping mall as a teenage hangout', *Childhood* 7, 3, 279–294.

Matthews, A. and Truscott, P. (1990) *Disability, Household Income and Expenditure: A follow-up survey of disabled adults in the Family Expenditure Survey*, DSS Research Report No. 2, London: HMSO.

Matthews, H. (2001) *Children and Community Regeneration: Creating better neighbourhoods*, London: Save the Children.

Matthews, H. and Limb, M. (undated) *Exploring the 'Fourth Environment': Young people's use of place and views on their environment*, ESRC award L129251031 www.regard.ac.uk

Matthews, M.H. (1992) *Making Sense of Place: Children's understanding of large-scale environments*, Hemel Hempstead: Harvester Wheatsheaf.

Maung, N. (1995) *Young People, Victimisation and the Police: British Crime Survey findings on experiences and attitudes of 12 to 15 year olds*, London: HMSO.

McCallum, I. (1993) *Testing 7 year olds – performance and context: Projecting school rolls and assessing performance*, London: London Research Centre.

McCann, J.B., James, A., Wilson, S. and Dunn, G. (1996) 'Prevalence of psychiatric disorders in young people in the care system', *British Journal of Psychiatry*, 31, 3, 1529–30.

McClure, G.M. (2000) 'Changes in suicide in England and Wales 1960–1997', *British Journal of Psychiatry*, 176, 64–67.

McClure, G.M. (2001) 'Suicide in children and adolescents in England and Wales, 1970–1998', *British Journal of Psychiatry*, 178, 469–74.

McCoy, D. and Smith, M. (1992) *The Prevalence of Disability Among Adults in Northern Ireland*, PPRU.

McCrum, J. (2001) *Homeless Families: Homeless children*, Belfast: Simon Community, Northern Ireland.

McGee, C. (2000) *Childhood Experiences of Domestic Violence*, London: Jessica Kingsley.

McGuigan, W.M. and Pratt, C.C. (2001) 'The predictive impact of domestic violence on three types of child maltreatment', *Child Abuse and Neglect*, 25, 869–83.

McKechnie, J. and Hobbs, S. (1998a) *Working Children: Reconsidering the debates*, Reflections on the work of the International Working Group on Child Labour, DCI, ISPCAN.

McKechnie, J. and Hobbs, S. (1998b) 'Working children: the health and safety issue', *Children and Society*, 12, 38–47.

McKechnie, J. and Hobbs, S. (2001) 'Work and education', in P. Mizen, C. Pole and A. Bolton (eds) *Hidden Hands: International perspectives on children's work and labour*, London: Routledge Falmer.

McMurray, R.G., Harrell, J.S., Deng, S., Bradley, C.B., Cox, L.M. and Bangdiwala, S.I. (2000) 'The influence of physical activity, socio-economic status, and ethnicity on the weight status of adolescents', *Obesity Research*, 8, 2, 130–39.

McQuiod, J. (1994) 'The self-reported delinquency study on Belfast, Northern Ireland', in J. Junger-Tas, *et al.* (ed.) *Delinquent Behaviour amongst Young People in the Western World*, Amsterdam: Kluger Publications.

McVicar, D. (2000) *Young People and Social Exclusion in Northern Ireland: Status 0 four years on*, Belfast: NIERC.

Meadows, S. and Dawson, N. (1996) *Teenage Mothers and Their Children: Factors affecting their health and development*, London: Department of Health.

Mehanni, M., Cullen, A., Kiberd, B., McDonnell, M., O'Regan, M. and Matthews, T. (2000) 'The current epidemiology of SIDS in Ireland', *Irish Medical Journal*, 93: 264–268.

Melrose, M., Barrett, D. and Brodie, I. (1999) *One Way Street? Retrospectives on Childhood Prostitution*, London: The Children's Society.

Meltzer, H. and Gatward, R. with Goodman, R. and Ford, T. (2000) *Mental Health of Children and Adolescents in Great Britain*, London: The Stationery Office.

Mental Health Foundation (1996) *Off to a Bad Start*, London: Mental Health Foundation.

Mental Health Foundation (1997) *Joint Policy Statement on Race and Mental Health, a briefing from the Mental Health Foundation*, London: Mental Health Foundation.

Mental Health Foundation (1999) *Bright Futures: Promoting children and young people's mental health*, London: Mental Health Foundation.

Meyrick, J. and Swann, C. (1998) *Reducing the Rate of Teenage Conceptions: An overview of the effectiveness of interventions*, London: Health Education Authority.

Middleton, S. and Loumidis, J. (2001) 'Young people, poverty and part-time work', in P. Mizen, C. Pole and A. Bolton (eds) *Hidden Hands: International perspectives on children's work and labour*, London: Routledge Falmer.

Middleton, S. and Shropshire, J. (1998) 'Earning your keep? Children's work and contributions to family budgets', in B. Pettit (ed.) *Children and Work in the UK*, London: Child Poverty Action Group.

Miles, G. and Eid, S. (1987) 'The dietary habits of young people', *Nursing Times*, 93, 50, 46–48.

Millham, S., Bullock, R., Hosie, K. and Haak, M. (1986) *Lost in Care: The problem of maintaining links between children in care and their families*, Aldershot: Gower.

Milner, J. and Blyth, E. (1999) 'Theoretical debates and legislative framework', in E. Blyth and J. Milner (eds) *Improving School Attendance*, London: Routledge.

Ministry of the Environment, Finland (2001) *Housing Statistics in the European Union* Delft, Ministry of the Environment, Finland/ Ministry of Housing, Netherlands. Accessible on http://www.euhousing.org/EU_Home.taf (correct 15/5/02)

Minty, B. (1987) *Child Care and Adult Crime*, Manchester: Manchester University Press.

Mirrlees-Black, C (1999) *Domestic Violence: Findings from a new BCS self-completion questionnaire*, London: Home Office.

Mitchell, R., Dorling, D. and Shaw, M. (2000) *Inequalities in Life and Death: What if Britain were more equal?*, Bristol: Policy Press.

Mittler, P. (2000) *Working Towards Inclusive Education: Social Contexts*, London: David Fulton.

Mizen, P., Bolton, A. and Pole, C. (1998) 'The paid employment of children in Britain: Sociological themes and issues'. Paper to Working Group 03, International Sociological Association World Congress, Montreal, Canada, August 1998.

Mizen, P., Pole, C. and Bolton, A. (eds) (2001a) *Hidden Hands: International perspectives on children's work and labour*, London: Routledge Falmer.

Mizen, P., Pole, C. and Bolton, A. (2001b) 'Why be a school age worker?', in P. Mizen, C. Pole, and A. Bolton (eds) *Hidden Hands: International perspectives on children's work and labour*, London: Routledge Falmer.

Mooney, A., Knight, A., Moss, P. and Owen, C. (2001) *Who Cares? Childminding in the 1990s*, London: Family Policy Studies Centre, for the Joseph Rowntree Foundation.

Morgan, M.Z. and Evans, M.R. (1998) 'Initiatives to improve a childhood immunisation uptake: a randomised controlled trial', *British Medical Journal*, 316, 1570–71.

Morrison, A., Stone, D.H. and the EURORISC Working Group (1999a) 'Unintentional injury mortality in Europe 1984–93: a report from the EURORISC Working Group', *Injury Prevention*, 5: 171–176.

Morrison, A., Stone, D.H. and Redpath *et al.* (1999b) 'Trend analysis of social economic differentials in deaths from injury in childhood in Scotland, 1981–1995', *British Medical Journal*, 318, 7, 1893.

Mortimore, J. and Blackstone, T. (1982) *Disadvantage and Education*, Aldershot: Gower.

Moss, P. (2001) *The UK at the Crossroads: Towards an early years European partnership*, Paper 2 in the Daycare Trust 'Facing the Future Policy Papers Series', London: Daycare Trust.

Motion, C. (2000) 'Breaking the cycle of homelessness in West Lothian: A study of repeat homelessness', Dissertation submitted for the Diploma in Housing Studies, Department of Applied Social Science, University of Stirling.

Mullender, A. (2000) *Reducing domestic violence . . . what works?*, London: Home Office.

Mumford, K. (2000) *Talking to Families in East London*, CASE Brief 19, London: London School of Economics.

Munn, P., Lloyd, G. and Cullen, M.A. (2000) *Alternatives to Exclusion from School*, London: Paul Chapman Publishing Ltd.

Munton, A.G., La Valle, A., Barreau, S., Pickering, K. and Pitson, L. (2001) *Feasibility Study for a Longitudinal Survey of the Impact of Out of School Childcare of Children*, DfES Research Report RR319, Nottingham: DfES Publications.

Myers, W. and Boyden, J. (1998) *Child Labour: Promoting the best interests of working children,* London: International Save the Children Alliance.

National Audit Office (2001a) *Improving Student Performance: How English further education colleges can improve student retention and achievement*, London: The Stationery Office.

National Audit Office (2001b) *Tackling Obesity in England*, Report by the Controller and Auditor General, HC220 Session 2000–2001, London: The Stationery Office.

National Childcare Strategy Task Force (2001) *Task Force Report*, 21 October 2001, http://www.wales.gov.uk/show.dbs

National Playing Fields Association (2000) *Best Play*, National Playing Fields Association.

National Runaway Switchboard (2001) *Runaway Prevention Curriculum*, National Runaway Switchboard.

NCH (2000) *Factfile 2000*, London: National Children's Homes.

NCH (2001) *Factfile 2001*, London: National Children's Homes.

Needleman, H. and Gastonis, C. (1990) 'Low level lead exposure and the IQ of children', *Journal of the American Medical Association*, 263.

Nettleton, S. and Burrows, R. (2000) 'When a capital investment becomes an emotional loss: the health consequences of the experience of mortgage possession in England', *Housing Studies*, 15, 3, 463–79.

Nettleton, S., Burrows, R., England, J. and Seavers, J. (2000) *Losing the Family Home: Understanding the social consequences of mortgage repossession*, York: York Publishing Services.

New TSN Unit (2000) *Making it Work. The second new TSN Annual Report*, http:www.newtsnni.gov.uk/making it work/action_plans/de_4.htm – accessed 12 February 2002.

New TSN Unit (2001) *Consultation with Travellers on the Recommendations of the Final Report of the PSI Working Group on Travellers*.

Newburn, T. (1999) *Disaffected Young People in Poor Neighbourhoods: A review of the literature*, Paper commissioned by Policy Action Team12, London.

Newburn, T. and Shiner, M. (2001) *Young People and Alcohol: A review of the literature*, York: Joseph Rowntree Foundation.

Newman, C. (1989) *Young Runaways: Findings from Britain's first safe house*, London: The Children's Society.

Newman, T. (2000) 'Workers and helpers: Perspectives on children's labour 1899–1999', *British Journal of Social Work*, 30, 323–38.

Newson, J. and Newson, E. (1989) *The extent of parental physical punishment in the UK*, London: Approach.

NHS Centre for Reviews and Dissemination (1996) 'Preventing unintentional injuries in children and young people', University of York: NHS CRD.

NHS Centre for Reviews and Dissemination (1997) 'Preventing and reducing the effects of unplanned teenage pregnancies', *Effective Health Care Bulletin*, 3, 1, 1–12.

NHS Centre for Reviews and Dissemination (2001) *Undertaking Systematic Reviews of Research on Effectiveness*, CRD Report Number 4 (2nd Edition), March 2001, University of York.

NHS Health Advisory Service (1995) *Child and Adolescent Mental Health Services: Together we stand: the commissioning, role and management of child and adolescent mental health services*, London: HMSO.

Nicoll, A., Ellimna, D. and Begg, N.T. (1989) 'Immunisation: Causes of failure and strategies and tactics for success', *British Medical Journal*, 299, 808–12.

NIHE (2001) *Homelessness Strategy and Services Review: Summary report*, Northern Ireland Housing Executive.

NISRA (1996) *Mid-year Estimates of Population, 1995*, Belfast: Demography and Methodology Branch, Northern Ireland Statistics and Research Agency.

NISRA (2000a) *The Annual Report of the Registrar General*, Belfast: General Register Office for Northern Ireland.

NISRA (2000b) *Community Statistics 1 April 1999 – 31 March 2000*, Northern Ireland Statistics and Research Agency, London: National Statistics.

NISRA (2001a) *The Annual Report of the Registrar General*, Belfast: General Register Office for Northern Ireland.

NISRA (2001b) *Report of the Promoting Social Exclusion Working Group on Travellers*, Belfast: New Targeting Social Need Unit. Accessible on www.newtsnni.gov.uk/consultation/travellers_in_ni.htm (correct 15/5/02).

NISRA (2002) *Young Persons' Behaviour and Attitudes Survey Bulletin. October 2000–November 2000*, Northern Ireland Statistics and Research Agency website. Tables also accessed via: www.ofmdfmni.gov.uk

Nobes, G. and Smith, M. (1997) 'Physical punishment of children in two-parent families', *Clinical Child Psychology and Psychiatry*, 2, 2, 271–81.

Nobes, G. and Smith, M. (2000) 'The relative extent of physical punishment and abuse by mothers and fathers', *Trauma, Violence and Abuse*, 1, 1, 47–66.

O'Brien, M. (1998) *Space for Children: Patterns of family life for the children of the 1990s*, Professional Lecture Series, London: University of North London.

O'Brien, M., Jones, D., Sloan, D. and Rustin, M. (2000) 'Children's independent spatial mobility in the urban public realm', *Childhood*, 7, 3, 253–77.

O'Dea, J. and Caputi, P. (2001) 'Association between socio-economic status, weight, age and gender and the body image and weight control practices of

6 to 19 year old children and adolescents', *Health Education Research*, 16, 5, 521–32.

O'Donnell, C. and White, L. (1998) *Invisible Hands: Child employment in North Tyneside,* London: Low Pay Unit.

O'Donnell, C. and White, L. (1999) *Hidden Danger: Injuries to children at work in Britain,* London: Low Pay Unit.

O'Keefe, D. (1994) *Truancy in English Secondary School,* London: HMSO.

O'Mahony, D. and Deazley, R. (2000) *Juvenile Crime and Justice*, Belfast: The Stationery Office.

OECD (1998) 'Recent labour market developments and prospects', *Employment Outlook*, June.

OECD (2001) *Society at a Glance: OECD Social Indicators*, Paris: OECD.

Office for National Statistics (2002) *Living in Britain: Results from the 2000 General Household Survey,* London: The Stationery Office.

Office for National Statistics (England and Wales) *Mortality Statistics,* ICD Codes E950–9 plus E980–9 minus E988.8.

OFSTED (1996) *Exclusions from Secondary Schools 1995/6,* London: The Stationery Office.

OFSTED (1999) *Raising the Attainment of Minority Ethnic Pupils,* London: Office for Standards in Education.

OFSTED (2001) *Improving Attendance and Behaviour in Secondary Schools*, London: Office for Standards in Education.

OFSTED (2002) *Standards and Quality in Education 2000/01,* London: Office for Standards in Education.

Oldman, C. and Beresford, B. (1998) *Homes Unfit for Children: Disabled children and their families,* Bristol and York: Policy Press and Joseph Rowntree Foundation.

Oliver, M. (1990) *The Politics of Disablement*, London: Macmillan.

ONS (1996) *Mid-1995 Population Estimates for England and Wales*, Population and Health Monitor PP1 96/2, London: Government Statistical Service.

ONS (1997) *Mortality Statistics: Childhood, infant and perinatal. Review of the Registrar General on deaths in England and Wales, 1999*, Series DH3 No. 28, London: The Stationery Office.

ONS (1998) *Mortality Statistics: Childhood, infant and perinatal. Review of the Registrar General on deaths in England and Wales, 1999*, Series DH3 No. 29, London: The Stationery Office.

ONS (1998a) *Key Health Statistics from General Practice 1996*, Series MB6 No. 1, London: Office for National Statistics.

ONS (1999) *Mortality Statistics: Childhood, infant and perinatal. Review of the Registrar General on deaths in England and Wales, 1999*, Series DH3 No. 30, London: The Stationery Office.

ONS (2000) *Mortality Statistics: Childhood, infant and perinatal. Review of the Registrar General on deaths in England and Wales, 1999*, Series DH3 No. 31, London: The Stationery Office.

ONS (2000a) 'Infant mortality: by social class, 1981, 1991, 1996 and 1997', *Social Trends Dataset*, London: ONS.

ONS (2000b) *Regional Trends, No. 35*, London: The Stationery Office.

ONS (2000c) *Annual Abstracts of Statistics: 2000*, Office for National Statistics, London: The Stationery Office.

ONS (2000d) 'Annual Update: morbidity and treatment data from general practice, 1998 (England and Wales)', *Health Statistics Quarterly*, 08, Winter 2000.

ONS (2000e) *Regional Trends 35: 2000 edition*, London: The Stationery Office.

ONS (2000f) *Social Focus on Young People*, London: Office for National Statistics.

ONS (2001a) *Mortality Statistics: Childhood, infant and perinatal. Review of the Registrar General on deaths in England and Wales, 1999*, Series DH3 No. 32, London: The Stationery Office.

ONS (2001b) *Health Statistics Quarterly*, Autumn, London: The Stationery Office.

ONS (2001c) *Children's Day Care Facilities at 31 March 2001, England* (Provisional Estimates), London: The Stationery Office.

ONS (2001d) *Regional Trends, 36: 2001 edition*, London: The Stationery Office.

ONS (2001e) *Report: Conceptions in England and Wales, 1999*, London: The Stationery Office.

OPCS (1988) *Occupational Mortality: Childhood Supplement 179–80, 1982–83*, Series DS, No. 8. London: HMSO.

Organisation for Security and Co-operation in Europe (2000) *Report on the Situation of Roma and Sinti in the OSCE Area*, The Hague: OSCE.

Osler, A., Watling, R., Busher, H., Cole, T. and White, A. (2001) *DfEE Research Brief No.244: Reasons for Exclusion from School*, Nottingham: DfEE Publications.

Oxley, H., Dang, T., Forster, M. and Pellizzari, M. (2001) 'Income inequalities and poverty among children and households with children in selected

OECD countries', in K. Vleminckx and T. Smeeding (eds) *Child well-being, child poverty and child policy in modern nations*, Bristol: Policy Press.

Packman, J. (1968) *Child Care Needs and Numbers*, London: Allen and Unwin.

Packman, J. and Hall, C. (1998) *From Care to Accommodation: Support, protection and control in child care services*, London: The Stationery Office.

Packman, J. with Randall, J. and Jacques, N. (1986) *Who Needs Care? Social work decisions about children*, Oxford: Blackwell.

Palmer, T. (2001) *No Son of Mine! Children abused through prostitution*, London: Barnardo's.

Parker, G. and Olsen, R. (1995) *A Sideways Glance at Young Carers*, Leicester: University of Leicester, Nuffield Community Care Studies Unit.

Parker, H. (1998) 'Low cost but acceptable – A minimum income standard for the UK: families with young children', Family Budget Unit in GCCNI (2001) *Hungry for Change – Community Action to tackle Food Poverty*, The Price of Being Poor Report 1, General Consumer Council Northern Ireland.

Parker, H., Aldridge, J. and Measham, F. (1998) *Illegal Leisure: The normalisation of adolescent recreational drug use*, London: Routledge.

Parsons, C. (1998) 'The costs of school exclusion', in N. Donovan (ed.), *Second Chances: Exclusion from school and equality of opportunity*, London: New Policy Institute.

Parsons, C. (1999) *Education, Exclusion and Citizenship*, London: Routledge.

Parsons, C. (2000) 'The third way to educational and social exclusion', in G. Walraven, C. Parsons, D. van Veen and D. Day (eds) *Combating Social Exclusion Through Education: Laissez-faire, authoritarianism or third way?*, Leuvan-Apeldoorn: Garant and European Educational Research Association.

Parsons, C. and Howlett, K. (2000) *Investigating the Reintegration of Permanently Excluded Young People in England*, Ely: Include.

Parsons, L. (1991) 'Homeless families in Hackney', *Public Health*, 105, 287–96.

Patterson, L. (1992) 'Social class in Scottish Education', in S. Brown (ed.) *Class, Race and Gender in Schools*, Glasgow: Scottish Council for Research into Education.

Pawson, H. (2000) *A Profile of Homelessness in Scotland*, Edinburgh: Scottish Homes.

Pawson, H., Third, H., Dudleston, A., Littlewood, M. and Tate, J. (2001) *Repeat Homelessness in Scotland*, Edinburgh: Scottish Homes.

Payne, J. (1998) *Routes at Sixteen: Trends and choices in the Nineties*, London: Department for Education and Employment.

Pettit, B. (ed.) (1998) *Children and Work in the UK*, London: Save the Children.

Pfeffer, C.R., Hurt, S.W., Peskin, J.R. and Siefker, C.A. (1995) 'Suicidal children grow up: ego functions associated with suicide attempts', *Journal of the American Academy of Child and Adolescent Psychiatry*, 34, 1318–25.

PHLS AIDS Centre and Scottish Centre for Infection and Environmental Health (2002) *Aids/HIV Quarterly Surveillance Tables: Cumulative UK data to end December 2001*, London: Public Health Laboratory Service.

PHLS, DHSSPS and the Scottish ISD(D)S Collaborative Group (2000) *Trends in Sexually Transmitted Infections in the United Kingdom, 1990–1999*, London: Public Health Laboratory Service.

Piachaud, D. (2001) 'Child poverty, opportunities and quality of life', *The Political Quarterly*, 72, 4, 446–53.

Pilgrim, S., Fenton, S., Hughes, T., Hine, C. and Tibbs, N. (1993) *The Bristol Black and Ethnic Minorities Health Survey Report*, Bristol: The University of Bristol.

Pinkerton, J. and McCrea, R. (1999) *Meeting The Challenge? Young People Leaving Care In Northern Ireland*, Aldershot: Ashgate.

Plass, P.S. and Hotaling, G.T. (1995) 'The intergenerational transmission of running away – childhood experiences of the parents of runaways', *Journal of Youth and Adolescence*, 24, 3.

Platt, S., Backett, S. and Kreitman, N. (1988) 'Social construction or causal ascription: distinguishing suicide from undetermined deaths', *Sociology Psychiatry and Psychiatric Epidemiology*, 23, 217–21 in K. Hill (1995) *The Long Sleep: Young people and suicide*, London: Virago Press.

Platt, S.D., Martin, C.I., Hunt, S.M. and Lewis, C.W. (1989) 'Damp housing, mould growth and symptomatic health state', *British Medical Journal*, 298, 1673–78.

Pleace, N., Jones, A. and England, J. (2000) *Access to General Practice for People Sleeping Rough*, York: University of York, Centre for Housing Policy

Pless Mulloli, T. (1999) *Do Particulates from Open Cast Mining Impair Children's Health?*, London: Department of Health.

Plowden Committee (1967) *Children and their Primary Schools: A report of the Central Advisory Council for Education*, London: HMSO.

Pond, C. and Searle, A. (1991) *The Hidden Army: Children at work in the 1990s*,

London: Birmingham City Council Education Department and the Low Pay Unit.

Prescott-Clarke, P. and Primatesta, P. (eds) (1999) *Health Survey for England 97, The Health of Young People '95–97*, London: The Stationery Office.

Pritchard, C. (1992) 'Children's homicide as an indicator of effective child protection: a comparative study of Western European statistics', *British Journal of Social Work*, 22, 663–84.

Provisional Results of the 2001 Pre-School and Day care Census. www.scotland.gov.uk/stats/bulletins/00107–00.asp

Quilgars, D. (2001a) 'Child homelessness', in J. Bradshaw (ed.) *Poverty: The Outcomes for Children*, London: Family Policy Studies Centre.

Quilgars, D. (2001b) 'Childhood accidents', in J. Bradshaw (ed.) *Poverty: The Outcomes for Children,* London: Family Policy Studies Centre.

Quinn, M.J. and Babb, P.J. (2000) 'Cancer trends in England and Wales', *Health Statistics Quarterly*, 08, 2000, 5–19.

Quinn, M.J., Babb, P.J., Kirby, E.A. and Brock, A. (2000) 'Report: registrations of cancer diagnosed in 1994–1997, England and Wales', *Health Statistics Quarterly*, 07, 2000, 71–82.

Quinton, D. and Rutter, M. (1988). *Parenting Breakdown: The making and breaking of inter-generational links*, Aldershot: Avebury.

Rabiee, P., Priestley and Knowles, J. (2001) *Whatever Next? Young disabled people leaving care*, Leeds: First Key.

Race Equality Unit (1996) 'Race, culture and the prevention of child abuse', in NCIPCA, *Childhood Matters: Vol 2. Background Papers*, London: The Stationery Office.

Raffe, D. (2000) *'Home International' Comparisons of Post-16 Education and Training*, Edinburgh: Centre for Educational Sociology, University of Edinburgh.

Rahman, M., Palmer, G. and Kenway, P. (2001) *Monitoring Poverty and Social Exclusion 2001*, York: Joseph Rowntree Foundation.

Rahman, M., Palmer, G., Kenway, P. and Howard, C. (2000) *Monitoring Poverty and Social Exclusion 2000*, York: Joseph Rowntree Foundation.

Raleigh, V.S. (1995) *Mental Health in Black and Minority Ethnic People: The fundamental facts*, London: The Mental Health Foundation.

Ramsay, M. and Partridge, S. (1999). *Drug Misuse Declared in 1998: Results from the British Crime Survey*, Home Office Research Study 197, London: Home Office.

Ramsay, M. and Spiller, J. (1997) *Drug Misuse Declared: Latest results of the*

British Crime Survey, Research Study No. 172, London: Home Office Research and Statistics Directorate.

Ramsay, M., Baker, P., Goulden, C., Sharp, C. and Sondhi, A. (2001) *Drug Misuse Declared in 2000: Results from the British Crime Survey*, London: Home Office, Research, Development and Statistics Directorate.

Randall, G. (1988) *No Way Home*, London: Centrepoint.

Randall, G. (1989) *Homeless and Hungry*, London: Centrepoint.

Randall, V. (2000) *The Politics of Child Daycare in Britain*, Oxford: Oxford University Press.

Rangasami, J.J., Greenwood, D.C., McSporran, B., Smail, P.J., Patterson, C.C. and Waugh, N.R. on behalf of the Scottish Study Group for the Care of Young Diabetics (1997) 'Rising incidence of type 1 diabetes in Scottish children: 1984–93', *Archives of Disease in Childhood*, 77: 210–13.

Raw, G. and Hamilton, R. (1995) *Building regulation and health*, Watford, Building Research Establishment.

Raws, P. (2001) *Lost Youth: Young runaways in Northern Ireland*, Belfast: The Children's Society.

Reading, R., Colver, A., Openshaw, S. and Jarvis, S. (1994) 'Do interventions that improve immunisation uptake also reduce social inequalities in uptake?', *British Medical Journal*, 308, 1142–44 (30 April).

Rees, G. (1993) *Hidden Truths: Young people's experiences of running away*, London: The Children's Society.

Rees, G. and Rutherford, C. (2001) *Home Run: Families and young runaways*, London: The Children's Society.

Rees, G. and Smeaton, E. (2001) *Child Runaways: Under 11s running away in the UK*, London: The Children's Society.

Rees, G. and Stein, M. (1999) *The Abuse of Adolescents within the Family*, London: National Society for the Prevention of Cruelty to Children.

Registrar General for Scotland (1996) *Mid-1995 Population Estimates Scotland*, Edinburgh: HMSO.

Reid, K. (1999) *Truancy and Schools*, London: Routledge.

Reidpath, D.D., Burns, C., Garrard, J., Mahoney, M. and Townsend, M. (in press) 'An ecological study of the relationship between social and environmental determinants of obesity', *Health and Place*.

Revell, K. and Leather, P. (2000) *The State of UK Housing*, Bristol and York: Policy Press and Joseph Rowntree Foundation.

Roberts, H. (1996) 'Child accidents at home, school and play', in B. Gillham and J. A. Thomson (eds) *Child Safety: Problems and prevention from preschool to adolescence*, London: Routledge.

Roberts, H. (2000) *What Works in Reducing Health Inequalities in Child Health*, London: Barnardo's.

Roberts, I. and Pless, B. (1995) 'Social policy as a cause of childhood accidents: the children of lone mothers', *British Medical Journal*, 311, 925–28.

Roberts, I. and Power, C. (1996) 'Does the decline in child injury mortality vary by social class? A comparison of class specific mortality in 1981 and 1991', *British Medical Journal*, 313, 784–86.

Roberts, K. (1995) *Youth and Employment in Modern Britain*, Oxford: Oxford University Press.

Robertson, M. and Walford, R. (2000) 'Views and visions of land use in the UK', *The Geographical Journal*, 166, 3, 239–54.

Rosano, A., Botto, L.D., Botting, B. and Mastroiacovo, P. (2000) 'Infant mortality and congenital anomalies from 1950 to 1994: an international perspective', *Journal of Epidemiology and Community Health*, 54: 660–666.

Rowe, J., Cain, H., Hundleby, M. and Keane, A. (1984) *Long Term Foster Care*, London: Batsford.

Rowe, J., Hundleby, M. and Garnett, L. (1989) *Child Care Now: A survey of placement patterns* (Research Series 6), London: British Agencies for Adoption and Fostering.

Rowlands, O. (1998) *Informal Carers*, London: The Stationery Office.

Royal Belfast Hospital/Queen's University Belfast (1990) *Child Sexual Abuse in Northern Ireland. A Research Study of Incidence*, Antrim: Greystone Books.

Royal Commission on Environmental Pollution (1997) *Transport and the Environment: Developments since 1994*, London: The Stationery Office.

Russell, D. (1984) *Sexual Exploitation*, Beverley Hills: Sage.

Rutter, M. and Smith, D.J. (1995) 'Towards causal explanations of time trends in psychosocial disorders of young people', in M. Rutter and D. J. Smith (eds) *Psychosocial Disorders of Youth*, New York: John Wiley & Sons.

Rutter, M., Giller, H. and Hagell, A. (1999) *Antisocial Behaviour by Young People*, Cambridge: Cambridge University Press.

Ruxton, S. (1996) *Children in Europe*, London: National Children's Homes.

Safe on the Streets Research Team (1999) *Still Running: Children on the streets in the UK*, London: The Children's Society.

Salmon, G., James, A. and Smith, D.M. (1998) 'Bullying in schools: Self reported anxiety, depression, and self-esteem in secondary school children', *British Medical Journal*, 317, 924–25.

Samaritans (2001) *Information Resource Pack 2001*, Slough: Samaritans – www.samaritans.org

Sammons, P. (1995) 'Gender, ethnic and socio-economic differences in attainment and progress: a longitudinal analysis of student achievement over nine years', *British Educational Research Journal*, 21, 4.

Sammons, P., West, A. and Hind, A. (1997) 'Accounting for variation in pupil attainment at the end of Key Stage 1', *British Educational Research Journal*, 23, 4, 490–511.

Sanford, L. (1991) *Strong at the Broken Places: Overcoming the trauma of childhood abuse*, London: Virago.

Saunders, L. and Broad, B. (1997) *The Health Needs of Young People Leaving Care*, Leicester: De Montfort University.

Save the Children (1996) *Breaking Barriers, Building Futures*, http://www.savethechildren.org.uk/development/reg_pub/uk_eur.htm – accesseed 21 January 2002.

Save the Children (2001) *Denied a Future? The Right to Education of Roma/Gypsy and Traveller Children in Europe*, London: Save the Children.

Schaffer, H. and Schaffer, E. (1968) *Child Care and the Family: A study of short term admission to care*, London: Bell and Sons.

School of Planning and Housing, Edinburgh College of Art/Heriot Watt University (1997) *Constraint and choice for minority ethnic home owners in Scotland*, Scottish Homes: Edinburgh.

Schuman, J. (1998) 'Childhood, infant and perinatal mortality, 1996: social and biological factors in deaths of children aged under three', *Population Trends*, 92: 5–14.

Schwartz-Kenney, B.M. *et al.* (2001) *Child Abuse: A global view*, London: Greenwood Press.

Scott, J. (1996) *Changing British Households: How are the children?* 'Paper presented to the conference European Societies or European Society?', Social Exclusion and Social Integration in Europe, Blarney, Ireland, March.

Scott, S., Harden, J., Jackson, S. and Backett-Milburn, K. (2000) *The Impact of Risk and Parental Risk Anxiety on the Everyday Worlds of Children*, ESRC Research Programme: Children 5–6: Growing into the 21st Century, Award Number L129251045.

Scottish Community Education Council (1994) *Being Young in Scotland*, SCEC.

Scottish Executive (1999) *Road Accidents Scotland 1999.*

Scottish Executive (2001a) *Attendance and Absence in Scottish Schools: 1997/98 to 1999/2000,* http://www.scotland.gov.uk/library3/education/aass-00.asp – accessed 28 October 2001.

Scottish Executive (2001b) *Child Protection Statistics for the Year Ended 31.3.00,* www.scotland.gov.uk/stats/bulletins

Scottish Executive (2001c) *Children Looked After in the Year to 31 March 2000,* News Release 28 March 2001 (www.scotland.gov.uk).

Scottish Executive (2001d) *Exclusions from Schools, 1999/2000.* http://www.scotland.gov.uk/stats/bulletins/00055.pdf – accessed 10 August 2001.

Scottish Executive (2001e) *Health in Scotland 2000,* http://www.scotland.gov.uk

Scottish Executive (2001f) *Learning with Care: The education of children looked after away from home by local authorities,* Astron for Scottish Executive.

Scottish Executive (2001g) *Men and Women in Scotland: A statistical profile,* Edinburgh: Scottish Executive.

Scottish Executive (2001h) *National Framework for the Prevention of Suicide and Deliberate Self-harm in Scotland* – www.show.scot.nhs.uk/sehd

Scottish Executive (2001i) *Number of Children Ceasing to be Looked After in the Year to 31ˢᵗ March 2000,* Edinburgh:Scottish Executive.

Scottish Executive (2001j) *Report of Advisory Group on Youth Crime,* Edinburgh: Scottish Executive.

Scottish Executive (2001k) *Statistical Bulletin: Criminal Proceedings in Scottish courts, 2000,* Edinburgh: Scottish Executive.

Scottish Executive (2001l) *Recorded Crime in Scotland,* 2000, Edinburgh: the Scottish Executive.

Scottish Executive (2002) *Scotland's Action Programme to Reduce Youth Crime,* Edinburgh: Scottish Executive.

Scottish Housing Executive (2001) *Housing Trends in Scotland: Quarter ending 30 June 2001,* Edinburgh: Scottish Housing Executive.

Scottish Office (1999) *Towards a Healthier Scotland,* London: The Stationery Office.

SEU (1998a) *Bringing Britain together: A national strategy for neighbourhood renewal,* Cm 4045, London: The Stationery Office.

SEU (1998b) *Truancy and School Exclusion,* London: The Stationery Office.

SEU (1999a) *Bridging the Gap: New opportunities for 16–18 year olds not in education, employment or training,* London: The Stationery Office.

SEU (1999b) *Teenage Pregnancy,* Cm 4342, London: The Stationery Office.

Shaffer, D. (1988) 'The epidemiology of teen suicide: an examination of risk factors', *Journal of Clinical Psychiatry*, 49, 35–41.

Shaffer, D., Gould, M.S. and Fisher, P. (1996) 'Psychiatric diagnosis in child and adolescent suicide', *Archives of General Psychiatry*, 53, 339–48.

Shah, R. and Hatton, C. (1999) *Caring Alone: Young carers in South Asian communities*, London: Barnardo's.

Sharples, P., Storey, A., Aynsleygreen, A. and Eyre, J.A. (1990) 'Causes of fatal childhood accidents involving head injury in Northern Region: 1979 – 1986', *British Medical Journal*, 301, 6762.

Shaw A., McMunn, A. and Field, J. (eds) (2000) *The Scottish Health Survey 1998 Volume No 1*, Joint Health Survey Unit.

Sheehan, T.J. (1998) 'Stress and low birth weight: a structural modelling approach using real life stressors', *Society of Science and Medicine*, 47: 1503–1512.

Shelter (2001) *Housing and Homelessness in England: the facts*, London: Shelter.

Sheppard, M. (1997) 'Double jeopardy: the link between child abuse and maternal depression in child and family social work', *Child and Family Social Work*, 2, 2, 91–107.

Shuttleworth, I. (1995) 'The relationship between social deprivation, as measured by individual free school meal eligibility, and educational attainment at GCSE in Northern Ireland: A preliminary investigation', *British Educational Research Journal*, 21, 4, 487–504.

Sidebotham, P. and the ALSPAC Study Team (2000) 'Patterns of child abuse in early childhood: a cohort study of the "children of the nineties" ', *Child Abuse Review*, 9, 311–20.

Simons, R. and Whitbeck, L. (1991) 'Running away during adolescence as a precursor to adult homelessness', *Social Services Review*, 65, 2, 224–47, June.

Sinclair, I. (1975) 'The influence of wardens and matrons on probation hostels', in J. Tizard, I. Sinclair, and R. Clarke (eds) *Varieties of Residential Experience*, London: Routledge.

Sinclair, I. and Gibbs, I. (1998) *Children's Homes: A study in diversity*, Chichester: Wiley.

Sinclair, I., Gibbs, I. and Wilson, K. (2000) *Supporting Foster Placements, Final report to the Department of Health*, York: Social Work Research and Development Unit, University of York.

Sinclair, R., Garnett, L. and Berridge, D. (1995) *Social Work Assessment with Adolescents*, London: National Children's Bureau.

Smaje, C. (1995) *Health, Race and Ethnicity: Making sense of the evidence*, London: Kings Fund Institute.

Smith, G. and Phillips, A. (1996) 'Passive smoking and health: should we believe Philip Morris's "experts"?', *British Medical Journal*, 1996, 313, 929–33, 12 October.

Smith, J., Gilford, S. and O'Sullivan, A. (1998) *The Family Background of Homeless Young People*, London: Family Policies Study Centre.

Smith, M. *et al.* (1995) 'Parental control within the family: The nature and extent of physical violence to children', in Department of Health, *Child Protection: Messages from Research*, London: HMSO.

Smith, R. (1998) *No Lessons Learnt: A survey of school exclusions*, London: The Children's Society.

Smith, T. and Noble, M. (1995) *Education Divides: Poverty and schooling in the 1990s*, London: Child Poverty Action Group.

Smyth, M. (1998) *Half the Battle: Understanding the impact of the troubles on children and young people*, Londonderry: Aberfoyle House.

Social Services Inspectorate (1994), *The Child, the Court and the Video*, London: Department of Health.

Social Services Inspectorate (1995) *Young Carers, Something to Think About. Report of Four SSI Workshops, May–July 1995*, London: Department of Health.

Social Services Inspectorate (1996) *Young Carers, Making a Start: Report of SSI fieldwork projects on families with disability or illness*, London: Department of Health.

Social Services Inspectorate (2001) *Key Indicators of Personal Social Services for Northern Ireland 2001*, Northern Ireland Statistics and Research Agency.

Social Services Inspectorate and OFSTED (1995) *The Education of Children who are Looked After by Local Authorities*, London: Department of Health and Office for Standards in Education.

Social Services Inspectorate Wales (2001) *Social Services Statistics Wales 2000*.

Social Work Daycare Services for Children In Scotland, Nov 1997, www.scotland.gov.uk/library/documents8/daycare-01.htm

Somerville, M., MacKenzie, I., Owen, P. and Miles, D. (2000) 'Housing and health: does installing central heating in their homes improve the health of children with asthma', *Public Health*, 114, 434–39.

Soni Raleigh, V. and Balarajan, R. (1995) 'The health of infants and children among ethnic minorities', in B. Botting (ed.) *The Health of our Children: The Registrar General's decennial supplement for England and Wales*, London: HMSO.

Soothill, K. *et al.* (1999) *Homicide in Britain: A comparative study of rates in Scotland and England and Wales*, Scottish Executive, Crime and Criminal Justice Research Findings, No. 36.

Speak, S. (2000) 'Children in urban regeneration: Foundations for sustainable participation', *Community Development Journal*, 35, 1, 31–40.

Spencer, N. (2000) *Poverty and Child Health*, 2nd Edition, Oxford: Radcliffe Medical Press.

Sport England (2000) *Young people and sport national survey 1999*, London: Sport England.

Sports Council for Wales (2001a) *Widening the Net? Young people's participation in sport 1999/2000*, Cardiff: Sports Council for Wales.

Sports Council for Wales (2001b) *Swings and Roundabouts? Primary school children's participation in sport 2000*, Cardiff: Sports Council for Wales.

Squires, T. and Busuttil, A. (1995) 'Child fatalities in Scottish house fires 1980–1990: A case of child neglect?', *Child Abuse and Neglect*, 19, 7, 865–73.

St Claire, L. and Osborn, A. (1987) 'The ability and behaviour of children who have been in care or separated from their parents', *Early Child Development and Care*, 28, Special Issue Monograph, 187–354.

Stallard, P., Velleman, R. and Baldwin, S. (1998) 'Prospective study of post-traumatic stress disorder in children involved in road traffic accidents', *British Medical Journal*, 317, 1, 619–23.

Stein, M. (1997) *What works in leaving care?*, Barkingside: Barnardo's.

Stein, M., Pinkerton, J. and Kelleher, P. (2000) 'Young people leaving care in England, Northern Ireland and Ireland', *European Journal of Social Work*, 3, 3, 235–46.

Stein, M., Rees, G. and Frost, N. (1994) *Running the Risk: Young people on the streets of Britain today*, London: The Children's Society.

Stiller, C.A. (1994) 'Population based survival rates for childhood cancer in Britain, 1980–91', *British Medical Journal*, 2, 1247–51.

Stillion, J.M., McDowell, E.E. and May, J.H. (1989) *Suicide Across the Life Span: Premature exits*, New York: Hemisphere.

Strachan, D.P. (1988) 'Damp housing and childhood asthma: validation of reporting of symptoms', *British Medical Journal*, 297, 1223–26.

Strand, S. (1999) 'Ethnic group, sex and economic disadvantage: associations with pupils' educational progress from baseline to the end of Key Stage 1', *British Educational Research Journal*, 25, 2, 179–202.

Sullivan, P.M. and Knutson, J.F. (2000) 'Maltreatment and disabilities: a population-based epidemiological study', *Child Abuse and Neglect*, 24, 10, 1257–73.

Sutherland, H. (2001) *Five Labour Budgets (1997–2001): Impacts on the distribution of household incomes and on child poverty*, Microsimulation Unit Research Note No. 41.

Sweeting, H. and West, P. (1996) 'The relationships between family life and young people's lifestyles', *Findings*, April.

Taylor, G. and Jones, S. (1990) *A Crying Shame: The child victims of homelessness*, London: The London Boroughs Association.

The Children's Society (2001) *National Playday 2001: Facts and statistics*, unpublished.

The Children's Society and The Children's Play Council (2001) *The Play Space Survey*, London: The Children's Society and The Children's Play Council.

Thomas, A. and Niner, P. (1989) *Living in Temporary Accommodation*, London: HMSO.

Thomas, S. (1995) 'Considering primary school effectiveness: an analysis of 1992 Key stage 1 results', *The Curriculum Journal*, 6, 279–95.

Thomson, H., Petticrew, M. and Morrison, D. (2001) 'Health effects of housing improvement: systematic review of intervention studies', *British Medical Journal*, 323, 187–90.

Todd, J., Currie, C., Smith, R. and Small, G. (2000) *Health Behaviour of Scottish School Children, Technical Report 3: Eating and activity patterns in the 1990s*, Edinburgh: Research Unit in Health and Behavioural Change, University of Edinburgh.

Townsend, P., Phillimore, P. and Beattie, A. (1988) *Health and Deprivation*. Beckenham: Croom Helm.

Trew, K. (1995) 'Psychological and social impact of the troubles on young people growing up in Northern Ireland', in W. McCarney (ed.) *Growing Through Conflict: The impact of 25 years of violence on young people growing up in Northern Ireland, Conference Proceedings*, Belfast: International Association of Juvenile and Family Court Magistrates.

TUC (1997) *Working Classes,* London: Trades Union Congress.

TUC (2001) *Class Struggles*, London: Trades Union Congress.

Tuthill, D.P., Stewart, J.H., Coles, E.C., Andrews, J. and Cartlidge, P.H. (1999) 'Maternal cigarette smoking and pregnancy outcome', *Paediatric and Perinatal Epidemiology*, 13: 245–253.

UKCCSG (2000) *Information about children's cancer*, United Kingdom Children's Cancer Study Group, http://www.ukccsg.org/children's_cancer.htm

UNICEF (2000*) A League Table of Child Poverty in Rich Nations*, Innocenti Report Card 1, Florence: UNICEF Innocenti Research Centre.

UNICEF (2001a) *A League Table of Child Deaths by Injury in Rich Nations*, Innocenti Report Card 2, Florence: UNICEF Innocenti Research Centre.

UNICEF (2001b) *A League Table of Teenage Births in Rich Nations*, Florence: UNICEF Innocenti Research Centre.

United Nations (1989) *The Convention on the Rights of the Child*, New York: United Nations and http://www.unhchr.ch/html/menu3/b/k2crc.htm

Utting, W. (1997) *People Like Us: Report of the review of safeguards for children living away from home*, London: Department of Health and the Welsh Office.

Van der Stoel, M. (2000) *Report on the Situation of Roma and Sinti in the OSCE Area*, The Hague: Organisation for Security and Co-operation in Europe.

Vernon, J. and Fruin, D. (1986) *In Care: A study of social work decision making*, London: National Children's Bureau.

Victor, C.R., Connelly, J., Roderick, P. and Cohen, C. (1989) 'Use of hospital services by homeless families in an inner-London health district', *British Medical Journal*, 229, 725–27.

Vostanis, P. and Cumella, S. (1999) *Homeless Children: Problems and needs*, London: Jessica Kingsley.

Vostanis, P. Grattan, E. and Cumella, S. (1998) 'Mental health problems of homeless children and families: A longitudinal study', *British Medical Journal*, 31, 6, 899–902.

Vulliamy, G. and Webb, R. (2000) 'Stemming the tide of rising school exclusions: problems and possibilities', *British Journal of Educational Studies*, 48, 2, 119–33.

Wade, J. and Biehal, N. with Clayden, J. and Stein, M. (1998) *Going Missing: Young people absent from care*, Chichester: John Wiley & Sons.

Wagner, J., Power, E.J. and Fox, H. (1988) *Technology-dependent Children: Hospital versus home care*, Office of Technology Assessment Task Force, J.P. Lippincott, Philadelphia.

Walker, A. (1996) *Young Carers and their Families: A survey carried out by the Social Survey Division of the Office for National Statistics on behalf of the Department of Health*, London: The Stationery Office.

Wallace, H.M., Goldstein, H. and Ericson, A. (1982) 'Comparison of infant mortality in the United States and Sweden', *Clinical Paediatrics*, 21: 156–162.

Walters, S. and East, L. (2001) 'The cycle of homelessness in the lives of young mothers: the diagnostic phase of an action research project', *Journal of Clinical Nursing*, 10, 171–79.

Warner, B.B., Kiely, J.L. and Donovan, E.F. (2000) 'Multiple births and outcome', *Clinics in Perinatology*, 27: 347–361.

Watson, L., Gamble, J. and Schonfield, R. (2000) *Fire Statistics United Kingdom 1999*, Home Office Statistical Bulletin 20/00, November.

Weaver, M. (2001) 'Labour tackles bed and breakfast homeless', *The Guardian*, 13 August 2001.

Wedge, P. and Mantle, G. (1991) *Sibling Groups and Social Work: A study of children referred for permanent substitute family placement*, Aldershot: Avebury.

Welsh Assembly (1999/2000/2001) *Key Publications: Statistics for Wales, Local Authority Child Protection Registers: Wales 1999/2000/2001*, www.wales.gov.uk/keypubstatisticsforwalesheadline/content/health

Welsh Assembly (2000) *A strategic framework for promoting sexual health in Wales*, Cardiff: Health Promotion Division.

Welsh Assembly (2001a) *National Statistics SDB 15/2001 Absenteeism From Secondary Schools In Wales, 1999/2000*.

Welsh Assembly (2001b) *National Statistics SDR 8/2001 Permanent Exclusions From Schools In Wales 2000*, http://www.wales.gov.uk/keypubstatisticsforwalesheadline/content/education/2001/hdw2001 – accessed 9 August 2001.

Welsh Assembly (2001c) *Social Services Statistics Wales 2001*, Cardiff: Statistical Directorate.

Welsh Assembly (2001d) *The Homeless Persons (Priority Need) (Wales) Order 2001, No. 607 (W.30)*, National Assembly for Wales.

Welsh Assembly (2001e) *Welsh Housing Statistics*, Cardiff: National Assembly for Wales.

West, P. and Sweeting, H. (1996) 'Nae Job, nae future. Young people and health in a context of unemployment', *Health and Social Care in the Community*, 4, 50–62.

West, P., MacIntyre., Annandale, E. and Hunt, K. (1990) 'Social class and health in youth: findings from the West of Scotland Twenty-07 Study', *Social Science and Medicine*, 30, 6, 665–73.

Wheway, R. and Millward, A. (1997) *Child's Play: Facilitating play on housing estates*, Coventry: Chartered Institute of Housing.

White, D., Raeside, R. and Barker, D. (2000) *Road Accidents and Children Living in Disadvantaged Areas: A Literature Review*, Scottish Executive Central Research Unit.

White, M. and Lissenburgh, S. (2001) *Factors Affecting or Restricting the Take-up of Childcare Among Working Mothers*, London: Policy Studies Institute.

Whiteford, P., Kennedy, S. and Bradshaw, J. (1996) 'The economic circumstances of children in ten countries', in J. Brannen and M. O'Brien (eds) *Children in Families: Research and policy*, London: Falmer.

Whitehead, M. and Drever, F. (1999) 'Narrowing social inequalities in health? Analysis of trends in mortality among babies of lone mothers', *British Medical Journal*, 318: 908.

WHO (2001) *1997–1999 World Health Statistics Annual (Table 1)*, World Health Organization, www3.who.int/whosis/whsa/whsa_table1

Wilcox, S. (2001) *Housing Finance Review*, 2000/2001, York: Joseph Rowntree Foundation.

Wilczynski, A. (1997) *Child Homicide,* London: Greenwich Medical Media.

Wilkinson, D. (1999) *Poor Housing and Ill Health: A summary of research evidence*, Edinburgh: The Scottish Office.

Wilkinson, R.G. (1994) *Unfair Shares: The effects of widening income differences on the welfare of the young*, Essex: Barnardo's.

Williamson, H. (1997) Status Zero Youth and the 'Underclass': Some considerations', in R. McDonald (ed.) *Youth, the Underclass and Social Exclusion*, London: Routledge.

Wilson, L. (1998) 'Dirty business', *Nursing Times*, 25, 94, 47, 71–5.

Woodroffe, C. *et al.* (1993) *Children, Teenagers and Health: The key data*, Milton Keynes: Open University Press.

Woodroffe, C., Glickman, M., Barker, M. and Power, C. (1993) *Children, Teenagers and Health: The key data*, Buckingham: Open University Press.

Woolley, H. and Amin, N. (1995) 'Pakistani children in Sheffield and their perception and use of public open spaces', *Children's Environments*, 12, 4, 479–88.

Wrate, R. and Blair, C. (1999) 'Homeless adolescents', in P. Vostanis and S. Cumella (eds) *Homeless Children: Problems and needs*, London: Jessica Kingsley.

Wynn, M. and Wynn, A. (2001) *New Evidence on the Nutrition of British School Children and Conclusions for School Meals,* unpublished paper.

Yuen, P. and Office of Health Economics (2001) *Compendium of Health Statistics* (13th Edition), London: Office of Health Economics.